Eye Diseases and Disorders

A Complete Guide

Eye Diseases and Disorders – A Complete Guide

Publisher: iConcept Press Ltd.

ISBN: 978-1-922227-324

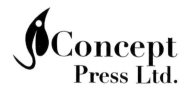

www.iconceptpress.com

Contents

Preface

According to the National Eye Institute (NEI), about 3.3 million Americans aged 40 or older are blind or have low vision and by 2020 this number could be 5.5 million – a 60Many eye diseases have no early symptoms. They may be painless, and you may see no change in your vision until the disease has become quite advanced. *Eye Diseases and Disorders - A Complete Guide* discusses eye diseases and disorders related contents, including risk, symptoms, treatment and recent research outcomes. This book is an indispensable reference book for busy primary care and specialist practitioners. It is also a concise encyclopaedia for students and researchers, making it an essential ophthalmology resource.

There are totally 11 chapters in this book. Chapter 1 presents features to enable readers (especially ophthalmologists) to identify skin diseases occurred around the eye more easily. It provides atlas-like guidance in alphabetical order, complemented with detailed, diagnostic text, written as a practical derm book for daily activity among ophthalmologists. Chapter 2 provides an up-to-date background on the current myopia research (focused mainly on the cellular/molecular level). Additionally, the common research techniques involved and the impacts contributed by different ocular cells on myopia is also discussed. Chapter 3 describes dry eye disease, a common ocular condition arises when the tear film does not adequately support biological functions of the ocular surface. This can arise due to extrinsic environmental stress, intrinsic cortical and endocrinological factors that reduce aqueous tear flow and/or increase tear film evaporation, leading to tear hyperosmolarity. Chapter 4 discusses the theory of Traditional Chinese Medicine (TCM) treatment for dry eye. This is an alternative to the conventional dry eye treatment, and addresses holistically any systemic disorder described by TCM theory.

Chapter 5 discusses diabetic retinopathy (DR), which is one of the major risk factors and a leading cause of preventable blindness worldwide. It is a vision-threatening disease presenting neurodegenerative features associated with extensive vascular changes. This chapter discusses ways to provide superior efficacy and safety profile for the treatment or prevention of DR. Chapter 6 discusses glaucoma, an irreversible blinding eye disease that is frequently associated with increased intraocular pressure. Elevated pressure arises from impaired aqueous humor outflow through the trabecular meshwork (TM) in the anterior segment of the eye. This chapter report alterations in mRNA levels of three HA synthase (HAS) genes in normal and glaucoma eyes. Confocal microscopy and immunostaining of HAS proteins in paraffin-embedded radial sections of human trabecular meshwork was also investigated. Chapter 7 discusses glaucoma in Nigeria as well as looks critically at a Nigerian study that compares quality of life in glaucoma patients to non-glaucoma patients using the GQL-15 and the NEIVFQ25 questionnaires. Chapter 8 discusses neurological examination and concludes that principles of diagnosis in neuro-ophthalmology are the same as in any other branch of neurology. A good history with a directed examination are essential for the accuracy. Neuro-ophthalmological disorders may occur as manifestations of more generalized neurological conditions.

Chapter 9 reviews the current strategy in the diagnosis and management of acanthamoeba keratitis, which is based on the available literature, personal comments of clinicians all over the world and authors' experiences. Chapter 10 reviews our understanding of the pathophysiology of fibrosis and its consequences in the anterior and posterior segment of the eye, and current treatment options to prevent blindness due to fibrosis. Chapter 11 discusses placental development. According to research, morphine consumption during pregnancy can be caused by defective development of the placenta. Placental development defects, delays in the development of the embryo nervous system, including the visual system.

Editing and publishing a book is never an easy task. Each chapter in this book has gone through a peer review, a selection and an editing process so as to guarantee its quality. Without the supports and contributions of the authors and reviewers, this book can never be able to complete. We would like to thank all of the authors in this book and all of the reviewers who participated in the reviewing process: Manal K Abdel-Rahman, Fatma A. Al-Mansouri, Ahmed Awadein, Dinesh Bhatia, Sanjoy K. Bhattacharya, Emmanuel S Buys, Stéphane Chabaud, Keji Chen, Russell W Chesney, Nikhil S. Choudhari, Michelle A. Clark, Cintia S. De Paiva, Andrzej Fertala, Andreas Frings, Agnes Fust, Feng Gao, Jinsong Hao, Maria C. Jimenez-Martinez, Tan Aik Kah, Jin Sook Kim, Akira Kobayashi, G. Phani Kumar, Jimmy S. M. Lai, Alex P. Lange, Kira L. Lathrop, Jacky W. Y. Lee, Paloma B. Liton, Yutao Liu, Santi M. Mandal, Sanjay Marasini, Simin Mashayekhi, Antonio Maturo, Bradley M Mitchell, Masoud Mozafari, Haruo Okado, Mohammad Pakravan, Donna M. Peters, Roman Pfister, Richard P. Phipps, Mark Pines, Howard Prentice, R Ramakrishnan, José M Ramírez, Sergio Claudio Sacca, Serena Salvatore, Rama Shankar, S K Sinha, Andrei Surguchov, Liping Tang, Shreya Thatte, Daniel Vaiman, Lei Wang and Yasuhiko Yamamoto. We hope that you, the reader, will find this book interesting and useful. Any advices please feel free and are always welcome to tell us.

iConcept Press Editorial Office

December 2015

Dermatological Diseases with Periocular Involvement ABC Alphabetical Dermatological Guide for Ophthalmologists

Anca Chiriac and Liliana Foia

1 Introduction

This chapter presents features to enable readers (especially ophthalmologists) to identify skin diseases occurred around the eye, more easily. It thus provides atlas-like guidance in alphabetical order, complemented with detailed, diagnostic text, written as a practical derm book for daily activity among ophthalmologists.

- **A.** Abscess Periocular, Achrochordon (Cutaneous Tag, Skin Tag) Palpebrarum; Acne; Actinic Keratosis; Acute Irritant And Allergic Contact Irritant Dermatitis; Addison's Disease; Alopecia; Atopic Dermatitis.

- **B.** Basal Cell Carcinoma; Behçet's Disease (Aphthosis Behçet, Behçet's Syndrome, Bipolar Aphthosis); Blue Nevus (Nevus Ceruleus, Nevus Bleu); Bowen Disease (Scc – Intraepidermal Squamous Cell Carcinoma - Bowen's Type); Bullous Impetigo (Impetigo Contagiosa); Bullous Pemphigoid; Burns.

- **C.** Café-Au-Lait Spot; Chalazion (Meibomian Cysts, Meibomian Gland Cyst, Tarsal Cyst); Chronic Actinic Dermatitis; Congenital Ichthyosiform Erythroderma; Cryptococcosis; Cutaneous Horn; Culicosis (Mosquito Bites); Cylindroma (Spiegler's Tumour, Turban Tumour; Dermal Eccrine Cylindroma, Tomato Tumour, Ancell-Spiegler Cylindroma, Poncet-Spiegler Tumour).

- **D.** Demodicidiosis; Dermatitis Solaris (Sunburn); Dermatofibroma (Nodulus Cutaneous, Fibroma Simplex, Dermatofibroma Lenticulare, Histiocytoma); Dermatomyositis; Discoid Lupus Erythematosus (Dle) (Lupus Erythematosus Chronicus Discoides); Drug Reactions.

- **E.** Ephelide; Eruptive Angiomatosis; Erysipelas of the Face; Erythema Infectiosum (Fifth Disease, Infectious Erythema).

- **F.** Factitial Dermatitis (Dermatitis Artefacta); Favre-Racouchot Syndrome (Nodular Elastosis with Cysts and Comedones; Elastoidosis Cutanea Nodularis Et Cystica).

- **H.** Hemangioma; Herpes Simplex/Zoster; Herpes Zoster.

- **L.** Lentigo Senilis/Maligna (Melanosis Circumscripta Precancerosa Dubreuilh; Melanotic Precancerosis); Lupus Vulgaris (Tuberculosis Cutis Luposa); Lyell Syndrome (Toxic Epidermal Necrolysis - TEN).

- **M.** Malignant Melanoma; Molluscum Contagiosum; Morphea Linear; Mycosis Fungoides.

- **N.** Nevus.

- **P.** Pemphigus; Cicatricial Pemphigoid; Psoriasis.

- **R.** Rosacea.

- **S.** Seborrheic Dermatitis; Seborrheic Keratosis; Sturge-Weber Syndrome.

- **T.** Tinea Faciei; Tuberous Sclerosis.

- **U.** Urticaria

- **V.** Vitiligo.

- **W.** Warts.

- **X.** Xanthelasma; Xanthogranuloma

Some of the most common terms used in dermatology such as papule, macule, pustule, nodule, vesicle and bula are presented and explained in Figure 1.

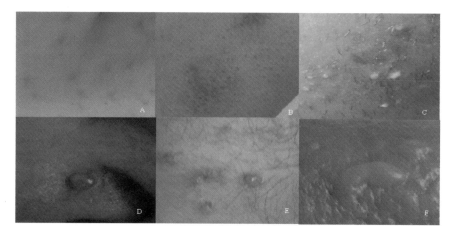

Figure 1: A. Papule: a small, circumscribed, solid, elevated lesion of the skin, less than 1 cm; B. Macule: flat, discolored area on the skin; C. Pustule: a small elevation of the skin containing pus; D. Nodule: a small collection of tissue that is palpable (1-2cm); E. Vesicle: a small blister (less than 5cm); F. Bula: a large blister.

2   A -

Abscess Periocular

The abscess periocular represents localized collection in the periocular area, in different stages of inflammation. Topical and/or systemic antibiotic administrations are recommended.

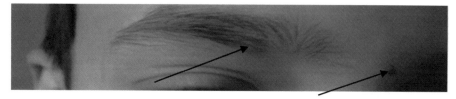

Figure 2: Abscess in the right eyebrow (left arrow); congenital melanocytic nevus (right arrow).

Achrochordon (Cutaneous Tag, Skin Tag) Palpebrarum

This disorder consists of benign pedunculated tumor of different size, most frequently asymptomatic (except the case of trauma-induced local inflammation), soft, mobile, no tender, often observed in obese subjects, especially in the neck region, axilla, inguinal region, rarely in the palpebral area (Gupta et al., 2008). The diameter can vary from 1mm to 1 cm or even more and the number increases by age.

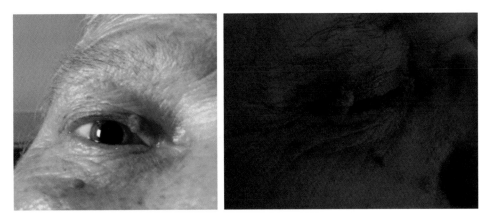

Figure 3: Achrochordon palpebrarum.

They are in general flesh – colored, but can turn into red or dark-brown when they are inflamed. Related to local trauma, although some opinions suggest an association with human papillomavirus infection, there are histologically characterized by acanthosis of the epidermis, chronic inflammation and fibrovascular structure (El Safoury et al., 2011).

There is no risk of malignancy, but the excision (classical, electrocautery or laser) is sometimes required for esthetic reasons or due to some irritation. Recurrence is very common.

Acne

Is a chronic inflammatory disease of the pilo-sebaceous units, common in teenagers (more than 90% of this age-ranged population being involved more or less); however the disease may onset in the twenties or later (Acne tarda) and persist for many years; it is characterized by comedones, papules, pustules, cysts, nodules and scars. Treatment considerations include the use of over-the-counter products, topical benzoyl peroxide, topical retinoids, topical antibiotics, oral antibiotics, hormonal therapy, and isotretinoin.

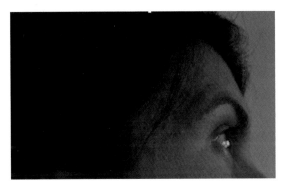

Figure 4: Acne tarda with papules and nodules along the eyebrow in a young woman.

Actinic Keratosis

Actinic keratosis (also known as solar keratosis, senile keratosis) presents as scaly, erythematous-yellowish or hyperpigmented, crusted lesions, localized on sun-exposed areas, multiple, flat or elevated, discrete or reaching a few cm in diameter. They might be noticed in elderly fair-skinned persons with excessive sun exposure during the first decades of life (Buinauskaite et al., 2013). Very recent studies have claimed the association of cutaneous human papillomavirus (HPV) infections with the onset of actinic keratosis (Schneider et al., 2013).

Histological: along with the epidermal changes, cellular atypia is the hallmark; actinic keratosis is premalignant and can potentially turn into squamous cell carcinoma. Progression rates of actinic keratosis to malignancy range from 0% to 0.075%/lesion/year, with a risk of up to 0.53% recurrence rate of between 15% and 53% per lesion; spontaneous regression rates range from 0% to 21%, with recurrences in 57% (Werner et al., 2013). Moreover, according to other opinions, actinic keratosis is regarded as keratinocytic intraepidermal neoplasia (Cohn, 2000).

Taking into consideration that no clinical criteria are settled in order to determine which lesion has the potential to undergo malignant switch, the most appropriate approach is to treat all visible actinic keratosis. Treatment plan include: cryotherapy, topical application of 5-flurouracil (Efudix) or Imiquimod cream 5%, 2.5% and 3.75% (Samrao & Cockerell, 2013); diclofenac 3% gel; laser; photodynamic therapy with 5-aminolevulinic acid (Buinauskaite et al., 2013; Lee & Weinstock, 2013); ingenol mebutate gel 0.015% or 0.05% (Abramovits et al., 2013).

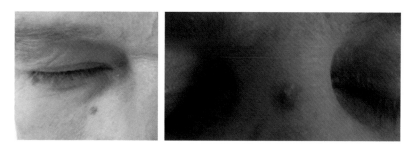

Figure 5: Actinic keratosis in the periorbital area and nose, respectively.

Acute Irritant and Allergic Contact Dermatitis

This is a common skin problem characterized by erythematous lesions and pruritus after contact with a foreign substance. The main features are presented in Table 1.

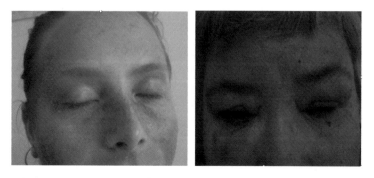

Figure 6: Acute irritant contact dermatitis and acute allergic contact dermatitis.

	Irritant contact dermatitis	Allergic contact dermatitis
Prevalence	Very common	Less frequent
Symptoms	Burning, pruritus, pain	Pruritus
Clinical aspects	Erythema, desquamation	Erythema, edema, vesicles, bullae
Sites	Site of direct contact	Site of contact and secondary lesions
Cause	Chemical irritants	Poison ivy, nickel and fragrances, Neomycin, metals (jewelry), cosmetics
Prior exposure	Not necessary	Essential (lesions appear after re-exposure)
Susceptibility	Everyone	Susceptible persons
Onset	Rapid onset (4-12 hours after contact)	Delayed onset (more than 24 hours after exposure)
Mechanism	Direct cytotoxic effects (non-immune-modulated irritation)	Type IV-T cell–mediated, delayed reaction, patch-test positive
Treatment	Avoidance of the substance	Antihistamines, topical steroids/orally desensitization

Table 1: Differential diagnosis between irritant and allergic contact dermatitis.

In chronic contact dermatitis the skin lesions are lichenified, with fissures, erythema, desquamation, pruritus.

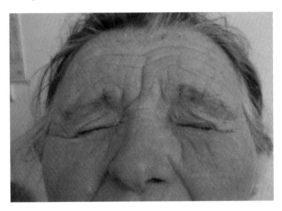

Figure 7: Erythema, lichenification, fissures, desquamation.

Addison's Disease

In adrenal insufficiency, hyperpigmentation (that must be differentiated from hemochromatosis, arsenic intoxication and metastatic melanoma) is intense, diffuse, distributed upon sun-exposed areas and axillae, perineum and nipples as well; it can also be associated with darkening of mucosa, hair, nails, scars, and palmar crease. Referring the patient to Endocrinology for evaluation and treatment is the best decision.

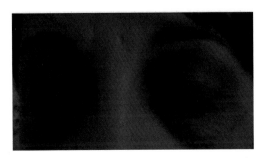

Figure 8: Hyperpigmentation of adrenal origin.

Alopecia

Alopecia represents a hair-loss pattern that can be classified into: non-cicatricial (with re-growth of hair) and cicatricial (permanent) alopecia.

- **Non-cicatricial Alopecia**

  o **Alopecia areata** (French: Pelade): rapid and complete hair loss in one or several patches on the scalp, beard, eyebrows, eyelashes or other hairy areas. Alopecia to-talis defines total loss of scalp hair, while alopecia universalis is commonly used for allover the body hair loss.

    Despite that several autoimmune diseases have been associated (autoimmune thyroiditis, pernicious anemia, Addison disease, vitiligo, atopic dermatitis), the eti-ology for this disorder remains still obscure. There is a genetic susceptibility and a possible abnormal cell-mediated immune mechanism. A spontaneous recovery may occur while sometimes it persists for life.

    Treatment options include: topical, intralesional, or systemic steroids, camou-flage in the form of wigs in unresponsive cases, 308-nm excimer laser, potassium channel openers drugs (minoxidil), contact irritants (anthralin, salicylic acid, di-phenylcyclopropenone), topical 8-methoxypsoralen plus targeted UVA photother-apy.

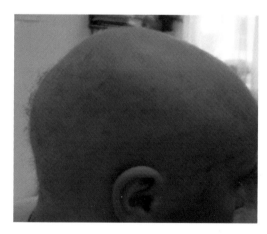

Figure 9: Alopecia areata.

  o **Alopecia Syphilitica**: affects the scalp but also eyebrows and eyelashes; the diag-nosis is made by serological investigations.

  o **Endocrinological Alopecia**: loss of eyebrows in the external parts, have been de-scribed during hypothyroidism. Trichotillomania is a practice of plucking or breaking hairs from the scalp or eyelashes, seen in children with neurological problems.

- **Cicatricial Alopecia** Cicatricial alopecia of inflammatory type might be induced by: discoid lupus erythematous, lichen planopilaris, sarcoidosis and folliculitis decalvans. Pseudopelade of Brocq (pseudo alopecia areata) also known as alopecia cicatrisata is a rare form of alopecia, a permanent hair-loss, mostly on the scalp.

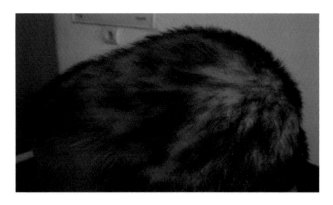

Figure 10: Cicatricial alopecia.

Atopic Dermatitis

Atopic dermatitis represents the dermatological manifestation of the atopic diathesis, associated to a variety of signs and symptoms. Its prevalence ranges from 1-25% (Naldi et al., 2009). Some of the patients develop atopic dermatitis within first year of life (60%), 85% by age 5; and is much rare in adults (Naldi et al., 2009; Williams et al., 1994). According to some opinions, the incidence of ocular complications in atopic dermatitis has varied from 25% to 40% (Kaujalgi et al., 2009). Ocular complications are varying from eyelid dermatitis: symmetrical, pruritic, erythematous, scaly plaques at the upper medial aspect of the eyelids to loss of eyelashes or eyebrows because of scratching or important xerosis and pruritus.

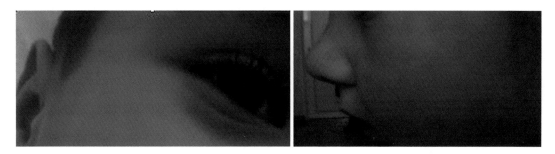

Figure 11: Atopic dermatitis: Dennie-Morgan lines (left picture); xerosis (right picture).

Dennie-Morgan lines are symmetrical folds of the lower lid, are commonly present from early life and can persist, needing to be differentiated from similar findings in Down syndrome. Atopic keratoconjunctivitis has a chronic evolution, is always bilateral, with high risk of corneal injuries and severe sequelae, sometimes turning to blinding (González-López et al., 2012). It is a challenge for treatment, often refractory to topical steroids and with good results to systemic or local cyclosporine (Cornish et al., 2010). Blepharitis, keratoconus, uveitis, anterior and posterior subcapsular cataract, retinal detachment are all signs during atopic dermatitis (Hogan, 1953). Treatment options include: emollients, topical corticosteroids, topical calcineurin inhibitors, phototherapy, very rare systemic corticosteroids, and educational programs.

3 B -

Basal Cell Carcinoma

It is the most common form of cutaneous malignancy; is a slowly growing tumor, localized on sun-exposed area (especially face: around the nose and inner canthus). It first appears as a small nodule further expanding, with central area exhibiting ulceration and leaving the characteristic rolled-edge.

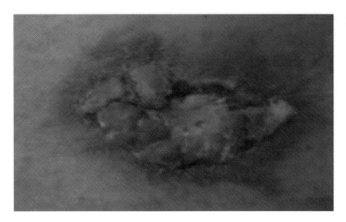

Figure 12: close-view of basal-cell carcinoma. The figure displays a large basal-cell carcinoma on the right malar area, surrounded by multiple actinic keratosis. It usually arises from basal keratinocytes, do not metastasize but can cause massive local destruction. The therapy includes: curettage, cryotherapy, surgery, topical application of 5-flurouracil (Efudix), or Imiquimod 5%.

Behçet's Disease (Aphthosis Behçet, Behçet's Syndrome, Bipolar Aphthosis)

Behçet's syndrome is rare, with still incompletely acknowledged etiology, described long time ago, over the traces of Old Silk Road, the ancient trade route from the eastern shores of the Mediterranean Sea, with a male predominance, and with differences between Eastern and Western population (in the West, ocular lesions being less common) (Zouboulis et al., 1997).

According to International Study Group criteria for classification of Behçet's disease, Behçet's syndrome is defined by the following criteria (International Study Group for Behçet's disease, 1990):

- Recurrent oral ulceration (aphthous or herpetiform) at least 3 times in a 12-month period, *with 2 of the following*:

    o   Recurrent genital ulceration

    o   Eye lesions: anterior or posterior uveitis, cells in vitreous through slit lamp examination, or retinal vasculitis

    o   Skin lesions: erythema nodosum, pseudo-folliculitis, papulopustular, acneiform nodules

    o   Positive pathergy test

- Additional clinical manifestations: stroke, aseptic meningitis, superficial or deep venous thrombosis, cerebral thrombosis, aortic, pulmonary aneurysms, arthralgias, arthritis, gastrointestinal involvement, history of a positive pathergy test and presence of HLA–B51.

Treatment in this case is quite challenging and includes: vitamins, antivirals, colchicine, topical and oral steroids, antibiotics (tetracycline, minocycline), immune modulators (thalidomide), pain relieving agents (lidocaine, benzocaine), zinc, quinolones, with deceiving results.

Blue Nevus (Nevus Ceruleus, Nevus Bleu)

It is a congenital or acquired melanocytic nevus, characterized by blue-gray appearance (Zouboulis et al., 1997), more frequently seen in Asian women (Baderca et al., 2013; Magarasevic & Abazi 2013).

Bowen Disease (SCC - Intraepidermal Squamous Cell Carcinoma - Bowen's Type)

"Bowen's disease" is known to refer to carcinoma in situ, but is a debatable designation. Excision is the rule.

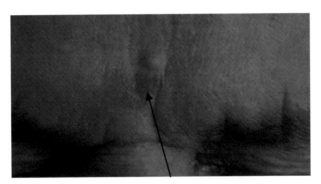

Figure 13: Bowen disease.

Bullous Impetigo (Impetigo Contagiosa)

It represents a superficial staphylococcal and/or streptococcal skin infection, most frequently seen in children. Bullous impetigo is highly contagious, caused by an epidermolytic toxin of *Staphylococcus aureus*, which produces cleavage under the stratum granulosum.

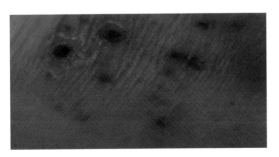

Figure 14: ruptured blisters, crusts in a case of bullous impetigo.

Clinically it appears as a thin-roofed, quickly ruptured blister, covered with a honey-colored crust, usually on the face and limbs. Impetigo may complicate pre-existing skin lesions - trauma, burns, insect bites, eczema, and atopic dermatitis (Habif, 2004).

In some cases cultures from fluid of intact bulla or crusted plaque may help identification of the causative agent. Only topical antibiotics are necessary, after cleaning with soap and water, because there is a scar-free healing due to the superficial infection.

In severe cases, like immunosuppressed patients, a short therapy with oral penicillin or erythromycin is strongly encouraged, in order to prevent post-streptococcal glomerulonephritis.

Bullous Pemphigoid

Cicatricial pemphigoid is a rare, chronic, sub-epidermal autoimmune vesiculobullous disease that affects primarily the mouth and eyes mucous membranes. The main mechanism consists of deposition of IgG, IgA, and C3 along the epithelial basement membrane zone, evidenced by direct immunofluorescence on biopsy of the conjunctiva. Indirect immunofluorescence identifies the specific IgA and IgG in the patient's serum.

Subsequent fibrosis induces ocular impairment: shrinkage of the conjunctiva, shortening of the fornices, symblepharon and cicatricial entropion (Matsuzaki et al., 1996). The mainstay therapy is represented by Dapsone (due to its anti-inflammatory and anti-fibrosis effect), followed by azathioprine and very rare steroids.

Burns

Skin injury caused by heat, chemicals, electricity, radiation, defines the burns (Herndon, 2012). There are classified in superficial-first degree when only the epidermis is involved, second degree when the injury affects the dermis also, third-degree when the damage extends to all layers of the skin and fourth-degree when it goes to muscle or bone.

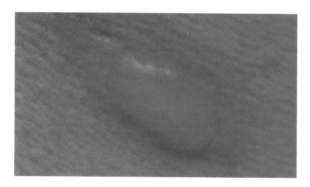

Figure 15: Second-degree burn (tense-blister).

4   C -

Café-au-Lait Spots

Neurofibromatosis type 1 (NF1) is an autosomal dominant neurocutaneous disease, characterized by neurofibroma, café-au-lait spots, axillary and inguinal freckling (ephelides), and Lisch nodules in the eye; occasionally, optic glioma and learning difficulties might be associated. NF1 is caused by mutation of the NF1 gene on chromosome 17q11.2 (Viskochil et al., 1990). The NF1 gene encodes for neurofibromin formation, which acts as a tumor suppressor protein.

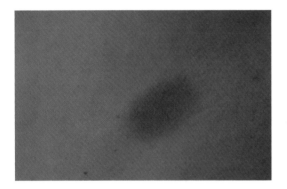 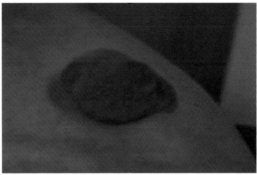

Figure 16: Café-au-lait spots.   **Figure 17:** Large neurofibroma on the cervical area.

Chalazion (Meibomian Cysts, Meibomian Gland Cyst, Tarsal Cyst)

It is a benign granulomatous inflammation within the eyelid, caused by retained meibomian secretions. It usually has a self-limiting evolution and a good prognosis even in recurrent forms.

Chronic Actinic Dermatitis

Chronic actinic dermatitis, also known as photosensitivity dermatitis and actinic reticuloid syndrome, is clinically described as dermatitis associated to abnormal photosensitivity to ultraviolet radiation, distributed mostly on sun-exposed areas.

It is frequently described in elderly men, skin manifestations varying from erythema with pruritus to more severe forms of chronic lichenified lesions (thickened dry skin). Phototesting confirms the abnormal reaction to the light; photopatch testing proves reactions to allergens (fragrances, sunscreens, other contact allergens).

Treatment plan includes: sun exposure avoidance, sun protection, emollients, topical steroids, immunosuppressive therapy (topical or systemic) and desensitization with photo-chemotherapy.

Congenital Ichthyosiform Erythroderma

It is clinically characterized by fine white-grayish scales distributed over the entire body, including face.

Cryptococcosis

Cutaneous cryptococcosis is a very uncommon disease. It appears usually secondary to hematogenous dissemination from a lung infestation in immunosuppressed patients (HIV-infected, organ transplantation, prolonged treatment with systemic corticosteroids). There have been identified 2 species and 4 serotypes of Cryptococcus: C. neoformans (var. grubii serotype A; var. neoformans serotype D) and C. gattii (serotype B and C) (Allegue et al., 2007).

The diagnosis is based on identifying the fungus through direct microscopic examination, histological analysis and microbiological culture. Azole is the best choice for treatment, but only for prolonged period (not less than 6 months), patient being under medical surveillance.

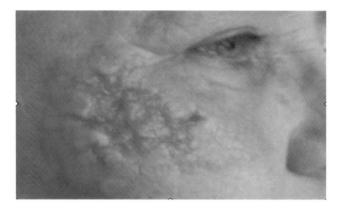

Figure 18: Cryptococcosis on the malar area.

Cutaneous Horn

It is a rare tumor, described on sun-exposed areas in elderly patients (Bondeson et al., 2001), on the face and trunk (even periorbital), composed of dead keratin on an underlying skin lesion that can be benign, premalignant or malignant (Nthumba, 2007). Excision is the rule, the histopathological report being mandatory.

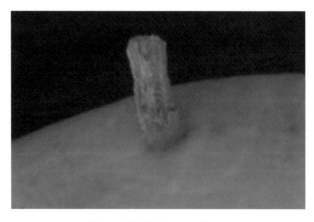

Figure 19: Cutaneous horn.

Culicosis (Mosquito Bites)

It represents erythematous papules and papulovesicles distributed on the face, trunk and limbs, with good response to antihistamines.

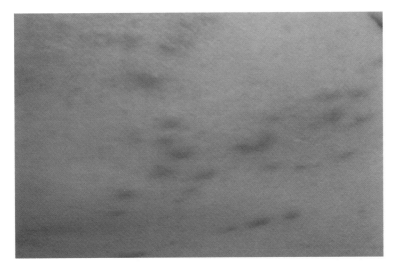

Figure 20: Papule-vesicles and excoriations on the face due to mosquito bites.

Cylindroma (Spiegler's Tumor, Turban Tumor, Dermal Eccrine Cylindroma, Tomato Tumor, Ancell-Spiegler Cylindroma, Poncet-Spiegler Tumor)

Cylindromas are benign, rarely malignant type, eccrine tumors, with two different clinical presentations: solitary and multiple. Solid cylindroma is a slow growing, benign tumor of the skin, while multiple cylindromas are inherited in an autosomal dominant pattern (Durani et al., 2001).

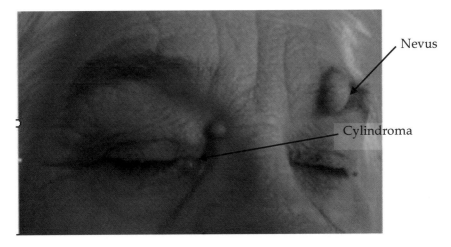

Figure 21: Cylindroma.

5   D -

Demodicidiosis (see Rosacea)

Dermatitis Solaris (Sunburn) (see Burns)

Dermatofibroma (Nodulus Cutaneous, Fibroma Simplex, Dermatofibroma Lenticulare, Histiocytoma)

Flesh colored nodule, sometimes tender, localized rarely on the face; a history of trauma or insect bite at the site is very common. It is benign and excision is the rule.

Dermatomyositis

It is a systemic autoimmune disease, part of a larger group of idiopathic inflammatory myopathies, characterized by muscle and skin involvement (Shinjo & Souza, 2013).

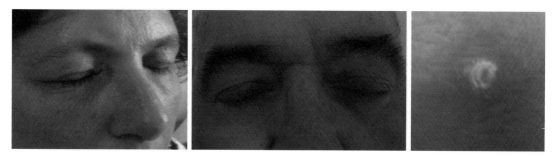

Figure 22: (from left to right) periorbital erythema, heliotrope erythema and calcinosis cutis.

Diagnosis is based on clinical picture:

- Typical skin rash: erythema in the periorbital area named heliotrope or blue-violet;

- Erythema and nodules on the dorsa of hands and fingers (Gottron's papules);

- Nail-fold hemorrhages, poikilodermic aspect of the skin on the neck and pre-sternal area

- Calcinosis cutis

Muscle weakness, increased levels of serum muscle enzymes (AST – aspartate transaminase, ALT- alanine transaminase, aldolase, creatin kinase), are also part of the missing puzzle for the proper diagnosis.

Dystrophic calcinosis represents abnormal deposition of calcium salts in affected skin, subcutaneous tissues, and muscles or tendons, with normal serum levels of calcium and phosphate (Shinjo & Souza, 2013). Myositis autoantigens comprise the well-defined aminoacyl-tRNA synthases, the Mi-2 helicase/histone deacetylase protein complex, and the signal recognition particle (SRP) ribonucleoprotein, together with novel targets such as TIF1-γ, MDA5, NXP2, SAE, and HMGCR (da Cunha et al., 2013).

Discoid Lupus Erythematosus (DLE) (Lupus Erythematosus Chronicus Discoides)

Lupus erythematosus is a spectrum of disorders, ranging from a benign pure cutaneous form (Discoid lupus erythematosus) to a severe, systemic, life-threatening disease with minimal skin involvement (Systemic lupus erythematosus - SLE). In between there are a number of clinical entities with progression from one form to another. Clinical spectrum is large, and linked to ocular area one can observe:

- Red, scaling plaques on the face, on sun-exposed-areas; scales are very adherent to the epidermis and hair-follicles (carpe-tack sign) (Discoid lupus erythematosus)
- Atrophic scars and alopecia on the scalp and eyebrows (DLE)
- Rash on the butterfly area, or more diffuse, determined by sun exposure (SLE)

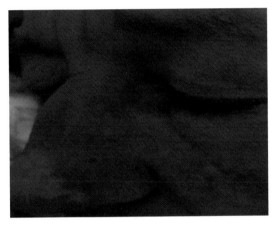

Figure 23: Erythema and scales, discrete atrophy over the nose, right in the inner part of the left eye.

Figure 24: Erythematous plaques malar area, right eyebrow, alopecia.

Drug Reactions

Cutaneous drug reactions are the most frequent adverse drug reactions. Although all types of skin manifestations can occur, maculopapular rash represent the majority (95%), followed by urticaria (5%) (Alanko et al., 1989). Any drug is capable of inducing adverse cutaneous reactions, most frequently involved being the antimicrobials and non-steroidal anti-inflammatory drugs (Chattergy et al., 2006).

- **Stevens Johnson Syndrome** Stevens-Johnson syndrome and toxic epidermal necrolysis are severe drug-induced cutaneous reactions, rare, but with high mortality. Toxic epidermal necrolysis is the most severe form, with epidermal detachment of > 30% of total body surface area; in Stevens Johnson syndrome, epidermal detachment is of < 10%, whereas involvement of 10% – 30% is defined as overlap syndrome (Fritsch & Sidoroff, 2000). The skin lesions are comparable to second-degree burns (Palmieri et al., 2002), and can be associated with major metabolic abnormalities, sepsis or multi organ failure. The treatment needs to be performed in intensive care units.

6 E -

Ephelide

Ephelides are small hyperpigmented macules, caused by increased melanin production. Ephelides are observed in genetically predisposed individuals, particularly fair-skinned people.

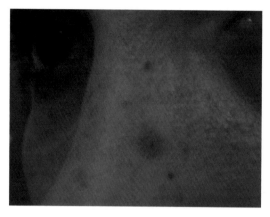

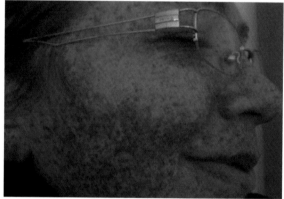

Figure 25: Ephelides constitutional Eruptive angiomatosis on the nose.

Figure 26: LEOPARD syndrome.

Eruptive Angiomatosis

Cutaneous angiomatosis is a large, diffuse, mainly superficial angioma, unique or multiple, especially on the face.

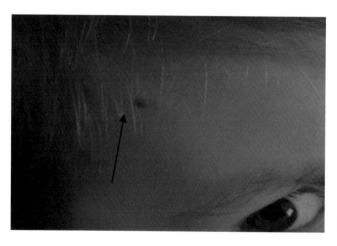

Figure 27: Superficial angioma.

Erysipelas of the Face

Facial erysipelas represents cutaneous streptococcal and *Staphylococcus aureus* infection, clinically characterized by sharply delineated, unilateral, intense erythematous (sometimes bullous), edematous area, especially on the face. It can be accompanied by fever, leukocytosis and lymphadenopathy. Antibiotics are prescribed from the first signs of infection: benzyl penicillin, erythromycin, flucloxacillin.

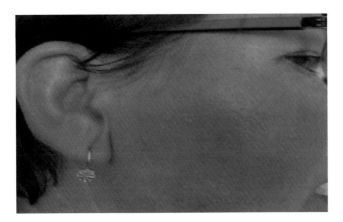

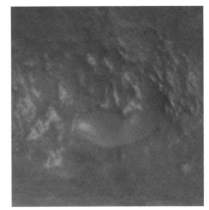

Figure 28: Erysipelas on the left hemifacies.

Figure 29: Bullae - close view.

Erythema Infectiosum (Fifth Disease, Infectious Erythema)

It is an infectious exanthema caused by parvovirus B19 that occurs in epidemics (Thammasri et al., 2013), during spring and summer especially in children. The erythema is quite characteristic: slapped cheek appearance.

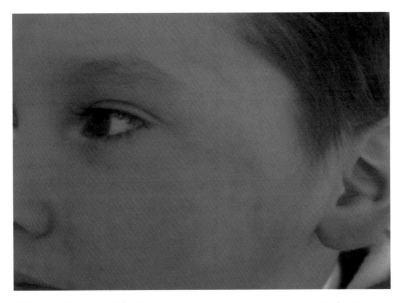

Figure 30: Slapped cheek appearance in a case of erythema infectiosum

7 F -

Factitial Dermatitis (Dermatitis Artefacta)

These conditions represent self-induced skin lesions as sign of emotional instability, psychiatric therapy being the rule.

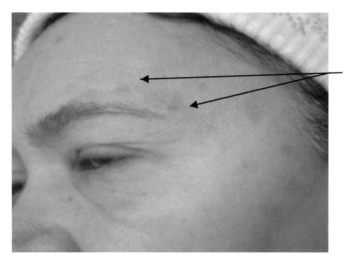

Figure 31: Atrophic scars around the ocular area.

Favre-Racouchot Syndrome (Nodular Elastosis with Cysts and Comedones; Elastoidosis Cutanea Nodularis Et Cystica)

It is a form of chronic actinic impairment of the skin after years of sun exposure; more frequently observed in men, in elderly, around the eyes. The lesions consist of giant comedones, cysts, wrinkles, deep furrows or yellowish discoloration of the skin. Dermabrasive methods or laser can be recommend for esthetic reasons.

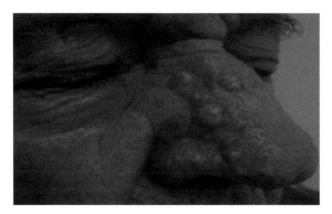

Figure 32: Giant comedones, cysts.

8   H -

Hemangioma

Periocular hemangioma is characterized by a benign proliferation of the vascular endothelium. They are not seen at birth, they develop during the first month of life, followed by a rapid proliferating phase (sometimes with ulceration). Slowly or spontaneously, they can regress through an involution phase; most described in girls, with no reported difference according to race. Based on the involvement degree, the classification made by Rootman distinguishes: superficial, subcutaneous, deep orbital or combined hemangioma (Rootman et al., 1988). They can be single, or multiple and of different size.

Superficial hemangioma affect the eyelid or conjunctiva and they are named strawberry hemangioma because of the intense red color; although bleeding, ulceration and infection may occur, the healing being spontaneous, with minimal scarring. If the lesion is posterior to the orbital septum, the clinical appearance is as subcutaneous bluish nodule (Hernandez et al., 2013).

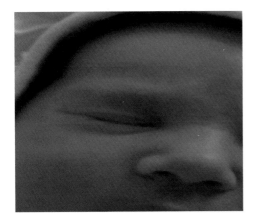 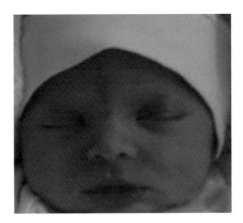

Figure 33: Hemangioma of the right palpebral area.   **Figure 34:** Hemangioma on the face.

If the diameter is higher than 1 cm, there is the risk of hemorrhages, obstruction of the visual axis, cosmetic problems and it raise the indication of therapy: surgical excision, laser, oral propranolol, topical timolol maleate, systemic or intralesional steroid, bleomycin, interferon alpha, vincristine, cyclophosphamide (Hernandez et al., 2013). Hemangiomas must be differentiated from vascular malformations (nevus flammeus, port wine stain) that are characterized by:

- Present at birth
- Macular area of erythema due to dilated superficial capillaries
- Trigeminal area involvement
- Lack of any tendency to spontaneous evolution
- Possible extension all over the face, in years

Herpes Simplex

It represents a cutaneous infection caused by Herpes virus hominis, type1 and 2, the latter being mostly associated with genital infection.

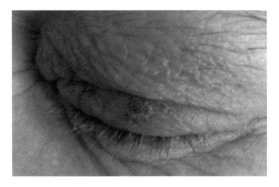
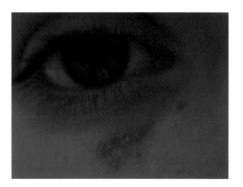

Figure 35: Herpes simplex on the left palpebral area.   **Figure 36**: Herpes simplex.

Clinical features are characteristic and easy to recognize even in atypical location (eyelid): group of small vesicles that persist for 3-6 days with spontaneous healing. If the infection touches the cornea there is the risk of scarring and ulceration and an immediate treatment is mandatory.

Recurrent forms are not rare and severe, cases being described in patients with AIDS. Therapeutic response to orally administered Acyclovir is better if the administration begins within first 72 hours; it lasts for 7 days and may be continuously in small doses in recurrent forms. Other options are: Valacyclovir or Brivudine, but more expensive.

Herpes Zoster

It is caused by Herpes virus varicellae. It appears as grouped small vesicles in a dermatome distribution, on an erythematous base, that can become infected. If the ophthalmic branch of trigeminal nerve is involved, ocular damage is reported. Post-herpetic neuralgia is frequently described in elderly, but not related to the intensity of clinical signs. Acyclovir is strongly recommended in higher doses up to 800mgx5/day for 7 days in severe cases. Neurologists must treat post-herpetic neuralgia.

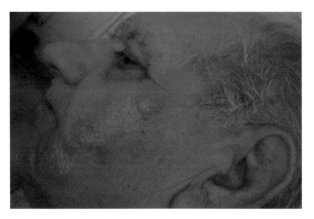

Figure 37: Herpes zoster to left hemifacies, with ocular involvement.

9   L -

Lentigo Senilis/Maligna (Melanosis Circumscripta Precancerosa Dubreuilh; Melanotic Precancerosis)

Lentigo senilis (Solar lentigo) known popular as liver spots, are benign, discrete hyperpigmented macules on sun-exposed areas (dorsa of the hands, face) observed in elderly persons. Melanosis circumscripta precancerosa Dubreuilh; Melanotic precancerosis) defines a plaque of similar clinical findings, localized mostly on the face, especially around the eyes. Photoprotection and follow-up are the indications.

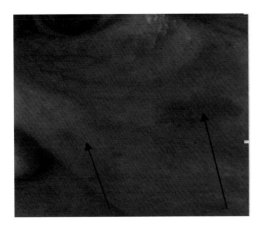

Figure 38: Lentigo senilis (left arrow) and melanosis Dubreuilh (right arrow).

Lupus Vulgaris (Tuberculosis Cutis Luposa)

It is the most diagnosed form of cutaneous tuberculosis, clinically pictured as a firm nodule on the face (apple jelly nodule on diascopy), with full diagnosis confirmation provided by biopsy (on histopathology report a tuberculoid granuloma is the hallmark) and culture. There is a good response to antituberculous drugs.

Figure 39: Lupus vulgaris on the right palpebral area.

Lyell Syndrome (Toxic Epidermal Necrolysis - TEN)

The Stevens–Johnson syndrome and toxic epidermal necrolysis represent two entities of the same drug-induced reaction syndrome, distinguished chiefly by severity and percentage of body surface involved. The incriminated drugs involved are mostly antibiotics and analgesics.

Stevens-Johnson syndrome is the less severe condition, detachment of the skin being less than 10% of the body surface; mucous membranes are affected in over 90% of patients, usually at two or more distinct sites (ocular, oral, and genital). Toxic epidermal necrolysis is a more severe form, in which more than 30% of the body skin is affected, the mucous membranes being also involved in all cases (Ameen et al., 2013).

10   M -

Malignant Melanoma

This disorder is represented by malign tumor of the melanocytic cells, displayed on sun-exposed areas. Early surgical excision is the first step of therapy, pursued by oncologic follow-up.

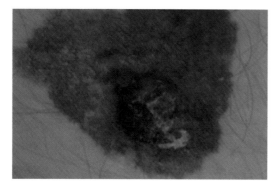

Figure 40: Malignant melanoma.

Molluscum Contagiosum

It is a DNA poxvirus infection, with an incubation period of 2 -7 weeks (Rao et al., 2013), clinically characterized by unique or multiple, round, translucid, dome shaped, flesh colored/pink papules with a central punctum. The lesions can be spread by autoinoculation, on the face, eyelids, around the mouth or on other parts of the body. Multiple lesions are seen in small children. The best therapeutic option resides in lesions removal by means of a curette followed by topical iodine applications upon the excised area.

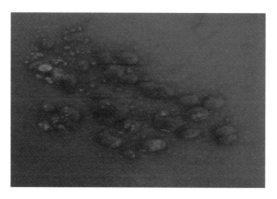

Figure 41: Close-view of a cluster of molluscum.

Morphea Linear

Linear morphea of the forehead or *en coup de sabre* is a variant of localized morphea (sclero-derma), usually present in children, as an indurated plaque that extend from the frontal hair-line to the face. Sclerosis can involve not only the skin but in rare cases, the muscles, bones or even brain, as well. There is a claimed etiologic relation with Borelli infection, but which is still controversial (Miller et al., 2012).

Mycosis Fungoides

It is a rare form of cutaneous lymphoma, clinically named "the great imitator" and diagnosed on histopathological grounds. Management of Mycosis fungoides is different, accordingly to the stage of the disease:

- Early stage: topical corticosteroids, phototherapy (psoralen plus ultraviolet A radiation or ultraviolet B radiation), topical chemotherapy, topical or systemic bexarotene, and radiotherapy;

- Advanced stage disease: retinoids(bexarotene), interferon-alpha, histone deacetylase inhibitors, the fusion toxin denileukin diftitox, systemic chemotherapy, extracorporeal photopheresis.

11   N -

Nevus

Banal or acquired melanocytic nevi are small (2-3 mm), with a brown uniform color, mostly appearing during the second life decade. Throughout maturation period they can become darker or they can loose pigment and transform into flash-colored nevi.

Halo nevi (Sutton nevi) are nevi with a depigmenting area around that usually disappear entirely in several months, a pale area of repigmentation occurring within years. There are commonly observed in children and no excision is necessary.

Congenital melanocytic nevi are present at birth, might be small, medium or giant, of different clinical aspect, and require a close follow-up for the risk of melanoma.

Atypical nevi are banal nevi with some characteristic features: larger than 4mm in diameter, irregular shape, color, or with sign of inflammation. They are difficult to distinguish from early melanoma and careful examination and specialized monitoring is compulsory.

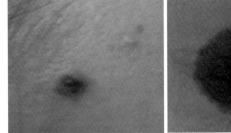 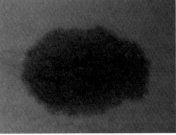 

Figure 42: Melanocytic nevi   **Figure 43:** Halo nevi   **Figure 44:** Congenital melanocyticnevi

12 P -

Pemphigus

Pemphigus vulgaris is an autoimmune bullous disease characterized by blistering of the skin and mucous membranes. Ocular involvement in pemphigus ranges from mild conjunctivitis to conjunctival blisters, erosions of the bulbar and palpebral conjunctiva (Palleschi et al., 2007). Diagnosis is based on clinical picture, histopathology (acantholysis), direct immunofluorescence (intercellular deposits of IgG and C3) and detection of anti-desmogelin 3 antibodies in patient's serum. The treatment requires high doses of prednisone and cyclophosphamide or izothiprine under strict medical surveillance (Olszewska et al., 2008).

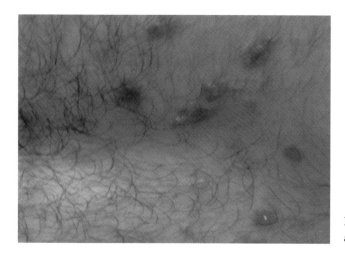

Figure 45: Pemphigus - blisters (vesicles and bullae) on the skin.

Cicatricial Pemphigoid

Mucous membrane pemphigoid is a systemic 'type 2' autoimmune disease, with ocular involvement in about 70% of cases (ocular cicatricial pemphigoid); it implicates conjunctiva in almost all cases, while clinical picture can vary from chronic conjunctivitis to end stage of progressive cicatrization and blindness. Even in early stage, diagnosis can be made based on immunoglobulin or complement deposition at the epithelial basement membrane of biopsied conjunctiva (Bernauer et al., 1997), or other mucous involvement. The mainstay of therapy is Dapsone due its anti-fibrosis and anti-inflammatory effect, followed by azathioprine, and rarely steroids.

Psoriasis

Psoriasis is a chronic inflammatory disease affecting skin, nails, and joints and with multiple comorbidities, psoriasis being thus now considered a systemic disease.

Along with typical erythematous scaly plaques that can be seen on the face and eyelids, ocular findings occur in approximately 10% of patients with psoriasis (Kilic et al., 2013), and include blepharitis, conjunctivitis, keratitis, xerophthalmia, corneal abscess, cataract, orbital myositis, symblepharon, chorioretinopathy, uveitis and entropion (Erbagci et al., 2003). Uveitis is a severe complication that is diagnosed in 7-20% of all psoriasis cases (Erbagci et al.,

2003). It is of great importance that ophthalmological examination should be carried out periodically in psoriatic patients! Treatment of psoriasis is very difficult and based on: corticosteroids, vitamin D analogue, coal tar, topical retinoids and methotrexate, biologic agents (infliximab, etanercept, adalimumab, ustekinumab) as systemic therapy, along with phototherapy.

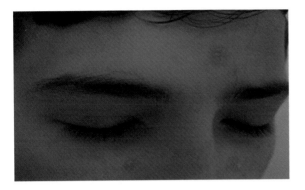 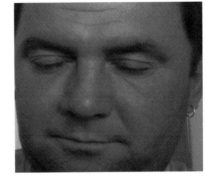

Figure 46: Small plaques psoriasis on the face.   **Figure 47:** Erythrodermic psoriasis (red man).

13 R -

Rosacea

Rosacea is a chronic skin disease that affects blood vessels and pilosebaceous units of the middle of the face (cheek, chin, nose, central forehead). Clinically there are 4 subtypes: erythematotelangiectatic, papulopustular, phymatous and ocular rosacea, and one variant granulomatous rosacea (phimatosis) (Wilkin et al., 2002). Patients with ocular rosacea may complain of foreign body sensation, dryness, itching, photophobia and tearing) (Baldwin, 2012). An ophthalmologic examination may reveal: blepharitis and meibomian gland dysfunction), chronic conjunctivitis, keratitis (Ghanem et al., 2003), iritis, episcleritis and scleritis (Oltz & Check, 2011).

Ocular rosacea improves with oral administered antibiotics: Doxycycline and Metronidazole, sometimes in prolonged administration. It is challenging, but very important as well, to link the two manifestations of the same disease: skin lesions and ocular problems.

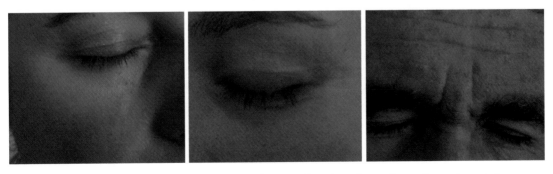

Figure 48: (from left to right) Rosacea erythematotelangiectatic, ocular and papulopustular.

14 S -

Seborrheic Dermatitis

Seborrheic dermatitis is a chronic inflammatory skin disease that mainly affects seborrheic areas of skin. An inflammatory response to the yeast *Pityrosporum ovale* has been thought to be important in the etiology of the condition (Chiriac et al., 2012). Excellent results may be achieved in this condition, by orally administered azoles.

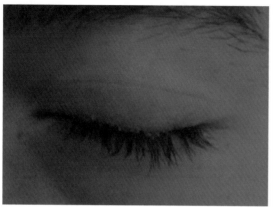
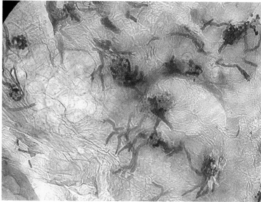

Figure 49: Seborrheic blepharitis.   **Figure 50:** Spores and hyphae of *Pityrosporum ovale*.

Seborrheic Keratosis

Known also under the name of seborrheic warts, the impairment is defined as benign proliferation of epidermal keratinocytes; it represents a constant observation, upon clinical examination especially in elderly. The term "wart" has been withdrawn in order to highlight the absence of human papilloma virus. Usually are multiple (sometimes tens), disseminated on cover parts of the body, with different hues of brown, of variable size. Incidental confusion is made with melanoma. The excision is routinely unnecessary, except esthetic demands or doubtful diagnosis.

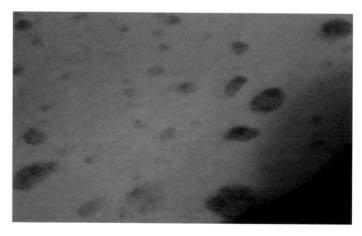

Figure 51: Seborrheic keratosis

Sturge-Weber Syndrome

Sturge-Weber syndrome is a rare congenital disorder characterized by: (1) Leptomeningeal hemangiomas (Leptomeningeal Angiomas); (2) Facial angiomas, typically in the ophthalmic (V1) and maxillary (V2) distributions of the trigeminal nerve. Ocular involvement may be present in the form of choroidal angioma, glaucoma, hemianopsia, or buphthalmos (enlargement of the coating of the eye) (Alexander & Norman, 1972).

15   T -

Tinea Faciei

Tinea faciei comprises cutaneous lesions due to dermatophytes, can be present on the face too, rarely on the palpebral area.

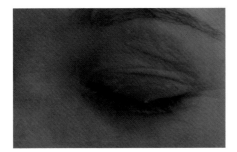   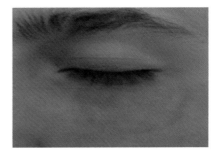

Figure 52: Tinea on the left palpebral area.   **Figure 53:** Tinea faciei.

The suspicion appears in front of an itchy, erythematous area, with raised advancing edges. Diagnosis is confirmed by revealing of the dermatophytes by direct examination of the scrapings taken from the edge; the isolation of the particular fungus is obtained by culture on Sabouraud medium. Treatment requires both topical and systemic approaches.

Tuberous Sclerosis

Tuberous sclerosis is a neurocutaneous syndrome characterized by abnormalities of the tegument and central nervous system. Diagnosis is based on evidence of existing two major features or one major plus two minor features (TSC Consensus Conference, 1998).

Major Features	Minor Features
Facial angiofibroma or forehead plaques	Multiple randomly distributed pits in dental enamel
Non-traumatic ungual or periungual fibroma	Hamartomatous polyps
Shagreen patch (connective tissue nevis)	Bone cysts
Multiple retinal nodular hamartomas	Cerebral white matter, radial migration lines
Cortical tuber	Gingival fibromas
Sub-ependymal nodule	Non-renal hamartoma
Sub-ependymal giant cell astrocytoma	Retinal achromic patch
Cardiac rhabdomyoma, single or multiple	"Confetti" skin lesions
Angiomyolipoma	Multiple renal cysts

Table 2: Major and minor features in the diagnosis of Tuberous sclerosis.

16   U -

Urticaria

The characteristic urticarial lesion is a rapidly developing raised wheal, unique or multiple, with transient course, commonly associated with pruritus. It is an emergency when signs of respiratory obstruction occur. Good response is obtained after administration of non-sedating antihistamines, short course of corticosteroids (7-10days).

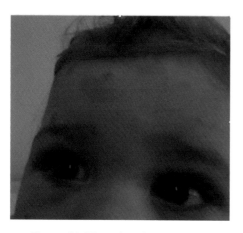 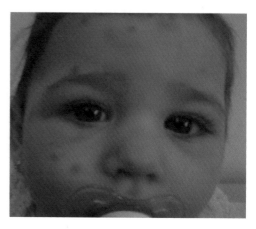

Figure 54: Hives (erythematous wheals) on the face (left) and right palpebral area (right)

17   V -

Vitiligo

Clinical definition: an area of acquired cutaneous depigmentation due to loss of normal mela-nocytes. The pathogenic mechanisms are complex, partially unknown, a strong association with autoimmune disorders such as pernicious anemia, thyroid diseases (autoimmune thy-roiditis), diabetes mellitus, Addison disease, being strongly incriminated. The ocular injuries occur frequently in vitiligo, an estimation of about 8.8% retinal impairment being stated in a recent study, although the percentage of ocular involvement is variable high (Shankar et al., 2012). Therapeutic attempt is based on topical corticosteroids, phototherapy (narrow band ultraviolet B), emollients, camouflage, grafting methods.

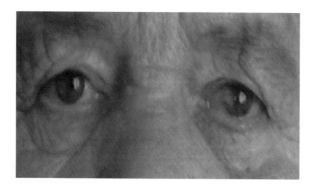

Figure 55: Vitiligo around the eyes.

18 W -

Warts

Warts are skin viral infections caused by human papilloma viruses (HPV) (more than 110 types being already described) (Schmitt et al., 2011). The virus is transmitted by direct contact, fewer strains of HPV being oncogenic.

 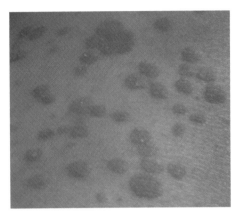

Figure 56: Verruca plana (plane warts).   **Figure 57:** Verruca vulgaris (common warts)

HPV phylogenetic tree is composed of five types (alpha, beta, gamma, mu, and nu papillomaviruses (Schmitt et al., 2011). Variable clinical manifestations are expressed on the skin, with different location, and related to a specific HPV. Plane and vulgaris warts that can be recognized on the face are due to non-oncogenic type alpha genus HPV (Schmitt et al., 2011). Although described in the literature as self-limiting, different somehow satisfying therapeutic methods have been tried: chemical destruction, cryotherapy, laser, surgical excision, curettage, electrocautery.

19 X -

Xanthelasma

White or yellow plaques of lipid deposits seen in the periorbital skin associated with hyper-lipidemias status, defines usually xanhelasma. The major concern is esthetic and excision is the choice.

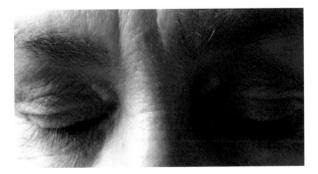

Figure 58: Xanthelasma.

Xanthogranuloma

This dermal pathology consists of yellowish, firm, round papule or nodule, with unknown etiology but with benign evolution, localized on the face, neck and trunk, especially in children. It is a form of histiocytosis (class IIa) derived from dermal dendrocytes (Sampaio et al., 2012). In cases where involution is not spontaneous, a surgical excision is widely accepted.

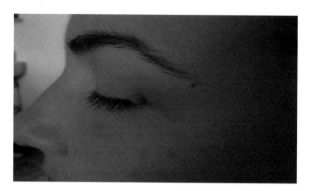

Figure 59: Palpebral localization of xanthogranuloma.

Authors

Anca Chiriac
Dermatology Department, Apollonia University, Iaşi, Romania
P. Poni Research Institute of Macromolecular Chemistry, Romanian Academy, Romania
Nicolina Medical Center, Iaşi, Romania

Liliana Foia
Surgical Department, Faculty of Dental Medicine, University of Medicine and Pharmacy "Gr. T. Popa", Iaşi, Romania

References

Abramovits, W., Oquendo, M., Vincent, K.D. & Gupta, A.K. (2013). PICATO (ingenol mebutate 0.015% and 0.05% gels): a novel treatment for actinic keratosis. Skinmed, 11(2), 111-115.

Alanko, K., Stubb, S. & Kauppinen, K. (1989). Cutaneous drug reactions: clinical types and causative agents. A five-year survey of patients (1981-1985). Acta dermato-venereologica, 69, 223–226.

Alexander, G.L., Norman, R.M. (1972). Sturge-Weber syndrome. In: Vinken P.J., Bruyn, G.W., editors. Handbook of clinical neurology.Vol.14. Amsterdam: Holland Publishing Company, pp. 223–240.

Allegue, F., Lis, M.P. & Pérez-Álvarez, R. (2007). Primary cutaneous cryptococcosis presenting as a whitlow. Acta Dermato-venereologica, 87, 443–444.

Ameen, K.H., Pinninti, R. & Jami, S. (2013). Aceclofenac induced Stevens-Johnson/toxic epidermal necrolysis overlap syndrome. Journal of Pharmacology and Pharmacotherapy, 4(1), 69-71.

Baderca, F., Mates, I. & Solovan, C. (2013). Unusual variant of blue nevus associated with dermatofibromas. Romanian Journal of Morphology and Embriology, 54(2), 413-417.

Baldwin, H.E. (2012). Diagnosis and treatment of rosacea: state of the art. Journal of Drugs in Dermatology, 11(6), 725-730.

Bernauer, W., Itin, P.H., Kirtschig, G. (1997). Cicatricial pemphigoid. Developments in Ophthalmology, 28, 46-63.

Bondeson, J. (2001). Everard home, John Hunter, and cutaneous horns: A historical review. American Journal of Dermatopathology, 23, 362–369.

Buinauskaite, E., Zalinkevicius, R., Buinauskiene, J. & Valiukeviciene, S. (2013). Pain during topical photodynamic therapy of actinic keratosis with 5-aminolevulinic acid and red light source: randomized controlled trial. Photodermatology Photoimmunology & Photomedicine, 29(4), 173-181.

Chattergy, S., Ghosh, A.P. & Barbhujia, Dey S.K. (2006). Adverse cutaneous drug reactions: A one year survey at a dermatology outpatient clinic of a tertiary care hospital. Indian Journal of Pharmacology, 38, 429–431.

Chiriac, A., Chiriac, A.E, Murgu, A. & Foia, L. (2012). Seborrheic dermatitis eyelid involvement (seborrheic blepharitis) in children not a rare clinical observation; Case report. Our Dermatology Online, 3(1), 52-53.

Cohn, B. (2000). From sunlight to actinic keratosis to squamous cell carcinoma. Journal of American Academy of Dermatology, 42, 143-144.

Cornish, K.S., Gregory, M.E. & Ramaesh, K. (2010). Systemic cyclosporine A in severe atopic keratoconjunctivitis. European Journal of Ophthalmology, 20(5), 844-851.

da Cunha, G.F., de Souza, F.H, Levi-Neto, M. & Shinjo, S.K. (2013). Chloroquine diphosphate: a risk factor for herpes zoster in patients with dermatomyositis/polymyositis. Clinics (Sao Paulo), 68(5), 621-627.

Durani, B.K., Kurzen, H., Jaeckel, A., Kuner, N., Naeher, H. & Hartschuh, W. (2001). Malignant transformation of multiple dermal cylindromas. British Journal of Dermatology, 145(4), 653–656.

El Safoury, O.S., Fawzy, M.M., Hay, R.M., Hassan, A.S., El Maadawi, Z.M. & Rashed, L.A. (2011). The possible role of trauma in skin tags through the release of mast cell mediators. Indian Journal of Dermatology, 56(6), 641-646.

Erbagci, I., Erbagci, Z., Gungor, K. & Beckir, N. (2003). Ocular Anterior Segment Pathologies and Tear Film Changes in Patients with Psoriasis Vulgaris. Acta Medica Okayama, 57, 299–303.

Fritsch, P.O., Sidoroff, A. (2000). Drug-induced Stevens-Johnson syndrome/toxic epidermal necrolysis. The American Journal of Clinical Dermatology, 1(6), 349–360.

Ghanem, V.C., Mehra, N., Wong, S. & Mannis, M.J. (2003). The prevalence of ocular signs in acne rosacea: comparing patients from ophthalmology and dermatology clinics. Cornea, 22(3), 230-233.

González-López, J.J., López-Alcalde, J., Morcillo Laiz, R., Fernández Buenaga, R. & Rebolleda Fernández, G. (2012). Topical cyclosporine for atopic keratoconjunctivitis. Cochrane Database System Review, 12, 9.

Gupta, S., Aggarwal, R., Gupta, S. & Arora, S.K. (2008). Human papillomavirus and skin tags: Is there any association? Indian Journal of Dermatology Venereology & Leprology, 74, 222–225.

Habif, T.P. (2004). Bacterial infections. Clinical dermatology: a color guide to diagnosis and therapy, 4.

Hernandez, J.A., Chia, A., Ouah, B.L. & Seah, L.L. (2013). Periocular capillary hemangioma: management practices in recent years. Clinical Ophthalmology, 7, 1227–1232.

Herndon, D. (2012). Chapter 4: Prevention of Burn Injuries, Total burncare (4th ed.). Saunders, 46.

Hogan, M.J. (1953) Atopic keratoconjunctivitis. American Journal of Ophthalmology, 36, 937-947.

International Study Group for Behçet's disease. Criteria for diagnosis of Behçet's disease [review]. (1990). Lancet, 335, 1078–1080.

Kaujalgi, R., Handa, S., Jain, A. & Kanwar, A.J. (2009). Ocular abnormalities in atopic dermatitis in Indian patients. Indian Journal of Dermatology Venereology & Leprology, 75, 148-151.

Kilic, B., Dogan, U., Parlak, A.H., Goksugur, N., Polat, M., Serin, D. & Ozmen, S. (2013). Ocular findings in patients with psoriasis. International Journal of Dermatology, 52(5), 554-559.

Lee, K.C. & Weinstock, M.A. (2013). Periocular actinic keratosis, keratinocyte carcinomas, and eyeglasses use. Department of Veterans Affairs, Topical Tretinoin Chemoprevention Trial Group. Journal of American Academy of Dermatology, 69(1), 165-167.

Magarasevic, L & Abazi, Z. (2013). Unilateral open-angle glaucoma associated with the ipsilateral nevus of ota. Case Reports in Ophthalmological Medicine. Epub.

Matsuzaki, T., Mashima, Y. Idei, T., Hashimoto, T. & Mashima, Y. (1996). Unilateral ocular cicatricial pemphigoid with circulating IgA and IgG autoantibodies reactive with the 180 kD bullous pemphigoid antigen. British Journal of Ophthalmology, 80(8), 769.

Miller, K., Lehrhoff, S., Fischer, M., Meehan, M. & Latkowski, J.A. (2012). Linear morphea of the forehead (en coup de sabre). Dermatology Online Journal, 18(12), 22.

Naldi, L., Parazzini, F. & Gallus, S. (2009). GISED study centers Prevalence of Atopic Dermatitis in Italian Schoolchildren: Factors Affecting its Variation. Acta Dermato-venereologica, 89, 122–125.

Nthumba, P.M. (2007). Giant cutaneous horn in an African woman: a case report. Journal of Medical Case Reports, 1, 170.

Olszewska, M., Komor, M., Mazur,M., Rogozinski, T. (2008). Response of ocular pemphigus vulgaris to therapy. Case report and review of literature. Journal of Dermatological Case Reports, 2(1), 1-3.

Oltz, M. & Check, J. (2011). Rosacea and its ocular manifestations. Optometry, 82(2), 92-103.

Palleschi, G.M., Giomi, B., Fabbri P. (2007). Ocular involvement in pemphigus. American Journal of Ophthalmology, 144(1), 149–152.

Palmieri, T.L., Greenhalgh, D.G., Saffle, J.R., Spence, R.J., Peck, M.D., Jeng, J.C., Mozingo, D.W., Yowler, C.J., Sheridan, R.L., Ahrenholz, D.H., Caruso, D.M., Foster, K.N., Kagan, R.J., Voigt, D.W., Purdue, G.F., Hunt, J.L., Wolf, S. & Molitor, F. (2002). A multicenter review of toxic epidermal necrolysis treated in U.S. burn centers at the end of the twentieth century. The Journal of Burn Care and Rehabilitation, 23(2), 87-96.

Rao, K., Priya, N., Umadevi, H. & Smitha, T. (2013). Molluscum contagiosum. Journal of Maxillofacial Pathology, 17(1), 146-147.

Rootman, J. Diseases of the Orbit. (1988). Philadelphia: JB Lippincott, 539–543.

Sampaio, F.M.S., Lourenço, F.T., Obadia, D.L. & do Nascimento, L.V. (2012). Case for diagnosis. Anais Brasileiros de Dermatologia, 87(5), 789-90.

Samrao, A. & Cockerell, C.J. (2013). Pharmacotherapeutic Management of Actinic Keratosis: Focus on Newer Topical Agents. American Journal of Clinical Dermatology, 4, 273-277.

Schmitt, M., de Konig, M.N., Eekhof, J.A., Quint, W.G. & Pawlita, M. (2011). Evaluation of a novel multiplex human papillomavirus (HPV) genotyping assay for HPV types in skin warts. Journal of Clinical Microbiology, 49(9), 3267-3267.

Schneider, I., Lehmann, M.D., Kogosov, V., Stockfleth, E. & Nindl, I. (2013). Eyebrow hair from actinic keratosis patients harbor the highest number of cutaneous human papillomaviruses. BMC Infectious Diseases, 13, 186-186.

Shankar, D.S., Shashikala, K. & Madala, R. (2012). Clinical patterns of vitiligo and its associated co morbidities: A prospective controlled cross-sectional study in South India. Indian Dermatology Online Journal, 3(2), 114-118.

Shinjo, S.K. & Souza, F.H. (2013). Update on the treatment of calcinosis in dermatomyositis. Revue Brazilian de Reumatologie, 53(2), 211-214.

Thammasri, K., Rauhamaki, S., Wang, L., Filippou, A., Kivovich, V., Marjomaki, V., Naides, SJ & Gilbert, L. (2013). Parvovirus B19 Induced Apoptotic Bodies Contain Altered Self-Antigens that are Phagocytosed by Antigen Presenting Cells. PLoS One, 12(8), 6.

Viskochil, D., Buchberg, A.M., Xu, G., Cawthon, R.M., Stevens, J., Wolff, R.K., Culver, M., Carey, J.C., Copeland, N.G., Jenkins, N.A., White, R. & O'Connel, P. (1990). Deletions and a translocation interrupt a cloned gene at the neurofibromatosis type 1 locus. Cell, 62(1), 187–192.

Werner, R.N., Sammain, A., Erdmann, R., Hartmann, V., Stockfleth, E. & Nast, A. (2013). The Natural History of Actinic Keratosis: A Systematic Review. British Journal of Dermatology. 2013, Epub.

Wilkin, J., Dahl, M., Detmar, M., Drake, L., Feinstein, A., Odom, R. & Powell, F. (2002). Standard classification of rosacea: Report of the National Rosacea Society Expert Committee on the classification and staging of rosacea. Journal of American Academy of Dermatology, 46(4), 584-587.

Williams, H.C., Purned, P.G.J., Pembroke, A.C. et al. (1994). The UK working party diagnostic criteria for atopic dermatitis. British Journal of Dermatology, 131, 401-416.

Zouboulis, C.C., Kotter, I., Djawari, D., Kirch, W., Kohl, P.K., Ochsendorf, F.R., Keitel, W., Stadler, R., Wollina, U., Proksch, E., Söhnchen, R., Weber, H., Gollnick, H.P., Hölzle, E., Fritz, K., Licht, T. & Orfanos C.E. (1997). Epidemiological features of Adamantiades-Behçet's disease in Germany and in Europe. Yonsei Medical Journal, 38, 411–422.

Myopia: Current Cellular Concepts on the Pathology and Mechanisms

Ping Kwan

1 Introduction

Belonging to the central nervous system (CNS), eyes are the primary visual organs in most of the well-known vertebrates (including birds and human). Due to the function of connecting the photonic world to the brain, eyes are also known as the "windows to the soul" or "mirror of systemic health" (due to the association of systemic pathology with retinopathy) (Foster and Khaw, 2009). As visual impairment significantly degrades the quality of life and even survival, vision health must not be overlooked. Among the common vision disorders (including macular degeneration, diabetic retinopathy, glaucoma and myopia) (Cooke Bailey et al., 2013), myopia (also known as near-sightedness or short-sightedness) is recognized as a refractive-error-associated visual disorder leading to a blurred distant vision (Cooke Bailey et al., 2013; Morgan et al., 2012). Although the consequence of myopia is commonly and readily managed by efficient vision aids (e.g. glasses, contact lenses and refractive surgery) (Morgan et al., 2012; Edwards, 1998), myopia has emerged as one of the major public health concerns world-wide (especially in Asia) due to: 1) of all refractive errors, high myopia has the most severe visual consequences; 2) the prevalence of myopia is increasing in developed countries; 3) World Health Organization (WHO) recognizes that myopia is a major cause of visual impairment if the refractive error is not fully corrected; and 4) people with moderate and high myopia are at a substantially increased risk of potentially blinding ocular pathologies (e.g. glaucoma and cataracts) which are not prevented by refractive corrections (Cooke Bailey et al., 2013; Morgan et al., 2012; Koh et al., 2013; Perera and Aung, 2010; Pan et al., 2013; Verhoeven et al., 2014). In 2002, it has been estimated that the prevalence of myopia in Asia was as high as 70-90%, in Europe and America 30-40%, and in Africa 10-20% (Fredrick, 2002). In 2011, a new study pointed out that myopia had become increasingly more common over the past 50 years, and was estimated to affect around 1.6 billion people worldwide, with numbers expected to climb to 2.5 billion by 2020 (Yu et al., 2011).

Despite the costs associated with myopia varies considerably from country to country and even within countries (please see table 1 for calculation model) (Edwards, 1998; Lim and Frick, 2010), the estimated costs (including professional services, eye-care products and other indirect costs related to loss of productivity) for the myopic population of the United States even in 1990 were US$4.8 billion (Edwards, 1998). Together with the social impacts (at least in Hong Kong, there are unaided vision requirements in some occupations including disciplined services and commercial aviation) (Edwards, 1998), it is imperative to investigate into different aspects of myopia (including the relevant cellular and molecular mechanisms) in order to provide insights for the development of better therapeutic/diagnostic management and even prophylactic interventions. This review will provide an up-to-date overview on the current concept of myopia (mainly focused on the cellular/molecular level). Additionally, the com-

Annual cost of myopia	= Number of paying myopes × **average amount spent per myope**	
	Or	
	= Population	× **myopia prevalence (%)**
		× **proportion of myopes having correction**
		× **proportion of myopes paying for correction**
		× **average amount spent per myope**

Table 1: model for calculating the economic cost of myopia. (Lim and Frick, 2010).

mon research techniques involved and the impacts contributed by different ocular cells on myopia will also be discussed.

2   Current Concept of Myopia

The concepts of near-sightedness and far-sightedness are commonly thought to be first identified by Aristotle (384-321 BC) and the term myopia (Greek: *myein* means "to close", *opos* means "the eye") was first coined by Galen (138-201 AD) (Rehm, 1981). The original meaning of the greek word "myopos" was "attempting to see clearly by partially closing the eyes" (Rehm, 1981). Since the 18th century, the concept of myopia is based upon the refractive error associated with the misalignment of image foci which are commonly believed to be shifted anteriorly towards the cornea and cannot be corrected by accommodation (figure 1) (Morgan *et al.*, 2012; Edwards, 1998). In other words, the recent definition of myopia is a refractive condition of the eye in which the images of distant objects are focused at some finite distances in front of the retina and cannot be corrected by accommodation (Morgan *et al.*, 2012; Edwards, 1998). In fact, the refractive status of the eye is a complex variable and is determined by the balance between the dioptric power of various ocular refractive elements (including cornea, aqueous humor, crystalline lens and vitreous body) and the ocular axial length (which is the most variable factor during development and with the strongest correlation with the refractive status) (Morgan *et al.*, 2012). Thus, assuming the overall ocular dioptric power is unchanged, longer eyes are more likely to be myopic than shorter eyes while shorter eyes could be more likely to be hyperopic than longer eyes (Morgan *et al.*, 2012). Additionally, retinal breaks and retinal detachment occur more frequently in eyes with increased ocular axial length (commonly measured in millimeters) as a result of lattice degeneration, increased frequency of posterior vitreous detachment, or macular hole formation (Jeganathan *et al.*, 2010; Khor, 2010; Mao *et al.*, 2011). In fact, it is commonly believed that ocular axial length is a major determinant of the ocular refractive error seen in myopic individuals (also known as myopes). Despite there are studies indicating that low myopes (subjects with low myopia) had similar ocular dimensions to emmetropes (subjects with normal vision) (Wildsoet, 1998), the importance of ocular axial length in myopia is well supported since the 19th century correlation studies which demonstrated that: 1) ocular axial length and ocular refractive error exhibited a strong linear correlation; 2) subjects with conus (clinically interpreted as a sign of excessive eye growth) had longer eyes; and 3) 50% of the variability in ocular refractive error was due to differences in ocular axial length while 25% of the variability was due to the cornea and another 20% was due to the crystalline lens (Wildsoet, 1998). Although myopia and ocular axial length have a very intimate relationship, it should be cautious that associations with myopia do not equal to associa-

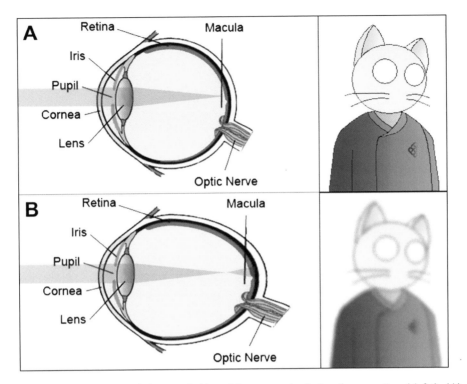

Figure 1: schematic optics of the eye (left) and its conceptual visual perception (right). (A) emmetropic eyes; and (B) myopic eyes. (Morgan *et al.*, 2012; Edwards, 1998).

tions with ocular axial length. For example, recent studies demonstrated that nuclear cataract was associated with myopia but not ocular axial length (Pan *et al.*, 2013).

Finally, it is noteworthy that myopia is commonly categorizes into different types and subtypes mainly according to the age of onset, severity of refractive errors and the main causative factor. For example, myopic conditions resulted mainly from a disproportionately increase of ocular axial length are coined as axial myopia (more common) while those resulted mainly from changes in ocular refractive elements (e.g. abnormal corneal curvature, abnormal density of crystalline lens and abnormal refractive index of ocular chamber media) are coined as refractive myopia (relatively less common) (Edwards, 1998; Perera and Aung, 2010; Khor, 2010). Regarding the severity classification of myopia, please refer to table 2. Other classifications of myopia will be discussed in later sections.

2.1 Pathology-based Myopia

As a consequence of imbalanced ratio of overall ocular dioptric power versus ocular axial length, myopia can also be induced by any pathophysiological processes that alter this ratio. Thus, these pathophysiologically induced myopic conditions may coin as the **pathological myopia** (also known as progressive myopia or degenerative myopia) (Edwards, 1998; Park *et al.*, 2013).

Pathological myopia was originally described as high myopia accompanied by characteristic degenerative changes in the ocular tunics with compromised visual function (Morgan *et al.*, 2012). Although not all highly myopic eyes develop pathological signs (degenerative changes), there is a trend that the prevalence of pathological signs increases with the severity

Phenotypes	Definition
Low (also known as mild) myopia	-03.00 D < SPH or SE < 00.00 D
Moderate myopia*	-05.00 D < SPH or SE ≤ -03.00 D
High myopia*	-10.00 D < SPH or SE ≤ -05.00 D
Very high (also known as extreme) myopia*	SPH or SE ≤ -10.00 D

Table 2: severity classification of myopia (in terms of refractive errors). SPH = sphere component/power; CYL = cylindrical component/power; SE = spherical equivalent refractive error (SPH + CYL/2); D = unit of lens power expressed in dioptres (1/focal length); * = it should be noted that some of the studies may use -6.00 D instead of -5.00 D as the boundary between moderate and high myopia while using -15.00 D instead of -10.00 D as the boundary between high and very high myopia. (Morgan *et al.*, 2012; Edwards, 1998; Khor, 2010; Li and Fan, 2010; Tsai *et al.*, 2008).

of refractive errors, deformations, age and the presence of other pathological features (Shih *et al.*, 2006; Morgan *et al.*, 2012; Flores-Moreno *et al.*, 2013). For example, high myopic patients with maculopathy were found older, had longer axial length and thinner SFCT (Hsu *et al.*, 2014).

Although some pathological complications (such as choroidal neovascularisation) are shared between myopia and pathological myopia (Wong *et al.*, 2014), it is commonly believed that the aetiology of pathological myopia is different from that of other forms of myopia (especially nearwork is not likely to be implicated in its onset or development) (Edwards, 1998). Since the suggestions made by Curtin in 1979 regarding the definition of physiological myopia, pathological myopia can be defined and diagnosed as a myopic condition in which the eye of regard has an ocular axial length longer than the emmetropic range while the temporal crescent is wider than one tenth of the optic disc diameter (Edwards, 1998). It should beware of that the presence of a significantly-wide temporal crescent is not always accompanied with a longer-than-emmetropic ocular axial length as recognized in 1967 by Otsuka who proposed that such partially matching condition shall be described as intermediate myopia (Edwards, 1998). Interestingly, temporal crescents are seen more frequently in Chinese eyes than in Caucasian eyes (Edwards, 1998).

Pathological myopia typically initiates around the pre-teen years and advances rapidly with characteristic fundus degenerations (Edwards, 1998; Wildsoet, 1998). Although the normal vision may or may not be attainable with correction lenses, ocular axial length is always abnormally large (Edwards, 1998). Additionally, posterior staphyloma (outward protrusion of posterior ocular tunics) is commonly considered as a pathognomonic feature of pathological myopia despite it is not common in highly myopic children (Morgan *et al.*, 2012; Lee, 2010). Recent studies have demonstrated that there was a high prevalence of beta peripapillary atrophy, retinal tessellation and peripheral retina degenerations in highly myopic eyes (Koh *et al.*, 2013). Although higher myopia is more likely leading to retinal degenerative changes, retinal degeneration per se can increase the susceptibility to myopia, at least in mice (Park *et al.*, 2013).

2.2   Accommodation-based Myopia

The state of ocular accommodation accounts for the variable dioptric power of the crystalline lens and is an important contributor to myopia (Edwards, 1998). As the shape/dioptric power of crystalline lens is regulated by cilliary muscles, spasm of the cilliary muscles may lead to a myopic shift even in emmetropic (Greek: *emmetros* means "well-proportioned", *opos* means "the eye") and hyperopic (Greek: *hyper* means "beyond", *opos* means "the eye") individuals (Edwards, 1998). Due to the dynamic properties of accommodation, myopia can only be accounted when the accommodative response is minimized (Rosenfield, 1998). As this myopic shift is caused by the failure to relax accommodation fully and can be relieved by the administration of cycloplegic drugs (muscarinic receptor antagonists, e.g. atropine) (Rosenfield, 1998; Forrester *et al.*, 2008d), such myopic condition is commonly known as **pseudomyopia** (also known as spurious myopia, false myopia, hypertonic myopia or functional myopia) (Edwards, 1998; Rosenfield, 1998). Although pseudomyopia can be caused by long periods of fine work at a short working distance, variations in the total amplitude and the subcomponents of accommodation seems unlikely to be the cause of nearwork-induced myopia (Edwards, 1998; Rosenfield, 1998). Regarding the accommodation amplitude, both emmetropic and myopic subjects exert only a small proportion (approximately 28% and 24%, respectively) of their total accommodation amplitude (Rosenfield, 1998). Regarding the accommodative subcomponents, please refer to Table 3 for details. It should be noted that although changes in blur-induced accommodation should not be regarded as a precursor to myopia development, the relative insensitivity to the presence of retinal blur may be an important factor in the aetiology of myopia (Rosenfield, 1998).

In addition to pseudomyopia, other accommodation-based myopic conditions included **anomalous myopias** (also known as empty field myopias) and **instrument myopia** which are induced mainly by light-intensity-associated mal-accomodation and optical-instrument-associated over-accommodation, respectively (Edwards, 1998). Within the anomalous myopia category, these temporary myopic states are further classified into: 1) **dark focus myopia** (induced by absence of light); 2) **night myopia** (induced by scotopic/low-ambient lighting levels); and 3) **twilight myopia** (induced by mesopic/medium-ambient lighting levels) (Edwards, 1998).

2.3   Astigmatism

Patients with myopia are often accompanied with astigmatism which further complicates the refractive error (Edwards, 1998). **Astigmatism** (Greek: *a* means "without", *stigmatos* means "a mark, spot or puncture") is a refractive condition wherein the non-uniform ocular dioptric powers hamper the sharp focus of images on the retina due to the resultant multiple misaligned image foci which cannot be corrected by changing viewing distance or accommodation (Kee, 2013; Packer *et al.*, 2011). To this day, astigmatism is generally classified into regular and irregular types (Packer *et al.*, 2011). **Regular types** feature orthogonal principal ocular meridians with symmetric dioptric power while **irregular types** feature a point-to-point variation in the angle separating the principal ocular meridians and in the magnitude of the dioptric power in each ocular meridian (Packer *et al.*, 2011). Regarding the details of ocular meridians and the tripartite nature of refraction, please refer to figure 2. Currently, there are many therapeutic options for managing astigmatism including corneal incisions, keratotomy and the use of toric intraocular lenses (Henderson *et al.*, 2011).

Despite the cause is not clear, astigmatism has been ascribed to a multi-factorial aetiology by human studies (Kee, 2013). Among the various factors, aberrant corneal structure is one of the important contributors to astigmatism as cornea contributes approximately 60% of the total dioptric power of the whole bio-optical system (Hauswirth *et al.*, 2008). In regard to the association with myopia, recent studies have indicated that while the "**with-the-rule**" astigma-

Accommodative subcomponents	Descriptions
Tonic accommodation	• Reflect the level of tonic innervation to the ciliary muscle • Emmetropic value > myopic value • Changes occur concurrently with myopic development
Proximally-induced accommodation	• Induced by the knowledge of apparent nearness of an object of regard • Emmetropic value > myopic value • The lowered value in myopes may be resulted from a reduced proximal gain factor
Convergent accommodation	• Induced by the output of the vergence system under closed-loop conditions with negative feedback mechanisms allowed to operate • No significant difference in the convergent accommodation versus convergence ratio among emmetropes and myopes
Disparity-induced accommodation	• Changes in the closed-loop accommodative response induced by the introduction of disparity stimuli • Emmetropic value > myopic value • Accomodative responses became equivalent between emmetropes and myopes after introducing a supplementary disparity stimulus
Blur-induced accommodation	• Changes in the accommodative response induced by the effects of retinal defocus • Emmetropic value > myopic value • Changes occur concurrently with myopic development

Table 3: relationship between various accommodative subcomponents and myopia. (Rosenfield, 1998).

tism predisposes the creation of myopia, both "**against-the-rule**" and **oblique** astigmatism have no influence on the creation of myopia (Czepita and Filipiak, 2005). Astigmatism has been found highly prevalent in both United States (around 28.4% of children) and Hong Kong (21.1% in preschool children) (Kleinstein *et al*, 2003; Fan *et al*, 2004).

3   Current Aetiological Concepts of Myopia

Body physiology is controlled by many different extracellular and intracellular molecular factors (including ions) that work together as different molecular cascades in an interlacing fashion (Kwan, 2013a; Kwan, 2013b; Kwan and Tse, 2013; Tse and Kwan, 2013). As the physiological state is the reflection of the underlying physiological pattern, pathological conditions are reflections of the aberrant changes of the corresponding physiological processes which further reflect the aberrant behaviour and/or changes of the underlying molecular factors and/or their associated molecular partners (Kwan, 2013a; Kwan, 2013b; Kwan and Tse, 2013; Tse and Kwan, 2013). Thus, myopia is a reflection of the aberrant physiological changes of the affected eye. In addition to the ocular pathophysiology, the mechanisms leading to such physiological changes or pathological consequences are also important targets for investigations. There are many epidemiological risk factors have been identified including nearwork, education/income, outdoor activity, age, race/ethnicity, nuclear cataract and family aggregation/genetics (Klein, 2010). Due to all physiological processes are affected by both **genetic** and

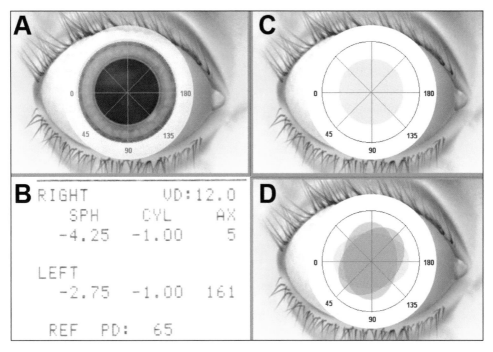

Figure 2: (A) principal ocular meridians: vertical axis (90-270°), horizontal axis (0-180°) and oblique axis (45-225°); (B) a prescription sample showing: the spherical component/power (SPH: primary indicator of ocular dioptric power where positive means convergent powers as seen in hyperopia while negative means divergent powers as seen in myopia), cylindrical component/power (CYL: one of the astigmatic indicators indicating the dioptric power of the astigmatic cylinder and is a separate entity from the spherical power), axis of the cylinder (AX: one of the astigmatic indicators), vertex distance (VD: distance between the back surface of a corrective lens and the front of the cornea) and pupillary distance (PD: distance between the centers of the pupils in each eye) of the right (also known as OD: oculus dexter) and left eye (also known as OS: oculus sinister); (C) an eye with non-astigmatic cornea; (D) an eye with astigmatic cornea: "with-the-rule" astigmatism (greatest dioptric power found around the vertical axis), "against-the-rule" astigmatism (greatest dioptric power found around the horizontal axis) and oblique astigmatism (greatest dioptric power found around the oblique axis). (Edwards, 1998; Gills *et al.*, 2011)

environmental factors (i.e. by nature and nurture) and considerably influenced by ageing (including both the schedules of tissue development and tissue senescence), all these epidemiological factors can broadly be discussed within three main categories: 1) **congenital**; 2) **ageing**; and 3) **environmental factors**.

3.1   Congenital Factors

Congenital myopia is commonly seen at birth and persists throughout life with prevalence of approximately 2% of all cases of myopia (Edwards, 1998; Wildsoet, 1998). If myopia develops after very early infancy, then it is termed acquired myopia (Edwards, 1998). Congenital myopia can be linked to premature birth and/or low birth weight (Wildsoet, 1998). Also, this myopic condition appears to be refractive in nature because the affected eye tends to be undersized with highly curved corneas (Wildsoet, 1998).

In the quest for myopia-associated genes, recent genome-wide association studies (GWAS) have identified at least 26 myopia-associated loci that involved in neurotransmission (e.g. GRIA4), ion transport (e.g. KCNQ5, CD55, CHNRG), retinoic acid metabolism (e.g. RDH5, RORB, CYP26A1), extracellular matrix remodeling (e.g. LAMA2, BMP2) and eye development (e.g. SIX4, PRSS56, CHD7) while the family-based linkage studies have identified at least 14 myopia-associated loci (e.g. MYP1, MYP2, MYP3) which are designated as MYP loci and numbered according to their time of discovery (Cooke Bailey *et al.*, 2013; Khor, 2010). In addition to whole genome investigation that involved introns, whole-exome investigation is also common in the investigation of myopia-associated genes. For example, a recent study has identified a novel missense variant of the CCDC111 gene as a potential susceptibility gene for high myopia by exome sequencing (Zhao *et al.*, 2013).

As inconsistent findings are not uncommon in genetic studies of complex traits (including refraction) (Klein, 2010), it is important to note that the potential importance of genes of modest effects (which are likely to interact with other genetic and environmental factors to influence the phenotype) can only be addressed meaningfully when the sample size is sufficiently large (Klein, 2010). Additionally, these genetic studies of myopia have also implied that the influences of some potential myopia-associated genes may be limited only to certain subtypes of myopia, for example: Pax6 is associated with very high myopia (Klein, 2010; Tsai *et al.*, 2008; Hewitt *et al.*, 2007). Interestingly, recent genetic studies indicated that although insulin-like growth factors (IGFs) play important roles in growth and development, IGF1 gene may not determine the susceptibility to high or very high myopia in Caucasians and Chinese (Miyake *et al.*, 2013). However, it should be noted that different single-nucleotide polymorphisms (SNPs) of the same gene may have different results in terms of their associations with myopia. For example, rs3735520 of hepatocyte growth factor (HGF) gene is associated with mild to moderate myopia but not with high or very high myopia while rs2286194 of the same gene is associated with high and very high myopia (Khor, 2010). SNPs of transforming growth factor-β (TGF-β) encoding gene TGFB1 and trabecular-meshwork inducible glucocorticoid response (TIGR) gene also have similar phenomenon (Khor, 2010).

With further relevance to the genes but in a more macroscopic aspect, the race/ethnicity background also influences the prevalence of myopia, for example: 1) adult Chinese in Singapore have a higher prevalence of myopia than similarly aged European-derived populations; and 2) Eskimos have a lower prevalence of myopia than Whites, Blacks and Chinese (Klein, 2010). Additionally, in Americans between the ages of 12 and 54, myopia has been found to affect Asian most (with prevalence = 18.5%), followed by Hispanics (13.2%) whereas Caucasians had the lowest prevalence of myopia (4.4%), which was not significantly different from African Americans (6.6%). For hyperopia, Caucasians had the highest prevalence (19.3%), followed by Hispanics (12.7%) whereas Asians had the lowest prevalence of hyperopia (6.3%) and were not significantly different from African Americans (6.4%). For astigmatism, both Asians and Hispanics had the highest prevalences (33.6% and 36.9%, respectively with no differences from each other), followed by Caucasians (26.4%) whereas African Americans had the lowest prevalence of astigmatism (20.0%) (Yu *et al.*, 2011).

It should beware of that race/ethnicity may contribute to the prevalence of myopia in ways other than the genetics, for example: sub-cultural/cultural influences in which the resultant behavior and living style may increase the risk of developing myopia (Klein, 2010; Perera and Aung, 2010).

3.2   Ageing Factors

Exerting considerable physiological changes to virtually all known cells, ageing and/or age per se is also an important contributor to myopia (Kwan, 2013a; Kwan, 2013b). For example, although recent school-based prevalence studies shown that myopia is more prevalent in Chinese female while the results in Iran shown the opposite, prevalence of myopia in both Chinese and Iranian students increased significantly with age (Hashemi *et al.*, 2014; You *et al.*, 2014). Most children are born hyperopic with normally distributed refractive errors which distribution narrows by emmetropisation during the first two years after birth (Morgan *et al.*, 2012; Mutti *et al.*, 2005). Considerable emmetropisation took place between 3 and 9 months of age (Mutti *et al.*, 2005), changes in ocular length (with associated scleral remodeling) and choroidal thickness are two most prominent ocular changes contributing to this process (Wallman and Nickla, 2010). If the eye elongates and/or its choroid thins beyond the normal range, the retina will be pulled backward and leading to a myopic shift (Wallman and Nickla, 2010). It should be noted that the growth rate of cornea and crystalline lenses may affect the development of this myopic shift as the corneal and lenticular growth increases the focal length of the far point plane (Wallman and Nickla, 2010). After the distribution narrowing of refractive errors, the cornea stabilises but refraction may still capable of becoming more myopic as ocular axial length can continue to increase for another two decades while the power of crystalline lenses decreases substantially up to the age of about 12 years before decreasing at a slower rate for most of adult life (Morgan *et al.*, 2012).

Myopia generally develops during the early to middle childhood years, but significant myopia can also develop in the late teenage years or early adulthood (Morgan *et al.*, 2012). To this day, there are three different forms of developmental myopia identified: 1) **early-onset myopia** (EOM; also known as youth-onset myopia) onsets prior to 15 years of age, and is clearly axial in nature while corneal steepening plays a negligible role in its development; 2) **late-onset myopia** (LOM; also known as young-adult myopia or early-adult-onset myopia) onsets at 15 years of age or later, and is also axial in nature while corneal steepening also plays a negligible role in its development; and 3) **late-adult-onset myopia** onsets after 45 years of age, and its development appears to be predominated by other ocular components (e.g. central/nuclear lenticular changes) (Edwards, 1998; Wildsoet, 1998; Rosenfield, 1998). Additionally, there is an accumulating body of evidences showing that the accommodation-vergence system in persons who develop myopia between the ages of about 18 and 25 years is different from that found in emmetropes and in persons who develop myopia in the pre-teens or early teens (Edwards, 1998). Thus, this evidence supports the view that the causes of these different types of myopia may be different. Finally, it would be worth noting that terms "**juvenile-onset**" and "**adolescent-onset**" can be used to describe myopia that starts before the age of about 18 years (Edwards, 1998). Further, both early-onset and late-onset myopia are affected by environmental factors (Edwards, 1998).

3.3   Environmental Factors

Although myopia is highly heritable, there is now increasing evidences suggesting that environmental factors may also play an important role in the development of myopia (Cooke Bailey *et al.*, 2013; Edwards, 1998). The idea of ocular growth and refractive status are actively influenced by visual environment can be traced back to 1866 when Cohn reported the association between myopia and formal schooling (Smith, 1998). To this day, nearwork, education/income and outdoor activity are recognized as representative environment-driven epi-demiological risk factors for myopia. Basis of the association between nearwork and myopia in both adult and children lies mainly on studies assessing the size/frequency of myopes in a population of interest with respect to a variable of investigation (usually being the intensity and/or nature of the nearwork, school work and/or reading) (Klein, 2010). Education factors (its effect usually not possible to separate from those of income) are implicated as reflections of nearwork activities and indeed recent studies of refraction indicated the presence of association between myopic refractive error and the level of educational achievement in both adult and children (Klein, 2010; Mirshahi *et al.*, 2014; You *et al.*, 2014). On the contrary, both adult and non-adult myopic refractive error was found inversely associated with the level of out-door activities (Klein, 2010; McKnight *et al.*, 2014). The inverse relationship between myopia and outdoor activities is, at least in part, attributed to the serum vitamin D level (Yazar *et al.*, 2014).

Besides, the effect of environment on myopia can also be seen in animal studies (Edwards, 1998). For example, depriving a young animal of form vision may induce deprivation myopia (also known as form-deprivation myopia) while using negatively powered ophthalmic lens to induce compensation in young animals may induce compensational myopia (also known as lens-compensation myopia) (Edwards, 1998). Finally, it is noteworthy that genetic programming may affect the two eyes differently or affect the susceptibility of two eyes to some environmental factor/factors differently (Edwards, 1998). Thus, both genetic and environmental factors may interact together and with each other to determine the overall physiological state and it has been suggested that unilateral myopia may be caused by such mechanism (Edwards, 1998).

4   Cellular Basis of the Eye and Myopia

Ocular tissues are originated from the optic sulci (also known as optic primordium) derived from the inner aspects of neural folds of the embryo around day 22 (Forrester *et al.*, 2008b). After the complex tissue development involving a delicate interaction between various developmental proteins and genes (important ocular developmental genes are listed in table 4) (Forrester *et al.*, 2008b), basic cellular structures of the eyes are established. Among the various ocular structures, retina is the main photoreceptive tissue transforming photonic energies into neural impulses that present to the brain as information (Forrester *et al.*, 2008a; Nicholls *et al.*, 2003). Details of the adult retinal structure are provided in Figure 3.

4.1   Waltz of the Ocular Neurons

To this day, there are many types of retinal cells have been identified (the commonly used markers for these cells are listed in table 5) (Forrester *et al.*, 2008a; Nicholls *et al.*, 2003). These cells are connected together and have arranged themselves into different layers within the retina (Forrester *et al.*, 2008a; Nicholls *et al.*, 2003). When light reaches retina, the photonic pattern of the visible electromagnetic wave is detected by the corresponding photoreceptors (located between the OLM and the RPE) (Forrester *et al.*, 2008a; Nicholls *et al.*, 2003). **Photoreceptors** are specialized retinal neurons which contain photoreceptive/visual pigments that are sensitive to a particular range of electromagnetic wavelengths (Forrester *et al.*, 2008a; Nicholls *et al.*,

Human gene	Expression Pattern	Ocular defects in humans with known mutations in related gene
PAX6	• Anterior neural plate • Optic sulcus/cup and stalk • Surface ectoderm (future lens and corneal/conjunctival epithelium) • Weakly expressed in mesenchymal cells	• Peter's anomaly • Anophthalmia • Anterior segment dysgenesis • Congenital glaucoma • Axenfeld-Rieger syndrome (aniridia)
PITX3	• Developing lens vesicle	• Peter's anomaly • Congenital cataract • Leucoma
CHD7	• Lens vesicle • Neuroectoderm	• CHARGE syndrome
MAF	• Lens vesicle • Lens placode • Primary lens fibres (transcription factors for alpha crystalline gene along with Sox1)	• Peter's anomaly • Defects in lens • Cornea and iris (coloboma)
FOXE3	• Lens placode	• Peter's anomaly • Posterior embryotoxon • Cataract
PITX2 FOXC1	• Periocular mesenchyme (presumptive cornea, eyelids, trabecular meshwork, extraocular muscle)	• Iridogoniodysgenesis • Axenfeld-Rieger syndrome • 50% develop juvenile glaucoma
SOX1, SOX2, SOX3	• Central nervous system • Sensory placodes • Sox2 in lens placode	• Anophthalmia without cataract
RX	• Anterior neural plate • Optic vesicle • Developing retina • Photoreceptors	• Anophthalmia
CRYA, CRYB, CRYG	• Lens	• Various forms of cataract

Table 4: list of genes important to ocular development. (Forrester *et al.*, 2008b).

of photoreceptive pigments and thus having a species-unique pattern of electromagnetic wavelength sensitivities (e.g. human are trichromatic while many bird species are tetrachromatic) (Wilkie *et al.*, 1998), photoreceptors are functionally and morphologically classified into two main types (rods and cones) (Forrester *et al.*, 2008a). **Rods** (approx. 115 million cells in human and predominantly found in the peripheral retina) are responsible for sensing contrast, brightness and motion, while **cones** (approx. 6.5 million cells in human and predominately found in the central retina with the highest density at the fovea) facilitate fine resolution, spatial resolution and color vision (Forrester *et al.*, 2008a). The cell bodies of rods and cones in the ONL are connected by an inner fibre to specialised expanded synaptic terminals, spherules and pedicles respectively (Forrester *et al.*, 2008a; Swaroop *et al.*, 2010).

Rod spherules lie more sclerad than the cone pedicles and have no apparent contact with other rod spherules but cone pedicles may be connected with each other by gap junctions

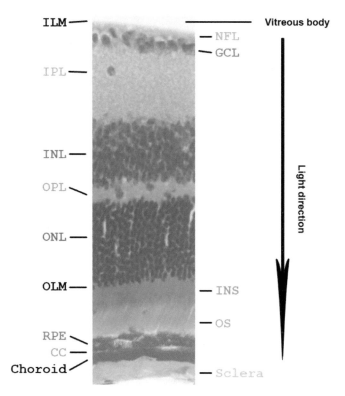

Figure 3: histology of a mouse retina. ILM = inner limiting membrane; NFL = nerve fibre layer; GCL = ganglion cell layer; IPL = inner plexiform layer; INL = inner nuclear layer; OPL = outer plexiform layer; ONL = outer nuclear layer; OLM = outer/external limiting membrane; INS = photoreceptor inner segment; OS = photoreceptor outer segment; RPE = retinal pigment epithelium; CC = choriocapillaris. (Forrester *et al.*, 2008a; Nicholls *et al.*, 2003)

(Forrester *et al.*, 2008a). Unlike rod spherules, cone pedicles have a pyramidal shape and are broader than their rod counterparts (Forrester *et al.*, 2008a). Both of these synaptic terminals are synapsed with bipolar and horizontal cells found in the INL (Forrester *et al.*, 2008a). In the electrophysiological perspective, functions of the photoreceptors can be estimated by the cornea-negative **a-wave** (Granit's PIII component) of the electroretinography (ERG), which reflects the photocurrent generated by light absorption in the outer segments of the photoreceptors (including a mix of rod and cone cells) and its response amplitude is correlated with both the severity of myopia and ocular axial length (Luu and Chia, 2010; Asi and Perlman, 1992; Frishman, 2013; Cone and Ebrey, 1965). ERG studies have shown that the response amplitudes of **short** (S), **medium** (M) and **long-wavelength sensitive** (L) **cone cells** are reduced in myopia in which L and M cone cells may be more affected than the S cone cells (Luu and Chia, 2010).

Bipolar cells are retinal interneurons (approx. 35.7 million cells in human) conveying signals from photoreceptors to the retinal terminal (i.e. last neuronal center in the retina along the afferent visual pathway) ganglion cells (Forrester *et al.*, 2008a; Nicholls *et al.*, 2003; Lin and Masland, 2005). Cell bodies of bipolar cells are oriented parallel to the photoreceptors in a radial fashion while their dendrites (pass outwards) and axons (pass inwards) make synapses with photoreceptors (also with horizontal cells) and ganglion cells (also with amacrine cells), respectively (Forrester *et al.*, 2008a). To this day, there are nine morphological subtypes of bi-

Cell Type	Markers
Rod cells	Reep6 (Keeley *et al.*, 2013); CtBP2 (Keeley *et al.*, 2013);
Cone cells	mCAR (Keeley *et al.*, 2013); CtBP2 (Keeley *et al.*, 2013); Red/Green Cone Opsin (Keeley *et al.*, 2013); Blue Cone Opsin (Keeley *et al.*, 2013);
Bipolar cells	PKC (Keeley *et al.*, 2013; Lin *et al.*, 2005); Syt2 (Keeley *et al.*, 2013); Cx36 (Lin *et al.*, 2005; Meyer *et al.*, 2014); VGluT1 (Meyer *et al.*, 2014);
Ganglion cells	β-tubulin 3 (Mi *et al.*, 2012b); Calb (Lee *et al.*, 2011); Calretinin (Lee *et al.*, 2011); SMI32 (Lee *et al.*, 2011; Lin and Peng, 2013); CD90.2/Thy-1.2 (Lin and Peng, 2013); Melanopsin (Lin and Peng, 2013); Cx36 (Meyer *et al.*, 2014);
Horizontal cells	NF150 (Keeley *et al.*, 2013); NGL2 (Keeley *et al.*, 2013); Calb (Keeley *et al.*, 2013; Lee *et al.*, 2011);
Amacrine cells	Calb (Lee *et al.*, 2011); Calretinin (Lee *et al.*, 2011); SMI32 (Lee *et al.*, 2011); Cx36 (Meyer *et al.*, 2014);
Neuroglia	
Müller cells/glia	CRALBP (Lindqvist *et al.*, 2010); GFAP (Mao *et al.*, 2011; Lindqvist *et al.*, 2010; Lee *et al.*, 2011); Vimentin (Mao *et al.*, 2011; Lindqvist *et al.*, 2010); GS (Mi *et al.*, 2012b); RAGE (Mi *et al.*, 2012b); SMI32 (Lee *et al.*, 2011); S100B (Zong *et al.*, 2010)
Astrocytes	GFAP (Mi *et al.*, 2012b; Lee *et al.*, 2011); ET1 (Mi *et al.*, 2012b); RAGE (Mi *et al.*, 2012b); S100 (Mansour et al., 2008);
Microglia	CD11b (Karlstetter *et al.*, 2014; Ellis-Behnke *et al.*, 2013); CD16/32 (Karlstetter *et al.*, 2014); CD36 (Karlstetter *et al.*, 2014); CD45 (Karlstetter *et al.*, 2014; Ellis-Behnke *et al.*, 2013); CD68 (Ellis-Behnke *et al.*, 2013); CX3CR1 (Karlstetter *et al.*, 2014); Coronin1a (Ellis-Behnke *et al.*, 2013); IBA1 (Ellis-Behnke *et al.*, 2013); HLA-DR (Ellis-Behnke *et al.*, 2013); F4/80 (Ellis-Behnke *et al.*, 2013);
Blood vessels	
Endothelial cells	PECAM1 (Mi *et al.*, 2012b); ET1 (Mi *et al.*, 2012b); RAGE (Mi *et al.*, 2012b);
Pericytes	α-SMA (Mi *et al.*, 2012b); NG2 (Mi *et al.*, 2012b);

Table 5: list of commonly used markers for retinal cells. Reep6 = receptor accessory protein 6; CtBP2 = C-terminal calcium binding protein 2; mCAR = mouse cone arrestin; Syt2 = Synaptotagmin 2; Cx36 = Connexin36; NF150 = neurofilament 150; NGL2 = netrin-G ligand 2; Calb = calbindin; CRALBP = cellular retinaldehyde-binding protein; GFAP = glial fibrillary acidic protein; GS = glutamine synthetase; RAGE = receptor for advanced glycation end products; ET1 = endothelin 1; IBA1 = ionized calcium-binding adapter molecule 1; HLA-DR = human leukocyte antigens-DR; PECAM1 = platelet endothelial cell adhesion molecule 1; (Keeley *et al.*, 2013; Mi *et al.*, 2012b; Mao *et al.*, 2011; Lindqvist *et al.*, 2010; Karlstetter *et al.*, 2014; Ellis-Behnke *et al.*, 2013; Lin *et al.*, 2005; Lee *et al.*, 2011; Lin and Peng, 2013; Meyer *et al.*, 2014).

polar cells have been identified in human and can be classified into three main categories: 1) **rod bipolar cells**; 2) **diffuse cone bipolar cells** (5 subtypes); and 3) **midget cone bipolar cells** (3 subtypes) (Forrester *et al.*, 2008a). It is worth noting that in the foveal region of the central retina one bipolar cell can receive stimuli from one cone cell and connects to one ganglion cell while in the peripheral retina one bipolar cell can receive stimuli from up to 50-100 rod cells (Forrester *et al.*, 2008a). Such structural arrangement suggests that the visual acuity is decreasing from the central retina to the peripheral retina (Forrester *et al.*, 2008a). However, the summation of stimuli from the rod cells is an important feature to the enhanced sensitivity of the rod system to low levels of illumination (Forrester *et al.*, 2008a). As the primary neurotransmitter in neurons of the retinal vertical pathway, glutamates are released by photorecep-tors, bipolar cells and ganglion cells (Perera and Aung, 2010; Kolb, 2009; Nelson and Con-naughton, 2012). Functionally, all bipolar cells belong to either ON or OFF types (ON bipolar cells depolarise while OFF bipolar cells hyperpolarise in response to light stimuli), each of which type can be further subdivided according to their temporal frequency of transmission (Lin and Masland, 2005; Nelson and Connaughton, 2012). In general, ON bipolar cells express metabotropic glutamate receptors (mGluRs) or glutamate transporters on their surface while OFF bipolar cells express only ionotropic glutamate receptors (iGluRs) (Nelson and Con-naughton, 2012).

Although ON bipolar cells commonly synapse with ON ganglion cells in the inner half of the IPL while OFF bipolar cells synapse with OFF ganglion cells in the outer half of the IPL, it is interesting to note that rod bipolar cells (commonly recognized as ON types in mammals) are generally believed to transmit their signals to the ON ganglion cells indirectly by overtak-ing the cone pathway through synapsing with AII amacrine cells by gap junctions (different types of ON cone bipolar cells seem to express different connexins at their gap junctions with AII amacrine cells) (Bloomfield and Dacheux, 2001; Lin and Masland, 2005; Nelson and Con-naughton, 2012; Lin et al., 2005). In the electrophysiological perspective, functions of the bipo-lar cells can be estimated by the ERG cornea-positive **b-wave** (Granit's PII component) which associates with potassium (K^+) current and reflects neural activities (particularly radially ori-ented cells) in the INL (Luu and Chia, 2010; Asi and Perlman, 1992; Frishman, 2013; Cone and Ebrey, 1965). As b-wave is a function of mixed cell types (at least in the case of mammalian retina, horizontal cells and Müller glia/cells are implicated), its interpretation of bipolar cell function needs to be cautious (Asi and Perlman, 1992; Frishman, 2013; Patil and Puri, 2009). Similar to the a-wave, response amplitude of b-wave is also correlated with both the severity of myopia and ocular axial length (Luu and Chia, 2010). However, due to the positive correla-tion between a-wave amplitude and b-wave amplitude, post-receptoral transmission function is usually determined by the amplitude ratio of b-wave versus a-wave (i.e. **b-/a-wave ampli-tude ratio**) (Luu and Chia, 2010). In myopia, the b-wave amplitudes are often reduced but the b-/a-wave amplitude ratios are often normal. Interestingly, among such normal amplitude ratios, the ratio value tends to be smaller in eyes with higher myopia suggesting myopic changes in the retinal signal transmission to some degree (Luu and Chia, 2010).

Horizontal cells are retinal association neurons which cell bodies are found mainly in the outer part of the INL while their processes are ramified in the OPL close to the cone pedi-cles and release inhibitory neurotransmitters (primarily GABA: γ-aminobutyric acid) (Forrest-er et al., 2008a). Overlapping between horizontal cells is considerable and any one area of reti-na may be served by up to 20 horizontal cells (Forrester et al., 2008a). To this day, there are three morphological subtypes (**HI, HII** and **HIII**) of horizontal cells identified in human while only two (**type A** and **type B**) identified in most species including the most extensively studied cats (Forrester et al., 2008a). Recent studies demonstrated that horizontal cells are important to the structural maintenance of photoreceptors in which rod cells are more affected than cone cells (Keeley et al., 2013). Clinically, the contribution of these cells to myopia is still unknown due to limited information available. However, pharmacological studies of myopia suggested that the activities of GABA-secreting cells (including horizontal cells and some subtypes of amacrine cells) may play an important role in the development of axial myopia due to their capability of releasing GABA which receptor signal interruption may inhibit the development of myopia (Chebib et al., 2009; Stone et al., 2003). In the electrophysiological perspective, functions of the horizontal cells can be estimated by the S-potential (also known as the horizontal cell response) of the intracellular recordings and/or by the ERG waveforms with the aid of appropriate pharmacological agents including tetrodotoxin citrate (TTX), N-methyl-D-aspartic acid (NMDA), 2-amino-4-phosphonobutyric acid (APB) and cis-2,3-piperidine-dicarboxylic acid (PDA) or 6-cyano-7-nitroquinoxaline-2,3-dione (CNQX) (Nishimura *et al.*, 2011; Patil and Puri, 2009; Chappell *et al.*, 2002).

Another type of retinal association neurons, **amacrine cells** are found mainly in the vitread or inner part of the INL while their processes are ramified in the IPL (where they terminate predominately in the synaptic complexes formed by the bipolar and ganglion cell processes) and release various neurotransmitters (GABA and dopamine, somatostatin or acetylcholine) depending on the subtype (Forrester *et al.*, 2008a). To this day, there are more than 25 different subtypes of amacrine cells identified in primates (including human) according to their morphology or their neurotransmitters (Forrester *et al.*, 2008a). Amacrine cells are commonly believed to play an important role (most probably inhibitory) in the modulation of signals reaching ganglion cells and are distinguishable as a consequence of their relatively larger size and oval shape (cell bodies are usually flask-shaped) (Forrester *et al.*, 2008a). Clinically, functions of the amacrine cells can be estimated by the ERG oscillatory potentials (OPs) which are small-amplitude wavelets (superimposed on the ascending limb of the b-wave) generated, possibly by local neural networks, in the inner retina involving bipolar cells, amacrine cells and ganglion cells (Asi and Perlman, 1992). Due to the contributions of more than one cell type to the OPs, together with the possible influence by the outer retinal functions and retinal circulations (Luu and Chia, 2010; Asi and Perlman, 1992), OP interpretation of amacrine cell function again needs to be cautious. In myopia, the importance of amacrine cell function is based on the capabilities of amacrine cells to release dopamine and glucagon in addition to their modulation of ocular growth (Luu and Chia, 2010; Fischer, 2011). In regard to the dopamine, this neurotransmitter is commonly found in the inner retina and is involved in the processing of amacrine cells and ganglion cells (Luu and Chia, 2010). Additionally, dopamine is important to the retinal luminance adaption and is associated with myopia development (Luu and Chia, 2010). In regard to the glucagon, this secreted peptide is expressed by a minor population of amacrine cells (known as the glucagon-expressing amacrine cells, GACs) and its synthesis is believed to be regulated by the early growth response 1 (EGR1) (Tong *et al.*, 2010; Fischer, 2011; Pagel and Deindl, 2011). Both the glucagon and the GACs are found to be essential to slow rates of ocular growth (Fischer, 2011). Back to the ERG studies, it has been shown that myopic eyes are associated with the presence of abnormal OPs and retinal adaptations (Luu and Chia, 2010). Despite there are many different possibilities, such abnormal OPs were suggested to be related to the changes in dopamine levels within the inner retina (Luu and Chia, 2010).

Ganglion cells (also known as RGCs: retinal ganglion cells) are the retinal terminal neurons (approx. 1.2 million cells in human) connecting the eyes to the cerebrum (Forrester *et al.*, 2008a; Mitchell and Lu, 2008). Cell bodies of the RGCs predominately found in the GCL despite they can be found occasionally in the INL (Forrester *et al.*, 2008a). Dendritic processes of the RGCs are synapsed with axons of the bipolar and amacrine cells predominately in the IPL while axons of the RGCs form the nerve fibre layer and are synapsed with cells in the lateral geniculate nucleus (LGN) of the thalamus (Forrester *et al.*, 2008a). Although RGCs are generally manifesting a large cell body, abundant Nissl substance (arrays of rough endoplasmic reticulum) and a large Golgi apparatus, they exhibit a great morphological diversity (18 subtypes in human; 25 subtypes in other mammalian species) and are classified into different categories (midget, parasol, bistratified and other ganglion cells) according to their cell body size, dendritic tree spread, branching pattern and branching level in the five strata of the IPL (Forrester *et al.*, 2008a; Baker, 2013; Sanchez, 2010). Among all RGCs, the majority of them are midget and parasol cells followed by the bistratified cells and then many other subtypes of RGCs (including the photosensitive subtypes) (Baker, 2013; Sanchez, 2010). Theoretically, each of the ganglion cells may receive stimuli from approximately 100 rod cells and 4 to 6 cone cells (Forrester *et al.*, 2008a). Similar to the bipolar cells, they are also classified into either ON or OFF functional types (Lin and Masland, 2005). It is interesting to note that some RGCs, cone axons and Müller cells (discuss in later section) in the macular area may contain xanthophyll (carotenoid) yellow pigments implicating their photo-sensing capabilities (Forrester *et al.*, 2008a).

Axons of the RGCs, **optic nerve fibres** in the eye commonly form bundles separated and ensheathed by ocular glial cells and oligodendrocytes before and after the lamina cribrosa, respectively (Forrester *et al.*, 2008a). While most subtypes of the RGCs project their axons to the LGN, some subtypes of RGCs project their axons to the superior colliculus (Sanchez, 2010). Only very few subtypes of RGCs project their axons to both of these cerebral structures (Sanchez, 2010). In regard to the LGN-projecting neurons, midget RGCs (also known as P-cells) connect with the parvocellular LGN neurons, parasol RGCs (also known as M-cells) connect with the magnocellular LGN neurons, and bistratified RGCs (also known as K-cells) connect with the koniocellular LGN neurons (Buck, 2004).

Clinically, RGCs are resistant to photoreceptor degeneration (Lin and Peng, 2013). Despite dramatic degeneration may induce disruption of normal retinal architecture and of outer retinal functions, RGCs are the only output cells of the retina and thus are important targets of investigation in neurodegeneration (including glaucoma and Alzheimer's disease) and neuroprotection studies (Mi *et al.*, 2012a; Chiu *et al.*, 2012; Mi *et al.*, 2012b; Lin and Peng, 2013). In the electrophysiological perspective, functions of the RGCs can be estimated by the microelectrode recordings and/or the ERG waveforms with the aid of appropriate pharmacological agents (e.g. TTX and NMDA) and/or surgical procedures (Nishimura *et al.*, 2011; Jensen, 2013; Nelson, 2007).

4.2   Thickness Matters

As more than 95% of all myopic conditions (including both youth-onset and adult-onset types) are due to an excessive ocular axial length (which is correlated to an enlarged vitreous chamber depth) (McBrien, 2010), knowing the mechanisms that lead to such structural changes in the affected eyes is clinically important. To this day, postnatal ocular growth is commonly believed to be constrained by the properties of the outer coat (sclera) of the eye (McBrien, 2010). Sclera is a fibrous connective tissue maintained by fibroblasts (major extracellular matrix-producing cell) and undergoes constant remodeling throughout life (McBrien, 2010). This highly organized ocular tunic plays major functional roles in: 1) protecting the delicate intraocular structures; 2) providing a stable base for ocular muscle contractions (ciliary muscles in accommodation, and extraocular muscles in accurate eye movements); and 3) allowing vascular and neural access to adjacent intraocular structures (McBrien, 2010).

In regard to myopia, thinning of sclera (particularly at the posterior pole of the eye) is identified as an important clinical feature (with subsequent development of posterior staphyloma occurred more frequently in pathological myopia while chorioretinal atrophy, lacquer cracks, choroidal neovascularization, foveoschisis, macular hole formation, lattice degeneration and posterior vitreous detachments occurred more frequently in high myopia) (McBrien, 2010; Wildsoet, 1998; Lee, 2010). In high myopes, scleral thickness at the posterior pole can be reduced up to 50% of those measured from the emmetropes (in human, the emmetropic scleral thickness at the posterior pole is approximately 1 mm) (McBrien, 2010). Maybe due to the structural organization of the sclera (its thickness gradually increases from anterior/equatorial to posterior reaching the maximum thickness at the posterior pole), the effect of scleral thinning is less marked in the anterior/equatorial ocular regions (McBrien, 2010). In addition to the scleral thinning, profound morphological changes in the scleral extracellular matrix have been noted and this view is further supported by the results from the biochemical and biomechanical assays showing that myopic eyes have lesser amount of biomarkers for collagen and glycosaminoglycans while being less resistant to mechanical deformation (McBrien, 2010).

As the major cell type in the sclera, fibroblasts are potential therapeutic targets and deserve attentions from both the clinical and scientific research levels. Scleral fibroblasts are flattened-spindle-shaped cells with long branching processes and localised between the collagen fiber bundle lamellae (McBrien, 2010). In addition to collagen, these cells also express a variety of other proteins including matrix metalloproteinase (MMP), tissue inhibitor of matrix metalloproteinase (TIMP) and all five types of muscarinic acetylcholine receptors (mAChRs) (McBrien, 2010). Interestingly, many scleral fibroblasts are found to express α-smooth muscle actin (α-SMA) and differentiate into myofibroblasts that have a high contractility and thus capable of rapid contractile responses to imposed tissue stress relieving tension within and limiting expansion of the surrounding matrix (McBrien, 2010). Further, myofibroblasts are capable of controlling their local environment through remodeling of the surrounding extracellular matrix (McBrien, 2010). Although the sclera contains a stable constant population of myofibroblasts, recent studies suggested an age-dependent increase in the proportion of myofibroblasts (McBrien, 2010).

Cell to cell communications within the scleral extracellular matrix is complex and involving a variety of molecular factors including members of the IGF, TGF-β and fibroblast growth factor (FGF) families (McBrien, 2010). In the recently proposed model for the axial myopia, it is suggested that the signal from the retina and/or choroid may affect the physiology of scleral fibroblasts and myofibroblasts leading to an altered proportion of these two cell types and an altered scleral biochemistry (e.g. reduced collagen synthesis, altered proteoglycans, increased MMP activity and increased collagen V/III to I ratio) (McBrien, 2010). Such biochemical changes may result in: 1) structural changes in the sclera (e.g. altered collagen fibres and scleral tissue loss) and subsequently changes in the scleral biomechanical properties ultimately leading to an increased scleral stress that further alters the scleral biochemistry; and 2) downregulation of both TGF-β and integrin, which further changes the cellular proportion of the scleral fibroblasts and myofibroblasts leading to a further change in the scleral biochemistry (McBrien, 2010). As a result, these series of scleral changes ultimately lead to the ocular elongation and thus the development of myopia (McBrien, 2010).

In regard to the scleral mechanical properties, there are several major determinants: 1) **scleral thickness**; 2) **scleral collagen fibril parameters** (both structural organization and rate of matrix turn over); and 3) **scleral hydration level** (determined by the hydrophilic carboyhydrates, particularly the glycosaminoglycans) (McBrien, 2010). All of these determinants are controlled by the physiology of fibroblasts/myofibroblasts. In the aforementioned retinoscleral signaling model of axial myopia, downregulation of TGF-β (as seen in the RPE, choroid and sclera) may represent a mechanism whereby the collagen production (as well as MMPs and TIMPs) by fibroblasts, proliferation of fibroblasts and differentiation of fibroblasts into myofibroblasts are hampered while downregulation of integrin (as seen in the early myopia development) may represent a mechanism whereby myofibroblasts disconnect from the scleral extracellular matrix releasing their mechanical influences on ocular ectasia and thus enhancing the capacity of the sclera to creep and the ocular growth (Khor, 2010; McBrien, 2010). As expression is affected by the TGF-β and mechanical stretch, TIGR gene product myocillin may be a potential target worth investigating (Khor, 2010). Additionally, HGF may also likely to play an important role in myopia development as this growth factor and its putative receptor cMET (member of the tyrosine kinase receptor family) are found in the eye (particularly in RPE, crystalline lens and cornea) where they trigger many cellular responses involved in cell division, migration, differentiation and survival of numerous cell types (Khor, 2010).

Next to the sclera is the choroid which is a vascular tunic lying between the sclera and the retina (Wildsoet, 1998). The functions of the choroid can be estimated by advanced imaging techniques (e.g. magnetic resonance imaging) and/or by ocular pressure waveforms (i.e. ocular pulses) (Wildsoet, 1998; Dastiridou et al., 2013). In myopia, the ocular pulse was found lower than that measured from the emmetropes while in moderate myopia the thickness of choroid at the posterior pole can be reduced up to 50% of those measured from the emmetropes (Wildsoet, 1998). In regard to the latter, such similarly with the case of sclera suggested a close association between these two tissues in which such coupling may be regulated by the biochemical interactions and by the traversing sclerochoroidal blood vessels that may act as anchorage points ensuring the choroid expands in parallel with local scleral changes (Wildsoet, 1998). Although the complete underlying mechanism remains unknown, choroidal thinning may involve stretching and detaching (Wildsoet, 1998). Both the choroidal thickness, level of fundus tessellation (clinical signs of stretching) and prevalence of optic nerve crescents (clinical signs of detaching) are well correlated with ocular axial length (Wildsoet, 1998; Flores-Moreno et al., 2013).

Similar and next to the choroid, retina also underwent a thinning process with stretching in myopia as evidenced mainly by but not limited to the stretching of RPE cells, straighter course of retinal blood vessels and rearrangements of the dendritic tree of the third order neurons (amacrine cells and RGCs) (Wildsoet, 1998; Flores-Moreno et al., 2013). Additionally, various retinal pathologies (e.g. lattice, paving-stone and pigmentary degenerations, and white with/without pressure) and visual function test results (e.g. impaired blue color discriminations and dark adaptations) may also serve as evidences of retinal thinning and stretching, respectively (Wildsoet, 1998).

After all, all three ocular tunics (i.e. retina, choroid and sclera) had become thinner in myopia (Flores-Moreno et al., 2013). However, it should be noted that although the retinal thickness (including macular region) was reported thinner in the myopic eyes, the foveal thickness was reported thicker and was positively correlated with the ocular axial length (Flores-Moreno et al., 2013). Recent studies using optical coherence tomography (OCT) found that subfoveal choroidal thickness (but not foveal thickness), mean macular choroidal thickness and outer retinal thickness (but not ONL thickness) are associated with and most predictive of visual acuity in highly myopic eyes without macular pathology (Flores-Moreno et al., 2013).

Finally, back to the molecular mechanisms, recent pharmacological studies have implied the importance of mAChRs in the development of myopia, particularly in the mediation of ocular growth (Tong et al., 2010). mAChRs (members of the G-protein coupled receptor superfamily) are expressed by both neuronal and non-neuronal cells (Tong et al., 2010). Among the five types of mAChRs, M_1, M_2 and M_3 receptors appeared to functionally dominate in mammalian retina (including RPE) while M_3 receptors are the predominant type found in human cornea, iris, ciliary body and epithelium of crystalline lens (Tong et al., 2010). All five types of mAChRs were found in the human sclera (also in sclera of tree shrews, mice and guinea pigs) (Tong et al., 2010). According to recent studies, mAChRs may mediate cell proliferations via intracellular pathways involving the mitogen activated protein kinases (MAPKs) and/or interactions with growth factor receptors (e.g. epidermal growth factor receptors) (Tong et al., 2010). Studies using mAChR antagonists have shown that there is also a relationship between mAChRs and the early-immediate genes (e.g. ZENK/EGR-1) (Tong et al., 2010). It is noteworthy that atropine (well-known mAChR antagonist that reduces myopia progression) can enhance the release of dopamine while inhibiting the release of growth hormone (Tong et al., 2010; Schwahn et al., 2000; Taylor et al., 1985).

4.3 Neuroglial Impacts

Glial cells (also known as glia or neuroglia) are important cellular housekeepers maintaining an optimal physiological environment for neuronal functions and survival. These neural cells usually aid brain functions by: 1) **providing a mass structure for the brain**; 2) **neuronal insulation**; 3) **developmental guidance**; 4) **environmental homeostasis**; 5) **neuroenergetics regulation**; 6) **neuronal nourishment**; and 7) **immune functions** (Verkhratsky and Butt, 2007a; Kettenmann and Ransom, 2005). Like retinal neurons, glial cells exhibit great morphological and functional diversity throughout the human body (e.g. myelinating glia, non-myelinating glia, developmental guiding glia and immunological microglia). Both glial cells and neurons are capable of expressing practically every type of neurotransmitter receptor known so far. Supported by findings that glia could communicate with neurons through gliotransmitters (specifically: glutamate, ATP and d-serine) (Verkhratsky and Butt, 2007a), both glial cells and neurons are mutually integrated into highly effective information processing units to form a functional neuronal-glial unit by wiring transmission and volume transmission (Verkhratsky and Butt, 2007b). Due to its dynamic interaction with neurons and blood vessels (Verkhratsky and Butt, 2007c; Kettenmann and Ransom, 2005; Takano et al., 2006), glia malfunctioning could directly affect neural functions. The most representative examples would be the demyelination seen in multiple sclerosis (MS) and Charcot-Marie-Tooth disease (CMT). Recent studies have also suggested that glia may play a causative role in common neurodegenerative diseases, including Parkinson's disease, Alzheimer's disease, amyotrophic lateral sclerosis (ALS) and ischemic stroke (Takano et al., 2006; Schubert et al., 2001; Holden, 2007; Jackson et al., 1999; Seifert et al., 2006; Filosa et al., 2006; Rao and Weiss, 2004; Teismann et al., 2003). Thus, the pathophysiological contributions of glial cells shall not be overlooked.

In retina, **Müller cells** (also known as Müller glia, MG) are the principal retinal glial cells and are considered analogous to the cerebral oligodendrocytes, radial glia and ependymal cells (Forrester et al., 2008a; García and Vecino, 2003; Wan et al., 2012; Fischer, 2011). These cells localized mainly in the INL and orient themselves radially with their processes extend through different retinal layers (from NFL to INS) (Forrester et al., 2008a; García and Vecino, 2003), in which MG extend: 1) smooth and sometimes rather long processes through the NFL ending in a basal end-foot lies adjacent to the ILM (which is a basal lamina at least partly produced by MG); 2) side branches into the IPL and OPL where they form sheaths around neuronal processes and synapses (particularly around the photoreceptor pedicles in the OPL); 3) lamellar processes in the nuclear layers to form structures enveloping the neuronal cell bodies;

and 4) apical microvilli (which length and number vary between species, probably inversely correlated to the degree of retinal vascularization) into the subretinal space between the inner segments of photoreceptor cells (near the ONL-INS interface) to form the OLM (García and Vecino, 2003). Interestingly, cilium is found on MG in some species (García and Vecino, 2003). Additionally, MG are connected to the neighbouring MG and photoreceptor cells (in INS) by specialised junctions (which are zonulae adhaerens or tight junctions in most vertebrate species but are intermediate junctions in many amphibian species; except human, frogs and toads in which are gap junctions instead) (García and Vecino, 2003). After all, MG are important in nourishing and maintaining the outer retina which lacks a direct blood supply (Forrester *et al.*, 2008a). In addition to neuronal cell bodies and their processes, MG processes also ensheaths blood vessels/capillaries on which these processes act as a communicating system for metabolic exchange between vasculature and neurons in much the same manner as postulated for brain astrocytes (Forrester *et al.*, 2008a; García and Vecino, 2003).

Recent studies have identified the neurogenic potential of MG. In damaged retinas, MG proliferate in the INL and express different embryonic retinal progenitor markers including Pax6, Chx10, Six3, transitin (nestin), Notch1, Hes1, Hes5, ascl1a, Sox2 and Sox9 (Fischer, 2011; Wang *et al.*, 2013a). Transcriptome of MG significantly overlaps with those of the retinal progenitors (Fischer, 2011). However, the neurogenicity of MG-derived progenitors is most likely limited by cellular factors (both intracellular and extracellular) as only <5% of these progenitors in damaged retinas may go on to form new neurons while the rest of the population appears to remain undifferentiated (Fischer, 2011). According to the chicken studies by Fischer and colleagues, daily sustained supply of both insulin and FGF2 can stimulate numerous MG to dedifferentiate, proliferate, become progenitor-like cells and produce a few new neurons (Fischer, 2011). It is noteworthy that the induction of progenitor-like cells requires the activation of both FGF receptors and MAPK signaling and the maintenance of Notch signaling at the baseline levels (Fischer, 2011). In regard to the Notch signaling, although this signaling likely maintains the progenitor-like qualities of MG; affects the neuroprotective functions of MG and is essential for MG to re-enter the cell cycle in response to acute retinal damage, Notch signaling inhibits neuronal differentiation of MG-derived progenitors (Fischer, 2011). In addition to the chicken studies, zebrafish studies by Wan and colleagues have found that heparin-binding epidermal-like growth factor (HB-EGF) is necessary and sufficient for stimulating MG dedifferentiation into a population of cycling multipotent progenitors in both injured and uninjured retinas (Wan *et al.*, 2012). HB-EGF exerts its effects via the EGFR/MAPK and Wnt/β-catenin signaling pathways regulating the expression of regeneration-associated genes (e.g. ascl1a and Pax6) and it is rapidly induced in MG at the damaged site of retina (Wan *et al.*, 2012). It is important to note that ascl1a and Wnt/β-catenin signaling are acting in a positive feedback manner in which ascl1a expression is necessary for β-catenin induction while Wnt signaling is necessary for ascl1a induction (Wan *et al.*, 2012). However, it should be careful that not all factors that induce MG proliferation will act in the same way for both uninjured and injured conditions. For example, ciliary neurotrophic factor (CNTF) can stimulate MG proliferation in the uninjured retinas but it seems to be more neuroprotective and inhibits MG proliferation in the injured retinas (Wan *et al.*, 2012; Kassen *et al.*, 2009).

In addition to the neurogenic potentials, MG are mechano-sensitive/responsive as reflected by their robust increase in intracellular calcium level during retinal stretch (for details of relevant gene expression changes, please refer to Wang *et al.*, 2013a, 2013b and 2013c), and also express the aforementioned TGF-β and dopamine which expression seems to associate with the activity of protein kinase C (PKC) (Mao *et al.*, 2011; Wang *et al.*, 2013a; Wang *et al.*, 2013b). Recent studies have shown that dopamine and one of its precursor enzymes tyrosine hydroxylase (TH) were downregulated in the guinea pig eyes with form-deprived myopia despite TGF-β and PKC were upregulated (Mao *et al.*, 2011).

Unlike in the brain, **astrocytes** are not the predominant glial cells in the retina but are predominantly located in the NFL, GCL, IPL and inner aspect of the INL (Forrester *et al.*, 2008a). On the other hand, both protoplasmic and fibrous subtypes of astrocytes are found in retina as in the cerebrum (Forrester *et al.*, 2008a). Retinal astrocytes commonly orient themselves perpendicular to the direction of the neuronal cell bodies and processes, and form irregular honeycomb scaffolds (perpendicular to the MG) between retinal neurons and blood vasculatures (Forrester *et al.*, 2008a). Both MG and retinal astrocytes are the essential components of the blood-retinal barrier and they are electrically coupled (by gap junctions) with each other (astrocyte-astrocyte, astrocyte-MG and MG-MG) (Forrester *et al.*, 2008a; García and Vecino, 2003; Robaszkiewicz *et al.*, 2010; Zahs and Ceelen, 2006; Reichenbach and Bringmann, 2013). It is noteworthy that chemical coupling between astrocytes may mediate the propagation of intercellular signals between glial cells (Forrester *et al.*, 2008a). After all, these glia couplings may facilitate the transport of key metabolites (e.g. glutamate, glutamine and lactate) into and out of glial cells by allowing them to diffuse between neighbouring cells in the glial syncytium (Forrester *et al.*, 2008a). Although both MG and retinal astrocytes have high K^+ membrane conductances, they may differ in their glycogen contents: while astrocytes have abundant glycogen in their cytoplasm, MG have only little intracytoplasmic glycogen (except in species with avascular retina) (Forrester *et al.*, 2008a).

Immunological housekeepers of the CNS, **microglia** (mesoderm-derived mononuclear phagocytes) are also present in the eyes where they localized predominately at the NFL-GCL interface and the INL-OPL interface (Forrester *et al.*, 2008a; Streit, 2005). These non-ectodermal glial cells are generally absent from the foveal pit and found more numerous in the peripheral retina (Forrester *et al.*, 2008a; Liu, 2007). Similar to their cerebral cousins, retinal microglia play an important role in tissue homeostasis and host defense (Forrester *et al.*, 2008a). The highly arborized processes of microglia are constantly on the move sampling their immediate microenvironment (Forrester *et al.*, 2008a). Upon tissue injury, microglia activate to become wandering macrophages and release both chemokines and cytokines (Forrester *et al.*, 2008a). Finally, it should beware of that although the term "perivascular microglia" refers to the subpopulation of microglia which located near a cerebral blood vessel, it should not be confused with the term "perivascular cells/macrophages" which refers to another type of cells not belonging to the CNS parenchyma as they are the components of the vascular wall and they separated from the CNS parachyma by a perivascular basement membrane (Forrester *et al.*, 2008a; Streit, 2005). Perivascular cells are so-called is mainly due to their localisation in the perivascular space (Forrester *et al.*, 2008a; Streit, 2005). Unlike microglia, these cells are not ramified despite they have an elongated shape (Streit, 2005).

As **oligodendrocytes** and myelin are not normally found in the mammalian retina, it has been hypothesized that **lamina cribrosa** (sieve-like structure in the human sclera) of the human eye may serve as a barrier to block the migration of oligodendroblasts that might otherwise enter the retina (Ffrench-Constant *et al.*, 1988). However, recent studies have identified novel glial cell types scattered across the IPL (Fischer, 2011). These novel glial cells express Nkx2.2, transitin, Sox2, Sox9 and vimentin but GFAP, S100β, glutamine synthetase and other glial markers (including Pax2, 2M6, CD45, RCA1 and lysosomal membrane glycoprotein) are not detectable (Fischer, 2011). Additionally, as these novel retinal glial cells are not associated with blood vessels and they do not upregulate GFAP in response to injury, they are coined as the non-astrocytic inner retinal glia (NIRG) to distinguish them from other well-documented retinal glial cells including both astrocytes and microglia (Fischer, 2011). Interestingly, although NIRG can upregulate transitin and proliferate within the IPL in response to the exposure of IGF1, such IGF1-mediated stimulation of NIRG is detrimental to the survival of retinal neurons and MG (Fischer, 2011). Further, as NIRG are found in the retinas of dogs and monkeys (implicating their presence in human retina) while there is no report regarding their presence in the rodent retinas, a species-unique character of these cells have been suggested (Fischer, 2011). Similarly, in the chicken studies by Rompani and colleagues, they have identified another novel type of retinal glial cells in the GCL based on their morphology and have coined them as the diacytes which express Olig2 but not GFAP and other well-established oligodendrocyte markers (Fischer, 2011; Rompani and Cepko, 2010).

Finally, proliferating retinal stem cells are also found at the far peripheral edge of the non-damaged retina (at the transition of neural retina to non-pigmented epithelium of the ciliary body) called the circumferential marginal zone (CMZ) (Fischer, 2011). The proliferation of these CMZ stem cells is affected by various growth factors (including insulin, IGF1, FGF2 and EGF) and is enhanced by form deprivation (Fischer, 2011). Interestingly, the proliferation of these CMZ stem cells is inhibited by glucagon which can be expressed by the bullwhip cells (unipolar neurons with large somata in the INL and neurites in the distal IPL) (Fischer, 2011). In regard to these bullwhip cells, their axons are commonly projected to and ramified within the CMZ and they are also capable of expressing substance P (Fischer, 2011). While these large bullwhip cells are commonly found in the ventral regions of the retina, their smaller cousins (minibullwhip cells) are commonly found in the dorsal regions of the retina (Fischer, 2011).

5   Conclusion

To this day, myopia is commonly recognized as an abnormal refractive condition affecting the quality of far vision and is affected by multiple risk factors involving both genetic and environmental factors in its aetiology. Myopia is commonly classified into different types and subtypes mainly according to their age of onset, severity of refractive errors and the main causative factor. Regardless of the diversity of myopia, since the underlying pathogenic mechanism is determined by a complex network of molecular interactions and cellular relationships, the complete mechanism underlying the aberrant physiological changes in the development and progression of various myopic conditions would only be better understood if the investigation is conducted at the cellular, molecular and genetics level.

After all, the most common myopic condition is that associated with abnormal ocular elongation, of which is linked to the development of refractive errors as well as degenerative changes that associated with higher myopic eyes. Although there are increasing evidences implicating the possibility of harnessing the neurogenic potential of endogenous retinal cells to restore vision and to treat sight-threatening diseases of the retina (of which MG as well as other retinal stem cells are potential targets), the current picture about the cellular/molecular mechanisms underlying myopia (particularly the ocular growth and the accompanying pathological complications) is still too elusive. Thus, further studies are required. Meanwhile, correction lenses and eye surgeries seem to be the most effective management for myopia at this stage.

Acknowledgement

I should like to thank Professor Sookja K. Chung and Professor Kwok-Fai So (Department of Anatomy, The University of Hong Kong) for their previous endorsement in my first eye research and providing me a post for studying glaucoma. I should also like to thank Dr. Chi-wai Do and Jeremy Guggenheim (School of Optometry, The Hong Kong Polytechnic University) for their opportunities to let me advance more in the field of ophthalmology. Finally, I should like to thank everyone who had helped reviewing and publishing this work. The author of this manuscript certifies that he complies with the guidelines for authorship and publishing in the Eye Diseases and Disorders - A Complete Guide (iConcept Press).

Authors

Ping Kwan

School of Pharmacy, Faculty of Medicine, The Chinese University of Hong Kong, Hong Kong (SAR) of China

Appendix

The author declares that he has no conflict of interest.

References

Asi H, Perlman I. (1992). *Relationships between the electroretinogram a-wave, b-wave and oscillatory potentials and their application to clinical diagnosis.* Doc Ophthalmol; 79(2):125-39.

Baker CI. (2013). *Chapter 4: Visual processing in the primate brain. In: Weiner IB, Nelson RJ, Mizumori SJY. Handbook of Psychology Volume 3: Behavioral Neuroscience. 2nd edition.* New Jersey: John Wiley and Sons, Inc; p81-114.

Bloomfield SA, Dacheux RF. (2001). *Rod vision: pathways and processing in the mammalian retina.* Prog Retin Eye Res;20(3):351-84.

Buck SL. (2004). *Chapter 55: Rod-cone interactions in human vision. In: Chalupa LM, Werner JS. The visual neurosciences.* US: MIT Press; p863-878.

Chappell RL, Schuette E, Anton R, Ripps H. (2002). *GABA(C) receptors modulate the rod-driven ERG b-wave of the skate retina.* Doc Ophthalmol; 105(2):179-88.

Chebib M, Hinton T, Schmid KL, Brinkworth D, Qian H, Matos S, Kim HL, Abdel-Halim H, Kumar RJ, Johnston GA, Hanrahan JR. (2009). *Novel, potent, and selective GABAC antagonists inhibit myopia development and facilitate learning and memory.* J Pharmacol Exp Ther; 328(2):448-57. doi: 10.1124/jpet.108.146464. Epub 2008 Nov 4.

Chiu K, Chan TF, Wu A, Leung IY, So KF, Chang RC. (2012). *Neurodegeneration of the retina in mouse models of Alzheimer's disease: what can we learn from the retina?* Age (Dordr); 34(3):633-49. doi: 10.1007/s11357-011-9260-2. Epub 2011 May 11.

Cone RA, Ebrey TG. (1965). *Functional independence of the two major components of the rod electroretinogram.* Nature; 206(987):913-5.

Cooke Bailey JN, Sobrin L, Pericak-Vance MA, Haines JL, Hammond CJ, Wiggs JL. (2013). *Advances in the genomics of common eye diseases.* Hum Mol Genet; 22(R1):R59-65. doi: 10.1093/hmg/ddt396. Epub 2013 Aug 19.

Czepita D, Filipiak D. (2005). *The effect of the type of astigmatism on the incidence of myopia.* Klin Oczna; 107(1-3):73-4.

Dastiridou AI, Ginis H, Tsilimbaris M, Karyotakis N, Detorakis E, Siganos C, Cholevas P, Tsironi EE, Pallikaris IG. (2013). Ocular rigidity, ocular pulse amplitude, and pulsatile ocular blood flow: the effect of axial length. Invest Ophthalmol Vis Sci; 54(3):2087-92. doi: 10.1167/iovs.12-11576.

Edwards MH. (1998). Chapter 1: Myopia: definitions, classifications and economic implications. In: Rosenfield M, Gilmartin B. Myopia and Nearwork. Butterworth-Heinemann; p1-12.

Ellis-Behnke RG, Jonas RA, Jonas JB. (2013). The microglial system in the eye and brain in response to stimuli in vivo. J Glaucoma; 22 Suppl 5:S32-5. doi: 10.1097/IJG.0b013e3182934aca.

Fan DS, Rao SK, Cheung EY, Islam M, Chew S, Lam DS. Astigmatism in Chinese preschool children: prevalence, change, and effect on refractive development. Br J Ophthalmol. 2004 Jul;88(7):938-41.

Ffrench-Constant C, Miller RH, Burne JF, Raff MC. (1988). Evidence that migratory oligodendrocyte-type-2 astrocyte (O-2A) progenitor cells are kept out of the rat retina by a barrier at the eye-end of the optic nerve. J Neurocytol; 17(1):13-25.

Filosa JA, Bonev AD, Straub SV, Meredith AL, Wilkerson MK, Aldrich RW, Nelson MT. (2006). Local potassium signaling couples neuronal activity to vasodilation in the brain. Nat Neurosci; 9(11):1397-1403.

Fischer AJ. (2011). Muller glia, vision-guided ocular growth, retinal stem cells, and a little serendipity: the Cogan lecture. Invest Ophthalmol Vis Sci; 52(10):7705-10, 7704. doi: 10.1167/iovs.11-8330.

Flores-Moreno I, Ruiz-Medrano J, Duker JS, Ruiz-Moreno JM. (2013). The relationship between retinal and choroidal thickness and visual acuity in highly myopic eyes. Br J Ophthalmol; 97(8):1010-3. doi: 10.1136/bjophthalmol-2012-302836. Epub 2013 Jun 13.

Forrester JV, Dick AD, McMenamin PG, Roberts F. (2008a). Chapter 1: Anatomy of the eye and orbit. In: Forrester JV, Dick AD, McMenamin PG, Roberts F. The eye: basic sciences in practice. 3rd edition. Saunders Ltd.; p1-108.

Forrester JV, Dick AD, McMenamin PG, Roberts F. (2008b). Chapter 2: Embryology and early development of the eye and adnexa. In: Forrester JV, Dick AD, McMenamin PG, Roberts F. The eye: basic sciences in practice. 3rd edition. Saunders Ltd.; p109-142.

Forrester JV, Dick AD, McMenamin PG, Roberts F. (2008c). Chapter 4: Biochemistry and cell biology. In: Forrester JV, Dick AD, McMenamin PG, Roberts F. The eye: basic sciences in practice. 3rd edition. Saunders Ltd.; p171-262.

Forrester JV, Dick AD, McMenamin PG, Roberts F. (2008d). Chapter 6: General and ocular pharmacology. In: Forrester JV, Dick AD, McMenamin PG, Roberts F. The eye: basic sciences in practice. 3rd edition. Saunders Ltd.; p319-350.

Foster P, Khaw KT. (2009). The eye: window to the soul or a mirror of systemic health? Heart; 95(5):348-9. doi: 10.1136/hrt.2008.158121. Epub 2009 Jan 8.

Fredrick DR. (2002). Myopia. BMJ; 324(7347):1195-9.

Frishman LJ. (2013). Chapter 7: Electrogenesis of the electroretinogram. In: Ryan SJ, Schachat AP, Wilkinson CP, Hinton DR, Sadda SR, Wiedemann P. Retina. 5th edition. Saunders; p177-201.

García M, Vecino E. (2003). Role of Müller glia in neuroprotection and regeneration in the retina. Histol Histopathol; 18(4):1205-18.

Gills JP, Wallace RB, Fine IH, Friedlander MH, McFarland MS. (2011). Chapter 7: Reducing pre-existing astigmatism with limbal relaxing incisions. In: Henderson BA, Gills JP, editors. A complete surgical guide for correcting astigmatism. 2nd edition. Thorofare, NJ: SLACK Incorporated; p55-72.

Hashemi H, Rezvan F, Beiranvand A, Papi OA, Hoseini Yazdi H, Ostadimoghaddam H, Yekta AA, Norouzirad R, Khabazkhoob M. Prevalence of Refractive Errors among High School Students in Western Iran. J Ophthalmic Vis Res. 2014 Apr;9(2):232-9.

Hauswirth SG, Hardten DR, Davis EA. (2008). Chapter 12: Indications for Penetrating Keratoplasty for Irregular Astigmatism. In: Wang M. Irregular Astigmatism: Diagnosis and Treatment. SLACK Incorporated; p117-127.

Henderson BA, Tehrani M, Mamalis N, Hoffman RS, Fine IH, Dick HB, Packer M. (2011). Chapter 1: Surgical correction of astigmatism. In: Henderson BA, Gills JP. A complete surgical guide for correcting astigmatism. 2nd edition. Thorofare, NJ: SLACK Incorporated; p3-10.

Hewitt AW, Kearns LS, Jamieson RV, Williamson KA, van Heyningen V, Mackey DA. (2007). PAX6 mutations may be associated with high myopia. Ophthalmic Genet; 28(3):179-82.

Holden C. (2007). Neuroscience. Astrocytes secrete substance that kills motor neurons in ALS. Science; 316(5823):353.

Hsu CC, Chen SJ, Li AF, Lee FL. (2014). Systolic blood pressure, choroidal thickness, and axial length in patients with myopic maculopathy. J Chin Med Assoc; 77(9):487-91. doi: 10.1016/j.jcma.2014.06.009. Epub 2014 Aug 5.

Jackson M, Steers G, Leigh PN, Morrison KE. (1999). *Polymorphisms in the glutamate transporter gene EAAT2 in European ALS patients.* J Neurol; 246(12):1140-4.

Jeganathan VSE, Saw SM, Wong TY. (2010). *Chapter 2.2: Ocular morbidity of pathological myopia. In: Beuerman RW, Saw SM, Tan DTH, Wong TY. Myopia: Animal Models to Clinical Trials. World Scientific Publishing Company; p97-120.*

Jensen RJ. (2013). *Effects of a metabotropic glutamate 1 receptor antagonist on light responses of retinal ganglion cells in a rat model of retinitis pigmentosa. PLoS One; 8(10):e79126. doi: 10.1371/journal.pone.0079126.*

Karlstetter M, Nothdurfter C, Aslanidis A, Moeller K, Horn F, Scholz R, Neumann H, Weber BH, Rupprecht R, Langmann T. (2014). *Translocator protein (18 kDa) (TSPO) is expressed in reactive retinal microglia and modulates microglial inflammation and phagocytosis.* J Neuroinflammation; 11(1):3. doi: 10.1186/1742-2094-11-3.

Kassen SC, Thummel R, Campochiaro LA, Harding MJ, Bennett NA, Hyde DR. (2009). *CNTF induces photoreceptor neuroprotection and Müller glial cell proliferation through two different signaling pathways in the adult zebrafish retina. Exp Eye Res; 88(6):1051-64. doi: 10.1016/j.exer.2009.01.007. Epub 2009 Feb 7.*

Kee CS. (2013). *Astigmatism and its role in emmetropization. Exp Eye Res; 114:89-95. doi: 10.1016/j.exer.2013.04.020. Epub 2013 May 2.*

Keeley PW, Luna G, Fariss RN, Skyles KA, Madsen NR, Raven MA, Poché RA, Swindell EC, Jamrich M, Oh EC, Swaroop A, Fisher SK, Reese BE. (2013). *Development and plasticity of outer retinal circuitry following genetic removal of horizontal cells. J Neurosci; 33(45):17847-62. doi: 10.1523/JNEUROSCI.1373-13.2013.*

Kettenmann H, Ransom BR. (2005). *Part 2: Functions of neuroglial cells. In: Kettenmann H, Ransom BR. Neuroglia. 2nd edition. New York: Oxford University Press; p251-417.*

Khor CC. (2010). *Chapter 3.3: TIGR, TGFB1, cMET, HGF, collagen genes, and myopia. In: Beuerman RW, Saw SM, Tan DTH, Wong TY. Myopia: Animal Models to Clinical Trials. World Scientific Publishing Company; p201-214.*

Klein BEK. (2010). *Chapter 1.1: Epidemiology of myopia and myopic shift in refraction. In: Beuerman RW, Saw SM, Tan DTH, Wong TY. Myopia: Animal Models to Clinical Trials. World Scientific Publishing Company; p3-22.*

Kleinstein RN, Jones LA, Hullett S, Kwon S, Lee RJ, Friedman NE, Manny RE, Mutti DO, Yu JA, Zadnik K; Collaborative Longitudinal Evaluation of Ethnicity and Refractive Error Study Group. *Refractive error and ethnicity in children. Arch Ophthalmol. 2003 Aug; 121(8):1141-7.*

Koh VT, Nah GK, Chang L, Yang AH, Lin ST, Ohno-Matsui K, Wong TY, Saw SM. (2013). *Pathologic changes in highly myopic eyes of young males in Singapore. Ann Acad Med Singapore; 42(5):216-24.*

Kolb H. (2009). *Neurotransmitters in the Retina. In: Kolb H, Nelson R, Fernandez E, Jones B. Webvision: The Organization of the Retina and Visual System [Internet]. Salt Lake City (UT): University of Utah Health Sciences Center; Retrieved from http://www.ncbi.nlm.nih.gov/books/NBK11546/ . Accessed 19-JAN-2014.*

Kwan P. (2013a). *Sarcopenia, a neurogenic syndrome? J Aging Res; 2013:791679. doi: 10.1155/2013/791679. Epub 2013a Mar 13.*

Kwan P. (2013b). *Sarcopenia: The gliogenic perspective. Mech Ageing Dev; doi:pii: S0047-6374(13)00082-1. 10.1016/j.mad.2013.06.001. [Epub ahead of print]*

Kwan, P. & Tse. (2013). *M.T. mTOR and its Physiological Impacts-Part I: An Overview. Journal of Biochemical and Pharmacological Research; 1(2): 124-137.*

Lee JH, Shin JM, Shin YJ, Chun MH, Oh SJ. (2011). *Immunochemical changes of calbindin, calretinin and SMI32 in ischemic retinas induced by increase of intraocular pressure and by middle cerebral artery occlusion. Anat Cell Biol; 44(1):25-34. doi: 10.5115/acb.2011.44.1.25. Epub 2011 Mar 31.*

Lee SY. (2010). *Chapter 2.4: The myopic retina. In: Beuerman RW, Saw SM, Tan DTH, Wong TY. Myopia: Animal Models to Clinical Trials. World Scientific Publishing Company; p137-148.*

Li YJ, Fan Q. (2010). *Chapter 3.4: Statistical analysis of genome-wide association studies for myopia. In: Beuerman RW, Saw SM, Tan DTH, Wong TY. Myopia: Animal Models to Clinical Trials. World Scientific Publishing Company; p215-235.*

Lim MCC, Frick KD. (2010). *Chapter 1.4: The economics of myopia. In: Beuerman RW, Saw SM, Tan DTH, Wong TY. Myopia: Animal Models to Clinical Trials. World Scientific Publishing Company; p63-80.*

Lin B, Jakobs TC, Masland RH. (2005). *Different functional types of bipolar cells use different gap-junctional proteins. J Neurosci; 25(28):6696-701.*

Lin B, Masland RH. (2005). *Synaptic contacts between an identified type of ON cone bipolar cell and ganglion cells in the mouse retina. Eur J Neurosci; 25(5):1257-70.*

Lin B, Peng EB. (2013). *Retinal ganglion cells are resistant to photoreceptor loss in retinal degeneration.* PLoS One; 8(6):e68084. doi: 10.1371/journal.pone.0068084. Print 2013.

Lindqvist N, Liu Q, Zajadacz J, Franze K, Reichenbach A. (2010). *Retinal glial (Müller) cells: sensing and responding to tissue stretch.* Invest Ophthalmol Vis Sci; 51(3):1683-90. doi: 10.1167/iovs.09-4159. Epub 2009 Nov 5.

Liu SQ. (2007). *Chapter 8: Embryonic organ development.* In: Liu SQ. Bioregenerative Engineering: Principles and Applications. New Jersey: John Wiley and Sons, Inc; p346–379.

Luu CD, Chia AWL. (2010). *Chapter 2.5: Retinal function.* In: Beuerman RW, Saw SM, Tan DTH, Wong TY. Myopia: Animal Models to Clinical Trials. World Scientific Publishing Company; p149-160.

Mansour H, Chamberlain CG, Weible MW 2nd, Hughes S, Chu Y, Chan-Ling T. (2008). *Aging-related changes in astrocytes in the rat retina: imbalance between cell proliferation and cell death reduces astrocyte availability.* Aging Cell; 7(4):526-40. doi: 10.1111/j.1474-9726.2008.00402.x. Epub 2008 Jun 28.

Mao JF, Liu SZ, Qin WJ, Xiang Q. (2011). *Modulation of TGFβ(2) and dopamine by PKC in retinal Müller cells of guinea pig myopic eye.* Int J Ophthalmol; 4(4):357-60. doi: 10.3980/j.issn.2222-3959.2011.04.06. Epub 2011 Aug 18.

McBrien NA. (2010). *Chapter 4.2: The mechanisms regulating scleral change in myopia.* In: Beuerman RW, Saw SM, Tan DTH, Wong TY. Myopia: Animal Models to Clinical Trials. World Scientific Publishing Company; p267-302.

McKnight CM, Sherwin JC, Yazar S, Forward H, Tan AX, Hewitt AW, Pennell CE, McAllister IL, Young TL, Coroneo MT, Mackey DA. (2014). *Myopia in Young Adults Is Inversely Related to an Objective Marker of Ocular Sun Exposure: The Western Australian Raine Cohort Study.* Am J Ophthalmol. pii: S0002-9394(14)00454-1. doi: 10.1016/j.ajo.2014.07.033. [Epub ahead of print]

Meyer A, Hilgen G, Dorgau B, Sammler EM, Weiler R, Monyer H, Dedek K, Hormuzdi SG. (2014). *AII amacrine cells discriminate between heterocellular and homocellular locations when assembling connexin36-containing gap junctions.* J Cell Sci; [Epub ahead of print]

Mi XS, Zhang X, Feng Q, Lo AC, Chung SK, So KF. (2012a). *Progressive retinal degeneration in transgenic mice with overexpression of endothelin-1 in vascular endothelial cells.* Invest Ophthalmol Vis Sci; 53(8):4842-51. doi: 10.1167/iovs.12-9999.

Mi XS, Feng Q, Lo AC, Chang RC, Lin B, Chung SK, So KF. (2012b). *Protection of retinal ganglion cells and retinal vasculature by Lycium barbarum polysaccharides in a mouse model of acute ocular hypertension.* PLoS One; 7(10):e45469. doi: 10.1371/journal.pone.0045469. Epub 2012 Oct 19.

Mirshahi A, Ponto KA, Hoehn R, Zwiener I, Zeller T, Lackner K, Beutel ME, Pfeiffer N. (2014). *Myopia and level of education: results from the gutenberg health study.* Ophthalmology; 121(10):2047-52. doi: 10.1016/j.ophtha.2014.04.017. Epub 2014 Jun 16.

Mitchell CH, Lu W. (2008). *Chapter 10: Retinal ganglion cells and glaucoma: Traditional Patterns and New Possibilities.* In: Civan MM. The Eye's Aqueous Humor. 2nd edition. Academic Press; p301-322.

Miyake M, Yamashiro K, Nakanishi H, Nakata I, Akagi-Kurashige Y, Tsujikawa A, Moriyama M, Ohno-Matsui K, Mochizuki M, Yamada R, Matsuda F, Yoshimura N. (2013). *Insulin-like growth factor 1 is not associated with high myopia in a large Japanese cohort.* Mol Vis; 19:1074-81. Print 2013.

Morgan IG, Ohno-Matsui K, Saw SM. (2012). *Myopia.* Lancet; 379(9827):1739-48. doi: 10.1016/S0140-6736(12)60272-4.

Mutti DO, Mitchell GL, Jones LA, Friedman NE, Frane SL, Lin WK, Moeschberger ML, Zadnik K. (2005). *Axial growth and changes in lenticular and corneal power during emmetropization in infants.* Invest Ophthalmol Vis Sci; 46(9):3074-80.

Nelson R. (2007). *Visual Responses of Ganglion Cells.* In: Kolb H, Nelson R, Fernandez E, Jones B. Webvision: The Organization of the Retina and Visual System [Internet]. Salt Lake City (UT): University of Utah Health Sciences Center; Retrieved from http://www.ncbi.nlm.nih.gov/books/NBK11550/ . Accessed 19-JAN-2014.

Nelson R, Connaughton V. (2012). *Bipolar Cell Pathways in the Vertebrate Retina.* In: Kolb H, Nelson R, Fernandez E, Jones B. Webvision: The Organization of the Retina and Visual System [Internet]. Salt Lake City (UT): University of Utah Health Sciences Center; Retrieved from http://www.ncbi.nlm.nih.gov/books/NBK11521/ . Accessed 23-JAN-2014.

Nicholls JG, Martin AR, Wallace BG, Fuchs PA. (2003). *Chapter 19: Transduction and signaling in the retina.* In: Yang XL, Tan DP, Ye B, Jiang ZY, Luo DG, Xu HP, Zhao JW, Li GL, Liu J, Huang H, Xu LY, Dong J, Jiang H, Shen Y, Chen L, Tian M, Lu XH, Liu DT, Yu YC. Neurobiology: From Neurons to Brain (ISBN-10: 7030109902). Ke xue chu ban she; p447-476.

Nishimura T, Machida S, Kondo M, Terasaki H, Yokoyama D, Kurosaka D. (2011). *Enhancement of ON-bipolar cell responses of cone electroretinograms in rabbits with the Pro347Leu rhodopsin mutation.* Invest Ophthalmol Vis Sci; 52(10):7610-7. doi: 10.1167/iovs.11-7611.

Packer M, Afshari NA, Alder BD. (2011). Chapter 2: Diagnosing astigmatism. In: Henderson BA, Gills JP, editors. A complete surgical guide for correcting astigmatism. 2nd edition. Thorofare, NJ: SLACK Incorporated; p11-20.

Pagel JI, Deindl E. (2011). Early growth response 1--a transcription factor in the crossfire of signal transduction cascades. Indian J Biochem Biophys; 48(4):226-35.

Park H, Tan CC, Faulkner A, Jabbar SB, Schmid G, Abey J, Iuvone PM, Pardue MT. (2013). Retinal degeneration increases susceptibility to myopia in mice. Mol Vis; 19:2068-79. eCollection 2013.

Patil B, Puri P. (2009). Chapter 4.4: Medical retina. In: Sundaram V, Barsam A, Alwitry A, Khaw PT. Oxford Specialty Training: Training In Ophthalmology - The Essential Clinical Curriculum. Oxford: Oxford University Press; p152-155.

Perera SA, Aung T. (2010). Chapter 2.3: Myopia and glaucoma. In: Beuerman RW, Saw SM, Tan DTH, Wong TY. Myopia: Animal Models to Clinical Trials. World Scientific Publishing Company; p121-136.

Rao SD, Weiss JH. (2004). Excitotoxic and oxidative cross-talk between motor neurons and glia in ALS pathogenesis. Trends Neurosci; 27(1):17-23.

Rehm DS. (1981). Chapter 5: A short history of myopia. In: Rehm DS. The Myopia Myth: The Truth About Nearsightedness and How to Prevent It. US: Intl Myopia Prevention Assn; p56-61.

Reichenbach A, Bringmann A. (2013). New functions of Müller cells. Glia; 61(5):651-78. doi: 10.1002/glia.22477. Epub 2013 Feb 26.

Robaszkiewicz J, Chmielewska K, Figurska M, Wierzbowska J, Stankiewicz A. (2010). Müller glial cells--the mediators of vascular disorders with vitreomacular interface pathology in diabetic maculopathy. Klin Oczna; 112(10-12):328-32.

Rompani SB, Cepko CL. (2010). A common progenitor for retinal astrocytes and oligodendrocytes. J Neurosci; 30(14):4970-80. doi: 10.1523/JNEUROSCI.3456-09.2010.

Rosenfield M. (1998). Chapter 5: Accomodation and myopia. In: Rosenfield M, Gilmartin B. Myopia and Nearwork. Butterworth-Heinemann; p91-116.

Sanchez F. (2010). Chapter 5: The external space. In: Sanchez F. The Master Illusionist: Principles of Neuropsychology. US: Xlibris; p109-169.

Schubert P, Ogata T, Marchini C, Ferroni S. (2001). Glia-related pathomechanisms in Alzheimer's disease: a therapeutic target? Mech Ageing Dev; 123(1):47-57.

Seifert G, Schilling K, Steinhäuser C. (2006). Astrocyte dysfunction in neurological disorders: a molecular perspective. Nat Rev Neurosci; 7(3):194-206.

Shih YF, Ho TC, Hsiao CK, Lin LL. (2006). Visual outcomes for high myopic patients with or without myopic maculopathy: a 10 year follow up study. Br J Ophthalmol; 90(5):546-50.

Smith EL 3rd. (1998). Chapter 4: Environmentally induced refractive errors in animals. In: Rosenfield M, Gilmartin B. Myopia and Nearwork. Butterworth-Heinemann; p57-90.

Stone RA, Liu J, Sugimoto R, Capehart C, Zhu X, Pendrak K. (2003). GABA, experimental myopia, and ocular growth in chick. Invest Ophthalmol Vis Sci; 44(9):3933-46.

Streit WJ. (2005). Chapter 5: Microglial cells. In: Kettenmann H, Ransom BR. Neuroglia. 2nd edition. New York: Oxford University Press; p60-71.

Swaroop A, Kim D, Forrest D. (2010). Transcriptional regulation of photoreceptor development and homeostasis in the mammalian retina. Nat Rev Neurosci; 11(8):563-76. doi: 10.1038/nrn2880.

Takano T, Tian GF, Peng W, Lou N, Libionka W, Han X, Nedergaard M. (2006). Astrocyte-mediated control of cerebral blood flow. Nat Neurosci; 9(2):260-7. Epub 2005 Dec 25.

Teismann P, Tieu K, Cohen O, Choi DK, Wu DC, Marks D, Vila M, Jackson-Lewis V, Przedborski S. (2003). Pathogenic role of glial cells in Parkinson's disease. Mov Disord; 18(2):121-9.

Tong LMG, Barathi VA, Beuerman RW. (2010). Chapter 5.1: Atropine and other pharmacological approaches to prevent myopia. In: Beuerman RW, Saw SM, Tan DTH, Wong TY. Myopia: Animal Models to Clinical Trials. World Scientific Publishing Company; p345-360.

Tsai YY, Chiang CC, Lin HJ, Lin JM, Wan L, Tsai FJ. (2008). A PAX6 gene polymorphism is associated with genetic predisposition to extreme myopia. Eye (Lond); 22(4):576-81. Epub 2007 Oct 19.

Tse, M.T. & Kwan, P. (2013). mTOR and its Physiological Impacts-Part II: Immunological Impact. Journal of Biochemical and Pharmacological Research; 1(2): 138-142.

Verhoeven VJ, Wong KT, Buitendijk GH, Hofman A, Vingerling JR, Klaver CC. (2014). Visual Consequences of Refractive Errors in the General Population. Ophthalmology. pii: S0161-6420(14)00641-1. doi: 10.1016/j.ophtha.2014.07.030. [Epub ahead of print]

Verkhratsky A, Butt A. (2007a). Chapter 1: Introduction to Glia. In: Verkhratsky A, Butt A. Glial Neurobiology. England: John Wiley and Sons, Inc; p4-12.

Verkhratsky A, Butt A. (2007b). Chapter 2: General Overview of Signalling in the Nervous System. In: Verkhratsky A, Butt A. Glial Neurobiology. England: John Wiley and Sons, Inc; p15-17.

Verkhratsky A, Butt A. (2007c). Chapter 3: Morphology of Glial Cells. In: Verkhratsky A, Butt A. Glial Neurobiology. England: John Wiley and Sons, Inc; p21-28.

Wallman J, Nickla DL. (2010). Chapter 4.1: The relevance of studies in chicks for understanding myopia in humans. In: Beuerman RW, Saw SM, Tan DTH, Wong TY. Myopia: Animal Models to Clinical Trials. World Scientific Publishing Company; p239-266.

Wan J, Ramachandran R, Goldman D. (2012). HB-EGF is necessary and sufficient for Müller glia dedifferentiation and retina regeneration. Dev Cell; 22(2):334-47. doi: 10.1016/j.devcel.2011.11.020.

Wang X, Fan J, Zhang M, Ni Y, Xu G. (2013a). Upregulation of SOX9 in Glial (Müller) cells in retinal light damage of rats. Neurosci Lett; 556:140-5. doi: 10.1016/j.neulet.2013.10.005. Epub 2013 Oct 11.

Wang X, Fan J, Zhang M, Sun Z, Xu G. (2013b). Gene expression changes under cyclic mechanical stretching in rat retinal glial (Müller) cells. PLoS One; 8(5):e63467. doi: 10.1371/journal.pone.0063467. Print 2013.

Wang X, Xu G, Fan J, Zhang M. (2013c). Mechanical stretching induces matrix metalloproteinase-2 expression in rat retinal glial (Müller) cells. Neuroreport; 24(5):224-8. doi: 10.1097/WNR.0b013e32835eb9d1.

Wildsoet CF. (1998). Chapter 3: Structural correlates of myopia. In: Rosenfield M, Gilmartin B. Myopia and Nearwork. Butterworth-Heinemann; p31-56.

Wilkie SE, Vissers PM, Das D, Degrip WJ, Bowmaker JK, Hunt DM. (1998). The molecular basis for UV vision in birds: spectral characteristics, cDNA sequence and retinal localization of the UV-sensitive visual pigment of the budgerigar (Melopsittacus undulatus). Biochem J; 330 (Pt 1):541-7.

Wong TY, Ohno-Matsui K, Leveziel N, Holz FG, Lai TY, Yu HG, Lanzetta P, Chen Y, Tufail A. (2014). Myopic choroidal neovascularisation: current concepts and update on clinical management. Br J Ophthalmol. pii: bjophthalmol-2014-305131. doi: 10.1136/bjophthalmol-2014-305131. [Epub ahead of print]

Yazar S, Hewitt AW, Black LJ, McKnight CM, Mountain JA, Sherwin JC, Oddy WH, Coroneo MT, Lucas RM, Mackey DA. Myopia is associated with lower vitamin D status in young adults. Invest Ophthalmol Vis Sci. 2014 Jun 26;55(7):4552-9. doi: 10.1167/iovs.14-14589.

You QS, Wu LJ, Duan JL, Luo YX, Liu LJ, Li X, Gao Q, Wang W, Xu L, Jonas JB, Guo XH. Prevalence of myopia in school children in greater Beijing: the Beijing Childhood Eye Study. Acta Ophthalmol. 2014 Aug;92(5):e398-406. Epub 2013 Oct 28.

Yu L, Li ZK, Gao JR, Liu JR, Xu CT. (2011). Epidemiology, genetics and treatments for myopia. Int J Ophthalmol; 4(6):658-69. doi: 10.3980/j.issn.2222-3959.2011.06.17. Epub 2011 Dec 18.

Zahs KR, Ceelen PW. (2006). Gap junctional coupling and connexin immunoreactivity in rabbit retinal glia. Vis Neurosci; 23(1):1-10.

Zhao F, Wu J, Xue A, Su Y, Wang X, Lu X, Zhou Z, Qu J, Zhou X. (2013). Exome sequencing reveals CCDC111 mutation associated with high myopia. Hum Genet; 132(8):913-21. doi: 10.1007/s00439-013-1303-6. Epub 2013 Apr 12.

Zong H, Ward M, Madden A, Yong PH, Limb GA, Curtis TM, Stitt AW. (2010). Hyperglycaemia-induced pro-inflammatory responses by retinal Müller glia are regulated by the receptor for advanced glycation end-products (RAGE). Diabetologia; 53(12):2656-66. doi: 10.1007/s00125-010-1900-z. Epub 2010 Sep 12.

Immunopathogenesis of Dry Eye Disease

Readon Teh and Louis Tong

1 Introduction

1.1 Immunity in Ocular Disease

The immune system is our body's natural biological defense system to prevent infection, disease or invasion by non-commensal microbes. Specialized collection of cells and molecules protect the body from numerous pathogenic microbes and environmental toxins. The immune system is a double edge sword. On one hand, it is required to limit the damage induced by offending agents, especially important in cases when the physical barriers (such as mucosal protection or eyelids) are compromised; on the other hand, overactive immunity is detrimental to host tissue. Chronic inflammatory processes in the cornea, the transparent tissue of the eye important for vision, can be particularly devastating. These result in corneal oedema, infiltration of immune cells, formation of myofibroblasts and scar tissue, and eventually vascularisation. All these result in a poorly reflective, opaque media, which cause deterioration of vision. In severe disease, there may be corneal ulceration, thinning and even perforation.

The ocular surface contains an immunological framework that limits host tissue damage when insulted by environmental trauma or pathogens, and to maintain tolerance against self-antigens. There are special properties of the ocular surface immune system, called the eye associated lymphoid tissue (EALT)(E. Knop & Knop, 2005; N. Knop & Knop, 2010), which shares similarities with the immune system in general. The EALT consists of LDALT (lacrimal drainage associated lymphoid tissue) and CALT (conjunctiva-associated lymphoid tissue). We will describe certain characteristics of this immune system which is unique to the ocular surface. These processes are key to the development of dry eye, ocular surface infections, allergies, chemical injury and cicatricial diseases. In severe cases, ocular surface inflammation is the cause of some of these devastating clinical syndromes.

Our understanding of immune responses in the cornea and ocular surface has been continuously evolving over the past decades. Although the ocular surface was once thought to be a site of immune privilege with the absence of cells that regulate immuno-inflammatory responses, current advances in literature have shown that there is a diverse family of cellular and molecular mediators from both innate and adaptive immunity in the ocular surface(Stern, Schaumburg, & Pflugfelder, 2013).Alterations of these finely balanced molecules can easily trigger inflammation and disease.

Knowledge in ocular immunity has led to advances in developing novel therapeutic agents that regulate ocular surface inflammation, and has been applied in the management of ocular surface disorders, or systemic diseases with ocular manifestations such as in autoimmune-mediated rheumatoid arthritis causing scleritis.

1.2 Dry Eye Disease and Ocular Surface Inflammation

One of the most common ocular surface disorders is dry eye disease (DED). DED is not merely due to reduced tear volume. It is a multi-factorial disease of the tear and ocular surface that arises when the pre-ocular tear film does not adequately support biological functions of the ocular surface. This arises due to environmental or endogenous stress, microbial insult or genetic factors (McDermott *et al.*, 2005). Acute inflammatory pathways of the ocular surface are triggered with tear dysfunction and hyperosmolarity, and this potentiates a chronic inflammatory cycle that is seen in DED. Such inflammatory pathways are driven by host ocular immunity.

Significantly, the overall prevalence of DED within the population ranges from 14.4% in a Caucasian cohort (Moss, Klein, & Klein, 2000) to 33% in an Asian cohort (Shimmura, Shimazaki, & Tsubota, 1999). Many risk factors have been identified; of greatest significance is that the prevalence of DED increases with age. Prevalence of DED among females is found to be greater than men across all age groups (Schaumberg, Dana, Buring, & Sullivan, 2009; Shimmura *et al.*, 1999). Other risk factors identified include systemic diseases like diabetes mellitus (Shimmura *et al.*, 1999), and lifestyle practices such as cigarette smoking (Schaumberg *et al.*, 2009), contact lens wear, prolonged viewing of electronic display screens (Uchino *et al.*, 2008), and low-humidity environments (Uchiyama, Aronowicz, Butovich, & McCulley, 2007).

Patients with DED experience varying severity of symptoms. Most patients complain of eye irritation, blurring of vision that fluctuates across the day and even photophobia. DED significantly reduces the quality of life among those affected. In fact, the impact of DED on patients was found to be equivalent to unstable angina, a life-threatening cardiac condition (Schiffman *et al.*, 2003).

Ophthalmologists who treat chronic DED patients have to manage the symptoms of ocular surface inflammation. The previous section mentioned the detrimental effects of inflammation on visual symptoms. Apart from reducing vision, the symptoms of inflammation also include redness, pain, swelling, oedema (chemosis) of the conjunctiva and eyelids. In DED, the irritaftive symptoms may be due to the release of pro-inflammatory cytokines(Lam *et al.*, 2009) and infiltration of inflammatory cells(Kunert, Tisdale, Stern, Smith, & Gipson, 2000) on the ocular surface, as well as stimulation of the nerve fibers innervating the ocular surface, resulting ocular surface tissue damage. Inflammation also leads to epitheliopathy, the key clinical sign identified in DED. Using dyes (such as fluorescein, lisamine green or rose bengal), defects in the ocular surface are visualised by observing irregular morphology and staining of the corneal or conjunctival epithelium. To prevent such damage of inflammation, components involving the innate and adaptive immune response have been described in a number of academic reviews(Stern et al., 2013). In addition to reviewing immune mechanisms in DED, we present new potential future molecular therapies.

2   Immunoregulation of the Ocular Surface

In the ocular surface, the major cell subtypes are distributed between the cornea and conjunctiva. Firstly, fibroblasts synthesize the stromal matrix that provides a framework for cellular organization. Secondly, corneal and conjunctival epithelium function as a cellular epithelial barrier(McCallum, Cobo, & Haynes, 1993). In addition, goblet cells found within the conjunctiva secrete mucous that lubricates the ocular surface (Shatos *et al.*, 2003).

2.1   Innate and Adaptive Immunity

The immune system can be broadly classified into two arms– innate and adaptive (Figure 1). These generally differ in the duration of response to invading pathogens, the cell-types in-

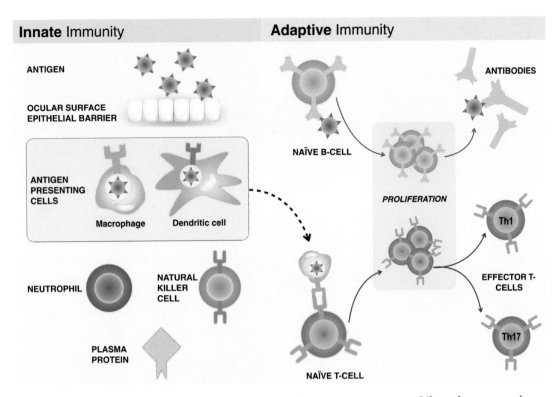

Figure 1: Components and of the ocular surface immune system. Like other mucosal tissues, the ocular surface immune system contains both innate and adaptive immunoregulatory arms that function to limit host tissue damage by external insult, and to maintain tolerance against self-antigens. Significant interaction between both arms of immunity occurs between antigen presenting cells (such as macrophages and dendritic cells) and naïve T-cells.

volved in mediating immune responses, and the specificity for targeted microbes.

Innate immunity consists of enzymes and cells that are always present within the host to target microbes at the site of infection. Other components of innate immunity consist of epithelial layers (acting as physical barriers lining the mucosa and skin), phagocytic leukocytes, antigen presenting cells (APCs), natural killer cells, circulating intra and intercellular chemical signals (cytokines) and antimicrobial substances, such as defensins and cathelicidin (LL-37)(L. C. Huang, Jean, & McDermott, 2005). Apart from these, other enzymatic components include those of lactoferrin, lysozyme and immunoglobulin A. The spectrum of immunity is not specific to any pathogen.

Adaptive immunity, on the other hand, consists of cells that have specific mechanisms to recognize and target an inflammatory response against a specific foreign microbe or antigen. The two arms of adaptive immunity include humoral immunity (mediated by immunoglobulins produced by mature cells of B-lymphocytic lineage), and cell-mediated immunity (mediated by T-lymphocytic cells). As their name suggests, APCs of innate immunity present antigens and interact with lymphocytic cells to initiate adaptive immunity against foreign antigens.

In the normal ocular surface, immunity is suppressed or relatively tolerant to host-tissue, non-pathogenic antigens and commensal bacterial flora. Immune tolerance is necessary to avoid unwanted ocular surface destruction(N. Knop & Knop, 2010), and is mediated by resident dendritic cells (inactive APCs), regulatory T-cells, suppressor T-cells and naïve B-cells. These cells can be found in various layers of the conjunctiva epithelia and stroma. For example, cluster of differentiation (CD)11c+ dendritic cells are found in corneal and conjunctival epithelium(Zheng, de Paiva, Li, Farley, & Pflugfelder, 2010).

Although the osmolarity of tears has not been measured *in vivo* in dry eye animal models, a study with cultured corneal epithelial cells has shown that hyperomsolarity is the cause of stress signaling and production of cytokines and proteases (Liu *et al.*, 2009). In addition, if hyperosmolar drops are given to mice for six times a day for two days, similar changes can be detected (Luo, Li, Corrales, & Pflugfelder, 2005). The hyperosmolar stimulation may be the trigger for loss of immune tolerance. In such a scenario, many components of the ocular immune system can be altered. In this more proinflammatory state, dendritic cells can load themselves with autoantigens (Mircheff *et al.*, 2005), mature, evade control by regulatory T-cells and subsequently migrate to regional draining lymph nodes, where it generates autoantigen-specific effector T-cell subtypes, thus giving rise to autoimmunity. Details will be specified elsewhere in this chapter.

2.2   A Model of Ocular Surface Inflammation in DED

Desiccating stress to the ocular surface (Figure 2) activates signaling pathways such as mitogen-activated protein kinase (MAPK) pathways including the p38, c-Jun N-terminal kinases (JNK) and extracellular signal regulated kinases (ERKs) (Luo *et al.*, 2004). These activated kinases initiate a protein phosphorylation signaling cascade that activates nuclear transcription factors such as nuclear factor kappa B (NFκB), activating protein 1 (AP-1) and activating transcription factor (ATF)(C. S. De Paiva, Pangelinan, *et al.*, 2009; Luo *et al.*, 2005), which causes increased production of pro-inflammatory mediators by ocular surface epithelium, the major ones being pro-inflammatory cytokines interleukin(IL)-1, IL-6 and TNF-α, chemokines and matrix metalloproteinases (MMPs)(D. Q. Li, Chen, Song, Luo, & Pflugfelder, 2004; D. Q. Li *et al.*, 2006; Luo *et al.*, 2004).The resulting pro-inflammatory milieu facilitates the activation and maturation of immature antigen-presenting cells (iAPC), consisting chiefly of dendritic cells and macrophages.

Activated APCs migrate to draining lymphatic tissue (such as regional lymph nodes and spleen) via afferent lymphatic vessels. They have the function of priming naïve T-cells in these lymphoid tissue, leading to differentiation and expansion into effector T_H1 (CD4+ helper T-cell) and T_H17 T-cell subtypes. Subsequently, T_H1 and T_H17 migrate via efferent blood vessels to the ocular surface, where they further release pro-inflammatory cytokines.

$T_H1$cells secrete interferon (IFN)-γ, which upregulates production of chemokines and cell adhesion molecules (CAMs) that further attract inflammatory cells to the ocular surface (including T_H17 subtype T-cells). In addition, T_H1 promotes maturation of ocular surface macrophages, thus giving rise to a positive immune feedback mechanism.

T_H17 secretes IL-17 on the ocular surface. IL-17 further worsens epithelial damage via stimulating production of matrix metalloproteinases (MMP). Also, IL-17 promotes lymphangiogenesis via increased production of vascular endothelial growth factor (VEGF). Increased lymphangiogenesis promotes the migration and trafficking of adaptive immune cells. A self-perpetuating cycle of inflammation develops, and this is the key of chronic inflammation in DED.

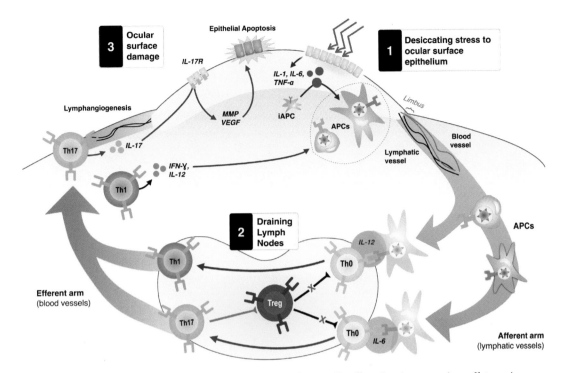

Figure 2: This diagram shows the processes leading to T-cell activation, a major cell type in the immunopathogenesis of dry eye. Desiccating stress to ocular surface epithelium triggers pro-inflammatory cytokine production, leading to maturation of antigen presenting cells (APCs). Mature APCs migrate to draining lymph nodes, where they polarize naïve T-cells (T_H0) to develop into T_H1 or T_H17 effector T-cell subtypes. T_H17 cells antagonize T-regulatory cell (Treg) function in draining lymph nodes, leading to loss of Treg suppression of cytotoxic T- cells. T-cells migrate via efferent blood vessels to the ocular surface, where they exert inflammatory effects, resulting in further epithelial apoptosis.

Many of the above immunological processes have only been studied in murine models of dry eye. There are several ways dry eye can be induced in mice. One of these methods involves the repeated injection of scopolamine (an anti-muscarinic agent) and fan blowing in a controlled environment chamber (Dursun *et al.*, 2002). The immunological landscape of this model will be described in subsequent sections.

3   Innate Immunity

3.1   Acute Inflammatory Proteins and Cytokines

Following desiccating stress to the ocular surface (Liu *et al.*, 2009; Luo *et al.*, 2005), epithelial cells release pro-inflammatory cytokines and chemokines (Corrales *et al.*, 2006; Luo *et al.*, 2004; Niederkorn *et al.*, 2006; Zheng, Bian, *et al.*, 2010). The early expression of pro-inflammatory cytokines, such as IL-1, IL-6 and TNF-α increases production of other pro-inflammatory cytokines, chemokines, and cell adhesion molecules (CAM) required for infiltration of innate immune cells, regulates activation of resident immature APCs and subsequent adaptive immunity players (Zheng, Bian, *et al.*, 2010).

IL-1 is a master regulator of other cytokines in the acute phase of inflammation. IL-1 receptor knockout in a murine model led to attenuation of the consequent pro-inflammatory cytokine milieu, including reduced IL-6 and TNF-α levels (Narayanan, Corrales, Farley, McDermott, & Pflugfelder, 2008). Interaction of IL-1 with TNF-α is vital for pro-inflammatory processes, such as upregulating expression major-histocompatibility molecules (MHC) class II on immature APCs (Hamrah, Liu, Zhang, & Dana, 2003), which is necessary for T-cell antigen presentation (Schaumburg *et al.*, 2011). Furthermore, this interaction increases chemokine production (Choi *et al.*, 2012; Yoon, De Paiva, *et al.*, 2007; Yoon *et al.*, 2010), promotes expression of endothelial adhesion molecules required for chemotaxis of inflammatory infiltrates (Pisella *et al.*, 2000), and production of matrix metalloproteinase (MMP)(D. Q. Li *et al.*, 2001). The MMPs result in breakdown of tight junctions causing ocular surface barrier dysfunction and inflammatory cell infiltration (Chotikavanich *et al.*, 2009).

IL-1 receptor antagonist (IL-1Ra) is a naturally occurring endogenous peptide that inhibits IL-1 activity, and serves to limit IL-1 mediated inflammation and tissue damage (Charles A. Dinarello, 2009). In the normal ocular surface, IL-1Ra is expressed abundantly in normal conjunctival and corneal epithelium (Gamache *et al.*, 1997; Heur, Chaurasia & Wilson, 2009; Kennedy *et al.*, 1995). In inflammatory DED, endogenous IL-1Ra production is elevated on the ocular surface (Dana, 2007; Stapleton *et al.*, 2008). Evaluation of tear protein markers has shown that IL-1Ra in tears of human dry eye patients correlated well with clinical signs and disease severity (corneal staining)(J. F. Huang, Zhang, Rittenhouse, Pickering & McDowell, 2012).

IL-1 blockade can reduce ocular surface barrier dysfunction. In a murine dry eye model, topical IL-1 receptor antagonist significantly reduced corneal fluorescein dye staining, a hallmark clinical finding of DED (Okanobo, Chauhan, Dastjerdi, Kodati, & Dana, 2012). In addition, there was decreased lymphangiogenesis and reduced expression of IL-1β cytokine. Over the central cornea, there was reduced infiltration of innate immune cells (such as neutrophils, monocytes and natural killer cells) as evidenced by significantly decreased CD11b+ leukocyte staining (CD11b is a marker of mononuclear phagocytes).

A recent randomized clinical trial showed that treatment with 2.5% Anankinra three times a day (a recombinant version of human IL-1 receptor antagonist approved for treatment of patients with rheumatoid arthritis) is sufficient in reducing the symptoms of dry eye in patients with refractory DED by 6 weeks. In addition, Anankinra is well tolerated by patients when compared to vehicle control treatment that does not contain active ingredient (Amparo *et al.*, 2013).

Inflammatory cells on the ocular surface, such as neutrophils, monocytes, as well as natural killer cells act in a concerted manner to cause tissue damage, and direct the innate immune response towards a chronic autoimmune inflammatory process driven mainly by adaptive immunity (Barabino *et al.*, 2010; Chan, Amankwah, Robins, Gray, & Dua, 2008; Zhang *et al.*, 2012). The role of the specific innate cell types will be further described.

3.2   Neutrophils and NETs (Neutrophil Extracellular Traps)

Neutrophils are the first line of defense in the innate immune response, and are classically labeled as the hallmark of acute inflammation. In DED, neutrophils are postulated to home in on the ocular surface, where they express cytokines that amplify innate immune responses by other cell types. α-defensins (also known as human neutrophil peptide) are a family of defensin proteins that are produced by neutrophils in response to pro-inflammatory states. It was found to be upregulated in patients with DED, suggestive of neutrophil involvement in the disease (Lo, Wu, Wu, & Shiea, 2010).

In addition to phagocytosis and secreting anti-microbial factors, neutrophils have been found to minimize damage to host cells via formation of an extracellular fiber network that binds pathogens, called neutrophil extracellular traps (NETs)(Brinkmann *et al.*, 2004). The main components of NETs are extracellular DNA, histones and neutrophil elastase. During ocular surface inflammation (such as DED), local reactive oxygen species (ROS) are generated (Tsubota *et al.*, 2012). The ROS may initiate a signaling cascade that leads to disintegration of nuclear and cellular membranes of neutrophils, and consequently the formation of extracellular traps (Wartha & Henriques-Normark, 2008). Since apoptosis has been found in DED (Yeh *et al.*, 2003), it is plausible that NETs exert apoptotic effects on epithelial cells, via cytotoxic extracellular histones and neutrophil elastase (Medina, 2009; Sonawane *et al.*, 2012).

Apoptosis of these cells releases extracellular DNA (eDNA) into the tear film. eDNA is a known DAMP that acts as a stimulus for the innate immune system's non-infectious inflammatory response. In a cohort of patients with severe dry eye, proteomic and genomic assessment of tear film found that neutrophils, NETs and eDNA are increased in tear film of dry eye (Sonawane *et al.*, 2012). Exfoliated cells found in the tear film also had increased eDNA induced signaling and production of inflammatory cytokines.

The tear film contains nucleases (such as lipocalin) (Versura *et al.*, 2010), which have an in vivo function of clearing presence of excess NETs and eDNA from the ocular surface, which suppresses inflammation (Yusifov, Abduragimov, Narsinh, Gasymov, & Glasgow, 2008). However, patients with dry eye have a reduced tear clearance and turnover, resulting in accumulation of NETs and eDNA (Sonawane *et al.*, 2012), causing a state of relative nuclease deficiency.

Dry eye has a compromised epithelial barrier due to destruction of tight junction proteases, but is not an epithelial wound healing disease per se. The clinical correlate to this is the staining of the ocular surface by dyes such as fluorescein. Wound healing is defective in neutrophil depleted mice, suggesting that neutrophils may have potential facilitatory role in the epithelial healing in DED as well. To induce a neutrophil defect, Gr-1 monoclonal antibodies against neutrophils were given to mice intraperitoneally. Subsequently, mechanical injury was induced in the cornea and relatively slower healing was observed by fluorescein staining and imaging (Marrazzo *et al.*, 2011). Although the use of Gr-1 monoclonal antibodies can improve wound healing situations, this may or may not be applicable to dry eye.

3.3   Natural Killer Cells

Natural killer (NK) cells are a subtype of cytotoxic lymphocytes in the innate immune system. They provide rapid response against infections, and direct apoptosis or cell lysis of infected cells. The cytokines associated with NK cell activity are IL-17 and IFN-γ. With acute desiccating stress in a murine model, depletion of NK cells reduces expression of IL-17 and other proinflammatory cytokines (such as IL-6 and IL-23), thus suppressing autoimmune pathogenic T_H17 response and reducing ocular surface epithelial barrier dysfunction (Zhang *et al.*, 2012). In human subjects with DED, there is increased expression of IL-17 mRNA transcripts on the conjunctival surface, which may suggest that IL-17 expressed by NK cells play a role in the pathogenesis of DED (C. S. De Paiva, Chotikavanich, *et al.*, 2009).

NK cells may have a protective or homeostatic role in the ocular surface. In desiccating stress, a reduction of NK cells in turn resulted in a reduction of IL-13, an immunosuppressive effect (C. S. De Paiva, J. K. Raince, *et al.*, 2011). Furthermore, NK cells may have a role in suppressing IFN-γ production, T$_H$17 differentiation and CD4+ T-cell infiltration (C. S. De Paiva, J. K. Raince, *et al.*, 2011; Zhang *et al.*, 2012). Desiccating stress induced a loss of this NK-mediated suppression and treatment with Cyclosporine A restores the role of NK/NKT in the ocular surface (C. S. De Paiva, J. K. Raince, *et al.*, 2011).

Although the details of NK cell involvement in the immunopathogenesis of DED remains to be elucidated, these findings suggest that it may be a potential therapeutic target for future therapy.

3.4   Monocytes

Monocytes are the bone marrow derived precursor cells of APCs. They replenish resident dendritic cells and macrophages on the ocular surface, and can rapidly differentiate to replenish APCs during ongoing inflammation (Kumar & Jack, 2006). The role of the resident APCs will be described in later sections. In DED, there is increased infiltration of monocytes on the ocular surface. Increased staining of cells expressing monocyte cell surface receptors CD11b and CD14 (Barabino *et al.*, 2010; Goyal, Chauhan, Zhang, & Dana, 2009) have been observed in murine experimental dry eye and DED patients. A later section will describe how monocytes bridge the innate and adaptive immune responses (Schaumburg *et al.*, 2011).

4   Tear proteins Involved in Inflammation

Tear proteomic profiling is useful to evaluate lacrimal gland function in relation to autoimmune disease or cellular apoptosis in dry eye-related ocular surface inflammation (Versura *et al.*, 2010). The tear proteome of dry eye patients is altered in comparison to healthy controls. Identification of novel biomarkers linked to disease activity in dry eye is useful in aiding the physician for prognosticating and monitoring of disease progression. Advances of proteomic science have enabled characterization and quantification of tear protein profiles.

4.1   Lactoferrin

Lactoferrin is a multifunctional protein that has antimicrobial activity and forms part of the innate immune defense at mucosal surfaces. It forms the main glycoprotein component of tears (Kawashima *et al.*, 2012), suppresses inflammation, exhibits anti-angiogenic and anti-oxidative properties, and promotes cellular growth and goblet cell differentiation (Baveye, Elass, Mazurier, Spik, & Legrand, 1999; Conneely, 2001; Dogru *et al.*, 2007; Kanyshkova, Buneva, & Nevinsky, 2001; Legrand, Elass, Carpentier, & Mazurier, 2005; Lindmark-Mansson & Akesson, 2000). In the eye, lactoferrin is produced by the lacrimal gland acinar cells (Gillette & Allansmith, 1980).

DED is a disease where components of the lacrimal functional are impaired. Not surprisingly, there is reduced lactoferrin in the tears of DED patients. Tear lactoferrin negatively correlates with severity of ocular surface staining in both primary DED and keratoconjunctivitis sicca secondary to Sjögren syndrome (Danjo, Lee, Horimoto, & Hamano, 1994; Ohashi *et al.*, 2003).

Dietary lactoferrin has been shown to reduce age-related lacrimal gland dysfunction in a murine model (Kawashima *et al.*, 2012). Notably, oral administration of lactoferrin for 1 month has been shown to be beneficial in a randomized controlled treatment trial of kerato-conjunctivitis sicca secondary to Sjögren syndrome. In this study, 10 patients given lactoferrin (270 mg/day) had improved tear film stability and reduced ocular surface epithelial inflammation (Dogru *et al.*, 2007) compared to 7 controls. There were no complications that arose from dietary lactoferrin supplementation. Therefore, dietary lactoferrin could be a viable form of therapy in DED. Although mechanisms underlying the anti-inflammatory properties of lactoferrin in DED are not well characterized, it is likely that this multifunctional protein exerts its effects via stabilizing the mucous tear layer and interfering with production of pro-inflammatory cytokines. Alternatively, the use of recombinant topical lactoferrin in treatment of DED can be a relatively safer therapy (Fujihara, Nagano, Nakamura, & Shirasawa, 1998).

4.2   Mucins in the Tear Film

Mucins, high molecular weight glycoproteins, are the key constituent of the mucous layer of the tear film and are produced by goblet cells and conjunctival epithelial cells. More importantly, mucins play a role in innate barrier defense against desiccating stress to the ocular surface by maintain lubrication and stabilizing both lipid and aqueous components of the tear film (Watanabe, 2002).

Ocular mucins can be classified into secreted (MUC2, MUC5AC, MUC5B, MUC7) or membrane associated (MUC1, MUC4, MUC16) subtypes (Ramamoorthy & Nichols, 2008; Spurr-Michaud, Argueso, & Gipson, 2007). MUC5AC, a gel-forming mucin, is synthesized by the goblet cells of healthy conjunctiva and forms a key component of the pre ocular tear film (Jumblatt, McKenzie, & Jumblatt, 1999). Changes in expression of gel-forming mucins alters viscoelastic properties of mucous and impairs the protective role of tear film (Watanabe, 2002). Loss of mucin barrier exposes ocular epithelium to environmental insult, leading to factors that trigger an immune response.

Certain mucin subtypes are deficient in corresponding dry eye subtypes. MUC5AC is deficient in Sjögren syndrome patients with keratoconjunctivitis sicca (Argueso *et al.*, 2002). An animal model of dry eye based on *Muc5ac* mucin pathology has been reported (Floyd *et al.*, 2012). *Muc5ac* knock-out mice demonstrate increased corneal staining, a clinical feature of DED. Interestingly, there is a compensatory increase in expression of *Muc5b* when compared to wild type mice. However this increase is unable to restore normal ocular surface function, suggesting that not all mucins share the same role and efficacy of protecting the ocular surface from inflammation. What regulates the production of MUC5AC from goblet cells? A novel epithelial factor, Spdef will be covered in the following segment.

4.3   Sterile-α-motif Pointed Domain Eepithelial-specific Transcription Factor

Sterile-α-motif pointed domain epithelial-specific transcription factor (Spdef) encoded for by the *SPDEF* gene, is required for conjunctival goblet cell differentiation (Marko *et al.*, 2013). In addition, Spdef is involved in the differentiation of goblet cells from precursor clara cells in the respiratory epithelia (Chen *et al.*, 2009; Park *et al.*, 2007). It also plays a role in the regulation of intestinal goblet and Paneth cell maturation (Gregorieff *et al.*, 2009). Since Spdef is involved in goblet cell differentiation within pulmonary and intestinal epithelia, it is likely to play a similar homeostatic and regulatory mechanism on the ocular surface.

In patients with dry eye secondary to Sjögren syndrome, there was increased expression of *SPDEF* mRNA expression in the conjunctival epithelia (Marko *et al.*, 2013). Furthermore, in

Spdef knockout (KO) mice, there was reduced production of *Muc5ac* on the ocular surface, which may affect the entire mucous layer (Marko *et al.*, 2013). Spdef KO mice also demonstrated a DED phenotype (increased corneal staining and ocular surface infiltration by pro-inflammatory cytokines IL-1 and TNF-α).

4.4   Transforming Growth Factor-β

Transforming growth factor (TGF)-β1 is produced by the human lacrimal gland, and is found in elevated levels in the ocular surface of patients with Sjögren syndrome-related keratoconjunctivitis sicca (Pflugfelder, Jones, Ji, Afonso, & Monroy, 1999; Zheng, De Paiva, Rao, *et al.*, 2010). *In vivo*, TGF-β is a regulatory molecule of the immune system – it blocks the proliferation of T-lymphocytes and B-lymphocytes, as well as increasing regulatory T-cell (Treg) proliferation and activity (Bettelli, Oukka, & Kuchroo, 2007; Veldhoen, Hocking, Flavell, & Stockinger, 2006; Wan & Flavell, 2007). In general, TGF-ß has a critical effect on induction of T_H effector cells, in particular T_H17(Wan & Flavell, 2007).

In a murine model of Sjögren syndrome, CD25 knockout mice demonstrated destruction of lacrimal gland architecture, with increased levels of TGF-β1 mRNA production (Rahimy *et al.*, 2010). If TGF-β is absent, or its signaling impaired at birth, mice subsequently demonstrated increased T-cell lymphoproliferation with autoimmunity (Dang *et al.*, 1995). Newly born TGF-β1 knockout mice die within 20 days due to significant generalized lymphocytic infiltration (Shull *et al.*, 1992), with extensive CD4+ infiltrates in their lacrimal and salivary glands that mimics the phenotype of keratoconjunctivitis sicca in Sjögren syndrome (McCartney-Francis *et al.*, 1996).Thus, TGF-β has a plausible regulatory role that prevents the progression of autoimmune dry eye disease.

On the other hand, disruption of TGF-β signaling in experimental DED mice improves ocular surface epithelial disease (C. S. De Paiva, E. A. Volpe, *et al.*, 2011). Experimental TGF-β receptor knockout mice subjected to desiccating stress exhibited reduced severity of dry eye phenotype as compared to wild type mice. This was assessed through improved corneal barrier function as observed on ocular surface staining, increased goblet cell density of ocular surface epithelium and reduced CD4+ T-cell infiltration in the conjunctiva. Furthermore, desiccating stress did not induce a T_H1 and T_H17 T-cell response, and there was failure to upregulate production of key cytokines (IL-17, IFN-γ) or matrix metalloproteinases (MMP-9) of inflammatory dry eye in the conjunctiva, thus strongly suggesting that TGF-β signaling is necessary in the progression of DED to involve T-lymphocytes of adaptive immunity.

TGF-ß is physiologically activated by dendritic cell derived thrombospondin-1 (TSP-1). In a murine model with knockout of TSP-1, there was less corneal barrier disruption, reduced loss of goblet cells and decreased T-cell infiltration of the conjunctiva, with no up-regulation of matrix metalloproteinases in the cornea and IL-17 in conjunctiva (Gandhi *et al.*, 2013). Thus TSP-1 could be an upstream target for mediating TGF-ß activity in DED.

4.5   Calgranulin A and B

Calgranulin A (S-100 calcium-binding protein A8) together with its dimerization partner, Calgranulin B (S-100 calcium-binding protein A9), are protein biomarkers that have positive correlation with increased severity of DED (Boehm *et al.*, 2013; L. Tong, Zhou, Beuerman, Zhao, & Li, 2011). These are potential diagnostic markers of DED severity when clinical findings may not correlate well with disease severity.

Calgranulin A and B are members of calcium-regulated cornified envelope proteins, which are involved in innate immunity, barrier function and stress signaling (Eckert *et al.*, 2004). In addition, Calgranulin A and B are found in abundance in neutrophils and are implicated in autoreactive diseases, such as rheumatoid arthritis (Nacken, Roth, Sorg, & Kerkhoff, 2003). Though its mechanism of action in dry eye is still unclear, we postulate that ocular surface neutrophilic infiltrates produce Calgranulin A and B as part of the pro-inflammatory cascade. These proteins are alarmins, which warn the local immune system of an existing insult. As such, these proteins may activate toll like receptors, the main receptors in the innate signaling pathways (Ehrchen, Sunderkotter, Foell, Vogl, & Roth, 2009). Activation of these pathways may correlate with the amount of inflammatory damage.

The actual role of Calgranulin A and B in triggering inflammation in the ocular surface has not been demonstrated so far. The association has however been described in a few ocular surface conditions (Louis Tong, Lan, Lim, & Chaurasia, 2013), and blocking Calgranulin A reduced inflammation in a model of corneal neovascularization (C. Li, Zhang, & Wang, 2010).

4.6 Matrix Metalloproteinases

Matrix metalloproteinases (MMP) are endopeptidases that are involved in degradation of extracellular matrix proteins, and tissue remodeling. In response to hyperosmolar stress, corneal epithelium produces MMP-1, MMP-3, MMP-9 and MMP-13 (D. Q. Li *et al.*, 2004). Cultured human corneal epithelial cells were stimulated *in vitro* by pro-inflammatory cytokines (IL-1β and TNF-α) seen in the acute inflammatory phase of DED to increase production of MMP-9 (D. Q. Li *et al.*, 2001).

Elevated levels of MMP-9 have been identified in the tears of dry eye patients, which correlated well with symptom severity, increased tear break up time and ocular surface staining (Chotikavanich *et al.*, 2009). A commercial test kit has been developed to assess for presence of MMP-9 as an early marker of DED (Kaufman, 2013). Knockout of MMP-9 attenuates the severity of experimental murine dry eye, demonstrating its role the immunopathogenesis of DED (Pflugfelder *et al.*, 2005). Doxycycline, a type of tetracycline antibiotic, has been shown to decrease production of MMP-9 by cultured human corneal epithelial cells (Kim, Luo, Pflugfelder, & Li, 2005; D. Q. Li *et al.*, 2001) and in murine experimental dry eye (Cintia S. De Paiva *et al.*, 2006), thus promoting ocular surface integrity.

5   Bridging Innate and Adaptive Immunity: Antigen Presenting Cells

5.1 Dysregulation of APC self-tolerance

Professional APCs (such as CD11c+ dendritic cells and CD11b+ macrophages) constitutively express human leukocyte antigen (HLA)-DR molecules, and influence T-cells to proliferate into T-effector or T-helper cells. HLA-DR is a MHC class II cell surface receptor involved in antigen presentation to T-cells. Hyperosmolar stress in DED increases the expression of HLA-DR (Versura, Profazio, Schiavi, & Campos, 2011). Both professional APCs as well as non-professional APCs (such as ocular surface epithelial cells and stromal fibroblasts) can upregulate HLA-DR expression and present antigens to T-cells (Ogawa *et al.*, 2003). This can dysregulate the tolerogenic nature of EALT (Mircheff *et al.*, 2005). Ocular surface APCs has been linked to subsequent activation of T-cells in adaptive immunity, and is subsequently described.

5.2   Dendritic Cells

In a murine dry eye model, CD11c+ dendritic cells accumulate within the ocular surface before CD4+ T-cell activation (Zhang *et al.*, 2012), and are localized to regional cervical lymph nodes within 24 hours of experimentally induced dry eye. This suggests that dendritic cells could be the key to T-cell activation within lymphoid tissue (such as lymph nodes) in DED.

A specific subtype of dendritic cell, the plasmacytoid dendritic cell, was initially described as interferon-producing-cells (IPC) before their dendritic cell nature was elucidated (Wildenberg, van Helden-Meeuwsen, van de Merwe, Drexhage, & Versnel, 2008). Circulating plasmacytoid dendritic cells express CD40, which binds to CD40L on T-lymphocytes to activate them. In the serum of patients with primary Sjögren syndrome, increased type 1 IFN-related genes were expressed in systemic monocytes. The expression levels of some of these IFN-related genes (IFI27 and IFITM1) in monocytes correlated to the CD40 expression in the peripheral dendritic cells. Therefore, inflammatory processes are driven not only locally, but also involve a systemic immune alteration.

5.3   Macrophages

Resident macrophages, the local equivalent of monocytes in the eye, are involved in production of chemokines that aid recruitment of inflammatory cells to the ocular surface. Animal models of DED have shown that macrophages produce increased chemokine ligand macrophage inflammatory protein (CCL) 3 and 4 (Yoon, De Paiva, *et al.*, 2007). These chemokines are able to recruit neutrophils and other inflammatory cells (such as lymphocytes) to the ocular surface, and upregulate the production of pro-inflammatory cytokines.

Apart from their role as APCs, macrophages have a synergistic effect with neutrophils to phagocytose cellular debris and produce growth factors and chemokines necessary for angiogenesis, downregulation of inflammation and wound closure (Willoughby, Moore, Colville-Nash, & Gilroy, 2000). In DED, macrophages could plausibly have a role in mediating corneal epithelial wound healing. Depletion of macrophages in mice which have undergone autologous corneal transplant led to impaired wound healing, as evidenced by irregularly distributed extracellular matrix, ingrowing of corneal epithelium into stroma, and even detachment of transplanted cornea (S. Li *et al.*, 2013). The role of macrophages as APCs and ocular surface repair cells needs to be further explored.

6   T-cell Differentiation and Homing in Dry Eye

T-cells have a central role in the immunopathogenesis of chronic dry eye (Zhou *et al.*, 2012). Activated CD4+ T-cells can be found in the ocular surface of DED(Stern et al., 2002), and blockade of T-cell activity decreases severity of DED (Kunert *et al.*, 2000). *In vivo*, the T-helper cell recruits macrophages, and assists B-cells in the production of immunoglobulins.

6.1   Major Histocompatibility Complex Class II

In order for T-cell activation to occur, antigen presentation must first take place. In DED, there is increased expression of cell-associated immunomodulatory molecules involved in antigen presentation. On the ocular surface of dry eyes, the following immunomodulatory molecules are expressed in greater quantity: HLA-DR, co-stimulatory molecules (CD40, CD40L, CD80,

CD86), Fas and FasL (Brignole *et al.*, 2000; Ogawa *et al.*, 2003; Rolando *et al.*, 2005; Tsubota, Fujihara, Saito, & Takeuchi, 1999; Tsubota, Fujita, Tsuzaka, & Takeuchi, 2003; Versura *et al.*, 2011).

HLA-DR is a MHC class II cell surface receptor found on APCs. When APCs have phagocytosed antigens, they process and present them on the cell surface complexed to HLA-DR. The cell surface antigens subsequently bind to the specific T-cell receptors found on naïve T_H0 T-lymphocytes. This APC-Tcell interaction requires co-stimulatory molecules, namely CD40, CD40L, CD80 and CD86 for full activation of the afferent immune response. These co-stimulatory molecules are found to be increased in mononuclear infiltrates and stromal fibroblasts on the ocular surface, which suggests that autoantigen presentation is likely to have occurred in the immunopathogenesis in DED (Ogawa *et al.*, 2003).

Fas is a death receptor that can induce cellular apoptosis when bound to its ligand, FasL. The presence of Fas and FasL on the ocular surface of DED patients suggests that cellular apoptosis has taken place, causing epitheliopathy and ocular surface damage (Tsubota *et al.*, 2003).

6.2 Cytokines and T-cell polarisation

Cytokines are small signaling molecules involved in cell signaling to achieve immunomodulation. These can be produced by APCs and lymphocytes after antigen presentation to T-cells (Boehm, Riechardt, Wiegand, Pfeiffer, & Grus, 2011). Some cytokines cause clonal proliferation of lymphocytes and polarize the development of precursor T-cells towards mature T_H1, T_H2 or T_H17 subtypes (C. A. Dinarello, 2007). Apart from these T-helper cells, naïve T_H0 cells can also differentiate into cytotoxic effector T-cells. Cytotoxicity may target ocular surface tissues to result in damage and release of further antigens to propagate the immune response.

DED typically elicits a T_H1 and T_H17 response (C. S. De Paiva, Chotikavanich, *et al.*, 2009), however the relative contributions of T_H1 and T_H17 cells remain unclear. The maturation of T_H1 cells is driven by IL-12 (Athie-Morales, Smits, Cantrell, & Hilkens, 2004; El Annan *et al.*, 2009), while IL-6 and TGF-β have been shown to promote the differentiation of T_H17 cells (Chauhan *et al.*, 2009). Interestingly, the maturation of T_H1 and T_H17 is not always synchronous, as TGF-β was found to suppress T_H1 mediated responses (Wan & Flavell, 2007). A growing pool of evidence suggests that T_H17 cells feature prominently in the immunopathogenesis of DED (Chauhan *et al.*, 2009; C. S. De Paiva, Chotikavanich, *et al.*, 2009).

6.3 T_H1 Axis

In DED, T_H1 is prominently featured on the ocular surface and is vital to ocular inflammatory processes (El Annan *et al.*, 2009). The most important experiment that suggests immune mediated disease in dry eye is the adoptive transfer of CD4+ effector T-cells in a murine model of dry eye to athymic mice (Niederkorn *et al.*, 2006). Even though recipient mice in adoptive transfer were not exposed to desiccating stress, they demonstrated evidence of ocular surface inflammation after receiving donor T-cells intra-peritoneally from DED mice. Furthermore, inflammation was restricted to the ocular surface and lacrimal gland in recipient mice. These findings suggest that donor mice subjected to desiccating stress had developed CD4+ T-cells that localized to the ocular surface and lacrimal gland, where they caused lacrimal gland dysfunction, goblet cell loss and inflammation.

T_H1 is a well characterized T-cell subset. T_H1 cells produce a cytokine milieu consisting of IFN-γ, IL-2, and TNF-α, which activates macrophages. The macrophages have phagocytic activity, which resulted in further antigen presentation and T_H1 differentiation. This propagates a vicious cycle of T_H1 activation. The next question is: where is the dominant site of antigen presentation? In a similar model of desiccating stress, (scopolamine and controlled environment), T-cells were activated within the draining lymph nodes of mice. CD69 (a transmembrane glycoprotein found on T-lymphocytes, NK cells and platelets) is the earliest cell membrane protein induced during lymphoid activation. CD40L, a marker of activated T-cells described above binds to CD40 on APCs as a co-stimulatory molecule. Both CD69 and CD40L expressing T-cells were found in the draining lymph nodes (El Annan *et al.*, 2009). These T-cells demonstrated a T_H1 cytokine phenotype (increased IFN-γ and IL12Rβ2, but no IL4R expression), and T_H1 chemokine phenotype (expression of CXCR3 and CCR5, but not CCR4).

6.4 T_H17 Axis

T_H17 is a novel T-cell subset that is different from the classically described T_H1 and T_H2 lineages. It is associated with autoimmune conditions, such as autoimmune uveitis and rheumatoid arthritis (Furuzawa-Carballeda, Vargas-Rojas, & Cabral, 2007; Yoshimura *et al.*, 2009). Activated T_H17 cells recruit neutrophils and macrophages, thus worsening inflammation. T_H17 cells also express cytokines IL-17, IL-23 and IFN-γ. The "signature" cytokine of this axis is IL-17 (Harrington *et al.*, 2005). In DED, there is significant increase of IL-17 concentration in the tears and ocular surface, which suggests that T_H17 cells have a role in the pathogenesis of DED.

IL-17 is potentially a novel target in the management of DED. In a murine model, it was found that the cervical lymph nodes contained T_H17 cells (Chauhan *et al.*, 2009; Zhang *et al.*, 2012). Reduced Treg activity unleashes further T_H17 expansion and migration to the ocular surface, which worsens DED. Neutralization of IL-17 *in vivo* resulted in marked decrease in the severity of DED. Taken together, this suggests that IL-17 promotes Treg-mediated suppression of T_H17 activity on the ocular surface.

What mediates the polarization of precursor T-Cells to differentiate into T_H17? It was found that NK cells in the ocular epithelial surface have a key role in promoting T_H17 activity in DED (Zhang *et al.*, 2012). NK cells produce a pro-T_H17 cytokine milleu when ocular surface is exposed to desiccating stress, as evidenced by increased expression of IL-17, IL-6, IL-23 and IFN-γ mRNA transcripts. In a murine model exposed to desiccating stress, depletion of NK cells was associated with less corneal barrier disruption, hallmark morphology of DED. Fewer T_H17 cells were found in the cervical lymph nodes of NK-depleted DED mice. In addition, there was reduced levels of cytokine IL-17, chemokine CCL20 (chemotatic for neutrophils) and MMP3/9.

6.5   Chemokines

Chemokines are type IV cytokines that coordinate the migration of responsive immune cells to sites of inflammation. Hence, chemokines are potential therapeutic targets in DED, as interfering with their activity can reduce recruitment of inflammatory cells to the ocular surface.

Blockade of monocyte chemotaxis to the ocular surface has been shown to improve both clinical and molecular manifestations of inflammatory dry eye. The C-C chemokine receptor type 2 (CCR2) mediates monocyte chemotaxis *in vivo*. Topical application of CCR2 antagonist to murine dry eye resulted in reduction of corneal staining, less infiltrates of monocytic cells and fewer pro-inflammatory cytokines on the ocular surface (Goyal *et al.*, 2009).

The chemotaxis of differentiated T-cells to the diseased tissue is the first step that localizes these cells to the ocular surface. The chemotaxis of T_H1 cells is mediated by CCL3 and CCL4 (Yoon, De Paiva, *et al.*, 2007). In a murine model, it was found that CCL3 and CCL4 were upregulated after desiccating stress was applied, and this corresponded with increased infiltration of ocular inflammatory cells.

In addition, chemotaxis of T_H17 cells is mediated by CCL20 (C. S. De Paiva, Chotikavanich, *et al.*, 2009) and CCR6 (Cintia S. De Paiva *et al.*, 2011). Disruption of CCR6/CCL20 binding with CCL20 neutralizing antibody in a murine dry eye model led to reduced T-cell migration and reduced T_H17 infiltration to the ocular surface, with improvement in clinical signs of DED (Dohlman *et al.*, 2013). Hence, agonists against these chemotatic agents are possible therapeutic targets to regulate chemotaxis of inflammatory cells to ocular surface in DED.

New evidence suggests that programmed-death-ligand 1 (PD-L1) expressed by hematopoietic and parenchymal cells, downregulates T-cell chemotaxis to the cornea in a murine DED model (El Annan *et al.*, 2010). Treatment of mice with anti-PD-L1 blocking antibody is associated with increased expression of chemokines and chemokine receptors for T-cell chemotaxis, as well as increased corneal T-cell infiltrates. In addition, blockade of PD-L1 signaling caused increased severity of DED phenotype as observed with corneal fluorescein staining. Apart from chemotaxis, PD-L1 also has a role in regulating peripheral T-cell tolerance (Keir *et al.*, 2006). Tissue-specific PD-L1 expression protects against corneal allograft rejection and ocular inflammation by inhibition of autoreactive and alloreactive T-cells (Shen, Jin, Freeman, Sharpe, & Dana, 2007; Yang *et al.*, 2009).

6.6   Homing of T-cells

The normal ocular surface is resistant to T-cell homing compared to other tissues in the body (Mott *et al.*, 2007). However, in DED, there is increased infiltration of T-lymphocytes within conjunctival and corneal epithelium (El Annan *et al.*, 2010; Stern *et al.*, 2002), where they exert pathogenic effects on the ocular surface. How do leukocytes home in to the ocular tissues?

First, circulating leukocytes must be slowed down in the capillaries of the inflamed area. The integrin α4β1 (or very late antigen VLA-4) on the leukocyte membranes binds to the vascular cell adhesion molecule VCAM-1 on the vascular endothelium. This is a critical interaction which would subsequently allows transmigration of the leukocyte through the capillary wall to the surrounding matrix of the diseased tissue (Postigo, Teixido, & Sanchez-Madrid, 1993). It has been shown that small molecule antagonists to VLA-4 can decrease the infiltration of T-cells in the conjunctiva in a mouse model of dry eye (Ecoiffier, El Annan, Rashid, Schaumberg, & Dana, 2008).

Lymphocyte diapedesis was also dependent on the interaction of intercellular adhesion molecule (ICAM-1) with integrin lymphocyte function-associated antigen (LFA-1). Experimental evidence for involvement of LFA-1 was from MRL/lpr mice which have systemic autoimmune disease causing ocular and lacrimal gland inflammation (Jabs, Lee, Burek, Saboori, & Prendergast, 1996). Injection of these mice with monoclonal antibodies against ICAM-1 or LFA-1 reduced ocular surface inflammation, evidenced by reduced T-cell activation and infiltration in the lacrimal glands (Gao *et al.*, 2004). Lifitegrast, a synthetic LFA-1 antagonist, has been used clinically to treat dry eye (Sun, Zhang, Gadek, O'Neill, & Pearlman, 2013).

6.7 Lymphangiogenesis

Recent evidence points towards corneal lymphangiogenesis as a key link between DED and adaptive immunity in corneal epithelium. In normal eyes, the conjunctiva is supplied by both blood and lymphatic vessels, whereas the cornea is relatively devoid of blood vessels and lymphatic drainage (Nakao, Hafezi-Moghadam, & Ishibashi, 2012). Desiccating stress in murine DED increased lymphatic vessel growth that is unaccompanied by hemangiogenesis within the cornea. There were significant increases in lymphangiogenic-specific growth factors (VEGF-D and VEGFR-3) six days after desiccating stress (Goyal *et al.*, 2010). Corneal lymphangiogenesis provided a route for APCs to come into contact with ocular antigens and was associated with presence of mature APCs in lymph nodes draining the ocular surface.

7 Regulation of T-cell Immunity

Two important regulatory systems exist in the T-cell mediated immune response.

7.1 Interaction with APC

The first type of regulation requires the role of APCs in CD4+ T-cell activation. APCs play a role in regulating T-cells apart from antigen presentation. This role has been described in a mouse model of autoimmune lacrimal keratoconjunctivitis, which mimics clinical and histopathological features of human dry eye disease (Schaumburg *et al.*, 2011). As mentioned in the mice experiments above, accumulation of mature dendritic cells correlates with CD4+ T-cell activation in cervical lymph nodes after exposure to desiccating stress (DS). APC depletion with liposome-encapsulated clodronate showed decreased levels of infiltrating DS-specific CD4+ T-cell. These results suggest that APC is necessary for the induction of infiltrative DS-specific T-cell response. Adoptive transfer of DS-specific CD4+ T-cells to naïve immunocompromised recipient mice without previous DS results in ocular surface inflammation and dry eye. Importantly, it was shown that the APC is required even in the recipient of this adoptive transfer for propagating the ocular surface inflammation. The damage resulting from adoptive transfer would be attenuated (less CD4+ T-Cell infiltration and more globlet cells retained) in APC depleted recipients. In the recipient mice, it is not known if the APC plays a regulatory role in T-cell homing or in the presentation of antigens released by secondary immunological damage.

7.2 Regulatory T-cells

Regulatory T-cells (Tregs) are T-cells that mediate tolerance against self-antigens and suppress immune responses. On the ocular surface, Tregs maintain a normal phenotype, and suppress immune-mediated inflammation. Abnormalities in Treg are implicated in systemic autoimmune diseases with ocular manifestations, such as Sjögren syndrome, rheumatoid arthritis and systemic lupus erythematosus (Bernard, Romano, & Granel, 2010).

The first type of T-regulatory cells described here are the CD4+CD25+FoxP3+ T-cells. In non-obese diabetic mice with Sjögren syndrome, there was reduced epithelial cell expression of CD25 (alpha chain of the IL-2 receptor) (Yoon *et al.*, 2008). The CD25 expressed on activated T-lymphocytes and B-lymphocytes, thymocytes and myeloid precursors has an immunomodulatory function. In mice with CD25 deletion (C. S. De Paiva *et al.*, 2010), there was increased infiltration of cytotoxic T-Cells (CD4+CD8+) in the conjunctiva and cornea, together with an elaboration of T_H1 and T_H17 cytokines. In vitro expanded CD4+CD25+FoxP3+ Treg cells, when transferred to T-cell deficient nude mice, suppressed ocular surface inflammation (Siemasko et al., 2008). Together, these findings suggest a suppressive role for IL-2R signaling mediated by CD25 on the differentiation of cytotoxic T effector cells.

CD25 can also be secreted into the plasma, resulting in soluble interleukin-2 receptor (sIL-2R). The role of sIL-2R is unclear, but the serum levels were higher in Sjögren syndrome patients, corresponding to a higher percentage of CD25+ lymphocytes, higher SSB (La) antibodies, and higher HLA-DR expression on epithelial cells. In this situation, the increased sIL-2R is an indicator of inflammatory lacrimal glandular involvement rather than suppression of ocular surface inflammation (Spadaro, Riccieri, Benfari, Scillone, & Taccari, 2001).

There is at least another class of Treg cells. Among the CD4+ cytotoxic T-cells with CD8+ expression, those that express the co-stimulatory molecule CD28 are effector T-cells. These interact with the T-cell receptor and the B7-2 (CD86) molecules on APCs. On the other hand, those CD8+ T-cells with no CD28 are Tregs and may have a negative modulatory role on the immune response. After transplantation of mesenchymal stromal cells in dry eye patients with graft versus host disease, there is an increase in the levels of such CD8+CD28-Tregs (Weng et al., 2012). This transplantation also resulted in the improvement of dry eye and higher levels of T_H1 cytokines (IL-2 and IFN-γ). CD8+CD28- Tregs have a role in regulating the balance between T_H1 (macrophage related) and T_H2 (B-cell related) responses.

In addition, CD8+ Treg suppress T_H17 related immune response to desiccating stress of the ocular surface. Depletion of CD8+ Tregs led to increase of IL-17A production by CD4+ T-cells subjected to desiccating stress. Adoptive transfer of CD4+ cells from CD8+ Treg-depleted mice to nude mice led to increased CD4+ T-cell infiltration and elevated IL-17A on the ocular surface with more severe corneal barrier disruption (Zhang et al., 2013).

Other classes of T-cells may play a role in dry eye. T-cells bearing the gamma delta T-cell receptor has been characterized in Sjögren syndrome (Gerli et al., 1993), where they have been found to be increased. These gamma delta T-cells may have a role in B cell help in the synthesis of immunoglobulins. In Sjögren syndrome (Narita et al., 1999), there is also the generation of NKT-cells (cells with intermediate expression of T-cell receptor and high expression of NK1.1) within salivary glands, although the function of these T-cells are still not well known in dry eye.

In T-cell mediated adaptive immunity, another type of regulation is by humoral immune system. Antibodies, secreted by plasma cells from the B-cell lineage are central to humoral immunity. These antibodies bind to circulating antigens (Stern et al., 2012). It has been postulated that DED has an autoimmune etiology, characterized by autoantigens associated with DED on the ocular surface. This will be explored in the next chapter.

8   Autoantigens in Dry Eye

Increasingly, more evidence points towards the etiology of DED being driven by autoantigens. The autoimmune regulator (AIRE) molecule is a transcription factor expressed in the thymus, which enables the body to rid itself of T-cells that are directed against autoantigens. In the absence of AIRE, self-antigens on the ocular surface are recognized by auto-reactive T-cells, which lead to inflammatory responses. This is demonstrated in AIRE knockout (KO) mice, which have ocular characteristics of Sjögren syndrome, such as increased corneal staining, decreased conjunctival globlet cell density and reduced saliva & tear production (Zhou *et al.*, 2012).

If there is an inciting antigen that initiates dry eye, it is not known. Nevertheless, it is hypothesized that the release of normally sequestered autoantigens from the damaged ocular surface as a result of dry eye can propagate further ocular surface inflammation (N. Knop & Knop, 2010). In established disease, it may be impossible to determine the original autoantigens from the secondary antigens.

Autoantigens have been implicated in DED secondary to Sjögren syndrome, a systemic autoimmune disease. Self-reactive antibodies targeting human muscarinic acetylcholine-receptor 3 (anti-m3AChR antibody) was frequently found in majority of Sjögren syndrome patients (Kovacs *et al.*, 2005). Anti-m3AChR antibody also reacted with membrane lacrimal gland acinar cells for Sjögren syndrome-related dry eye (Bacman, Berra, Sterin-Borda, & Borda, 2001), which is suggestive of the presence of autoantigens within lacrimal glands.

Passive transfer of anti-muscarinic IgG antibody was able to block muscarinic function and shown to induce autoimmune exocrine disease seen in Sjögren syndrome. Mice that received anti-muscarinic IgG antibody from Sjögren syndrome patients, unlike those that receive IgG from control patients, developed salivary gland pathology such as xerostomia (Robinson *et al.*, 1998). Furthermore, chronic antagonism of muscarinic acetylcholine-receptor 3 leads to proteolytic packaging of autoantigens into endosomes, where they can be secreted and processed by ocular surface APCs (Rose *et al.*, 2005). Taken together, these findings suggest the importance of autoantibody-autoantigen mediated pathogenesis of dry eye in Sjögren syndrome.

Kallikrein 13 (Klk13) was previously identified as an autoantigen in a murine dry eye model (Figure 3) (Takada, Takiguchi, Konno, & Inaba, 2005). Expression of Klk13 was identified in corneal, conjunctival and lacrimal gland cells after desiccating stress (Stern *et al.*, 2012). Significantly, expression of autoantigen corresponded with the development of autoantibodies specific for Klk13 *in vivo*, which suggests that autoantibodies are involved in the pathogenesis of dry eye. Passive transfer of anti-Klk13 autoantibody to nude mice was sufficient to induce ocular surface inflammation, through mechanisms such as a pro-inflammatory cytokine response (IL-6, IL-12, IL-17, TNF-α and IFN-γ) and increased infiltrates of neutrophils within ocular surface tissue. Goblet cell density was also reduced as a result of passive autoantibody transfer. Complement protein C3b was found within ocular surface tissue of nude mice receiving autoantibody, while complement depletion in nude mice reduced the severity of DED-like inflammation. These strongly suggest that in DED, autoantibodies produced against autoantigens function via activation of complement system, and also through antibody-mediated recruitment of neutrophils (and other innate immune cells). In this situation, the activation of B-cells appears to be T-cell independent, suggesting that B-cells are able to recognize and bind to autoantigen via B-cell receptors.

9   Conclusion

New evidence outlining the role of inflammatory mediators in the immunopathogenesis of DED has opened up new avenues for diagnosis and therapeutic strategies of this multifactorial disease (Table 1). Nevertheless, research in understanding the immunopathogenesis of DED

Immune Processes or Mediators	Inhibitors or Treatment *	Citation
IL-1	IL-1 receptor antagonist (eg: Anankinra)	(Amparo et al., 2013; C. A. Dinarello, 2011; Narayanan et al., 2008; Okanobo et al., 2012)
IL-2	Cyclosporine (0.05% ophthalmic emulsion of cyclosporine) Cyclokat (0.10% ophthalmic emulsion of Cyslosporine, delivered as a positively charged emulsion)	(Kymionis, Bouzoukis, Diakonis, & Siganos, 2008; Yavuz, Bozdag Pehlivan, & Unlu, 2012) (Buggage et al., 2012; Lallemand, Daull, Benita, Buggage, & Garrigue, 2012)
IL-6	IL-6 receptor antagonist (e.g: Tocilizumab)	(Maini et al., 2006; Yoon, Jeong, Park, & Yang, 2007)
IL-12	Anti-IL-12 antibody	(Mannon et al., 2004; Matthys et al., 1998)
IL-17	Anti-IL-17 antibody	(Chauhan et al., 2009; C. S. De Paiva, Chotikavanich, et al., 2009; Zheng, de Paiva, Li, et al., 2010)
TNF-α	Anti-TNF-α monoclonal antibody (e.g: Infliximab) Omega-3 fatty acid / alpha linolenic acid (ALA)	(Z. Li, Choi, Oh, & Yoon, 2012; Yoon, Jeong, et al., 2007) (Babcock, Helton, Hong, & Espat, 2002; Erdinest, Shmueli, Grossman, Ovadia, & Solomon, 2012; N. Li, He, Schwartz, Gjorstrup, & Bazan, 2010; Macri, Giuffrida, Amico, Iester, & Traverso, 2003; Rashid et al., 2008)
LFA-1	Anti-LFA-1 monoclonal antibody (e.g: Odulimomab)	(Gao et al., 2004; Whitcup, Chan, Kozhich, & Magone, 1999)
LFA-1: ICAM-1 interaction	Anti-ICAM-1 receptor antagonist (e.g: Lifitegrast)	(Semba et al., 2011; Sun et al., 2013)
VEGF	Anti-VEGF-A monoclonal antibody (e.g: bevacizumab) Anti-VEGF-C antibody	(Goyal, Chauhan, & Dana, 2012; Goyal et al., 2010)
Matrix Metalloproteinase 9	Doxycycline	(Cintia S. De Paiva et al., 2006; Kim et al., 2005; D. Q. Li et al., 2001)
Mucin Deficiency	Mucin secretagogues (e.g: Rebamipide)	(Kinoshita et al., 2012; Urashima, Okamoto, Takeji, Shinohara, & Fujisawa, 2004)
T-cells	Cyclosporine Tacrolimus	(Kymionis et al., 2008; Yavuz et al., 2012) (Moscovici et al., 2012; Sanz-Marco, Udaondo, Garcia-Delpech, Vazquez, & Diaz-Llopis, 2013)
B-cells	Rituximab	(Meijer et al., 2010)
NK/NKT cells	Cyclosporine A	(C. S. De Paiva, J. K. Raince, et al., 2011)
HLA-DR expression	Gamma-linolenic acid (GLA) and omega-3 (n-3) polyunsaturated fatty acids	(Sheppard et al., 2013)

* Corticosteroids inhibit multiple targets through effects on transcription factors (Comstock & DeCory, 2012).

Table 1: New avenues and therapeutic strategies of controlling inflammation in DED.

has been limited by practical and ethical considerations. Immune studies in humans have been hampered by difficulty in obtaining sufficient numbers of immune cells from the ocular surface, without resorting to ethically objectionable means. Although majority of immunology studies conducted in mice may not be fully applicable to human DED due to differences in immune systems between species, understanding both mechanistic and therapeutic differences will be useful in guiding future research in dry eye treatment (Barabino, 2004). Further research is necessary to elucidate the common and unique immunology in dry eye related to various systemic autoimmune diseases.

In current clinical practice, only cyclosporine eye drops, low dose glucocorticoid eye drops for short duration and oral tetracyclines are routinely used in the management of dry

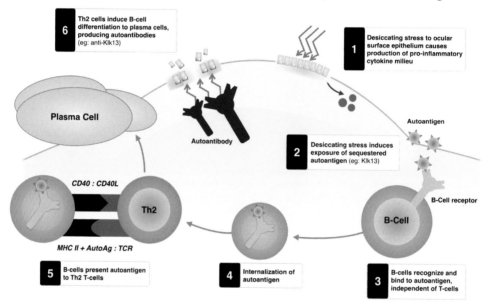

Figure 3: Proposed role of autoreactive B-cells in the immunopathogenesis of DED. Desiccating stress causes the release of autoantigens from damaged ocular surface epithelial tissue. The pro-inflammatory cytokine milieu causes dysregulation of B-cell self-tolerance; B-cells bind to autoantigen, internalize it, and subsequently present autoantigen to T_H2 T-helper cells. B-cell:T_H2 interaction results in B-cell differentiation into plasma cells that produce autoantibodies. Autoantibodies can either cause complement-mediated damage, or recruit immune cells to exert pathogenic effects.

eye ("Management and Therapy of Dry Eye Disease: Report of the Management and Therapy Subcommittee of the International Dry Eye WorkShop (2007)," 2007). A better understanding of the interplay between innate and adaptive immune mediators of inflammatory dry eye is necessary to advance ocular surface science. New therapeutic strategies in animal models hold great promise for newer, safer and more effective treatment modalities in human dry eye.

Acknowledgement

Funding: Grant NMRC/CSA/045/2012 from National Medical Research Council (NMRC), Singapore.

Authors

Readon Teh
Yong Loo Lin School of Medicine, National University of Singapore, Singapore

Louis Tong
Ocular Surface Research Group, Singapore Eye Research Institute, Singapore

References

Amparo, F., Dastjerdi, M. H., Okanobo, A., Ferrari, G., Smaga, L., Hamrah, P., . . . Dana, R. (2013). Topical interleukin 1 receptor antagonist for treatment of dry eye disease: a randomized clinical trial. JAMA Ophthalmol, 131(6), 715-723. doi: 10.1001/jamaophthalmol.2013.195.

Argueso, P., Balaram, M., Spurr-Michaud, S., Keutmann, H. T., Dana, M. R., & Gipson, I. K. (2002). Decreased levels of the goblet cell mucin MUC5AC in tears of patients with Sjogren syndrome. Invest Ophthalmol Vis Sci, 43(4), 1004-1011.

Athie-Morales, V., Smits, H. H., Cantrell, D. A., & Hilkens, C. M. (2004). Sustained IL-12 signaling is required for Th1 development. J Immunol, 172(1), 61-69.

Babcock, T. A., Helton, W. S., Hong, D., & Espat, N. J. (2002). Omega-3 fatty acid lipid emulsion reduces LPS-stimulated macrophage TNF-alpha production. Surg Infect (Larchmt), 3(2), 145-149. doi: 10.1089/109629602760105817.

Bacman, S., Berra, A., Sterin-Borda, L., & Borda, E. (2001). Muscarinic acetylcholine receptor antibodies as a new marker of dry eye Sjogren syndrome. Invest Ophthalmol Vis Sci, 42(2), 321-327.

Barabino, S. (2004). Animal Models of Dry Eye: A Critical Assessment of Opportunities and Limitations. Invest Ophthalmol Vis Sci, 45(6), 1641-1646. doi: 10.1167/iovs.03-1055.

Barabino, S., Montaldo, E., Solignani, F., Valente, C., Mingari, M. C., & Rolando, M. (2010). Immune response in the conjunctival epithelium of patients with dry eye. Exp Eye Res, 91(4), 524-529. doi: 10.1016/j.exer.2010.07.008.

Baveye, S., Elass, E., Mazurier, J., Spik, G., & Legrand, D. (1999). Lactoferrin: a multifunctional glycoprotein involved in the modulation of the inflammatory process. Clin Chem Lab Med, 37(3), 281-286. doi: 10.1515/cclm.1999.049.

Bernard, F., Romano, A., & Granel, B. (2010). [Regulatory T cells and systemic autoimmune diseases: systemic lupus erythematosus, rheumatoid arthritis, primary Sjogren's syndrome]. Rev Med Interne, 31(2), 116-127. doi: 10.1016/j.revmed.2009.03.364.

Bettelli, E., Oukka, M., & Kuchroo, V. K. (2007). T(H)-17 cells in the circle of immunity and autoimmunity. Nat Immunol, 8(4), 345-350. doi: 10.1038/ni0407-345.

Boehm, N., Funke, S., Wiegand, M., Wehrwein, N., Pfeiffer, N., & Grus, F. H. (2013). Alterations in the tear proteome of dry eye patients--a matter of the clinical phenotype. Invest Ophthalmol Vis Sci, 54(3), 2385-2392. doi: 10.1167/iovs.11-8751.

Boehm, N., Riechardt, A. I., Wiegand, M., Pfeiffer, N., & Grus, F. H. (2011). Proinflammatory cytokine profiling of tears from dry eye patients by means of antibody microarrays. Invest Ophthalmol Vis Sci, 52(10), 7725-7730. doi: 10.1167/iovs.11-7266.

Brignole, F., Pisella, P. J., Goldschild, M., De Saint Jean, M., Goguel, A., & Baudouin, C. (2000). Flow cytometric analysis of inflammatory markers in conjunctival epithelial cells of patients with dry eyes. Invest Ophthalmol Vis Sci, 41(6), 1356-1363.

Brinkmann, V., Reichard, U., Goosmann, C., Fauler, B., Uhlemann, Y., Weiss, D. S., . . . Zychlinsky, A. (2004). Neutrophil extracellular traps kill bacteria. Science, 303(5663), 1532-1535. doi: 10.1126/science.1092385.

Buggage, R. R., Amrane, M., Ismail, D., Lemp, M. A., Leonardi, A., & Baudouin, C. (2012). THE EFFECT OF CYCLOKAT® (UNPRESERVED 0.1% CYCLOSPORINE CATIONIC EMULSION) ON CORNEAL INVOLVEMENT IN PATIENTS WITH MODERATE TO SEVERE DRY EYE DISEASE PARTICIPATING IN A PHASE III, MULTICENTER, RANDOMIZED, CONTROLLED, DOUBLE-MASKED, CLINICAL TRIAL. Invest Ophthalmol Vis Sci, 53(E-Abstract 576).

Chan, J. H., Amankwah, R., Robins, R. A., Gray, T., & Dua, H. S. (2008). Kinetics of immune cell migration at the human ocular surface. Br J Ophthalmol, 92(7), 970-975. doi: 10.1136/bjo.2007.131003.

Chauhan, S. K., El Annan, J., Ecoiffier, T., Goyal, S., Zhang, Q., Saban, D. R., & Dana, R. (2009). Autoimmunity in dry eye is due to resistance of Th17 to Treg suppression. J Immunol, 182(3), 1247-1252.

Chen, G., Korfhagen, T. R., Xu, Y., Kitzmiller, J., Wert, S. E., Maeda, Y., . . . Whitsett, J. A. (2009). SPDEF is required for mouse pulmonary goblet cell differentiation and regulates a network of genes associated with mucus production. J Clin Invest, 119(10), 2914-2924. doi: 10.1172/jci39731.

Choi, W., Li, Z., Oh, H. J., Im, S. K., Lee, S. H., Park, S. H., . . . Yoon, K. C. (2012). Expression of CCR5 and its ligands CCL3, -4, and -5 in the tear film and ocular surface of patients with dry eye disease. Curr Eye Res, 37(1), 12-17. doi: 10.3109/02713683.2011.622852.

Chotikavanich, S., de Paiva, C. S., Li de, Q., Chen, J. J., Bian, F., Farley, W. J., & Pflugfelder, S. C. (2009). Production and activity of matrix metalloproteinase-9 on the ocular surface increase in dysfunctional tear syndrome. Invest Ophthalmol Vis Sci, 50(7), 3203-3209. doi: 10.1167/iovs.08-2476.

Comstock, T. L., & DeCory, H. H. (2012). Advances in Corticosteroid Therapy for Ocular Inflammation: Loteprednol Etabonate. International Journal of Inflammation, 2012. doi: 10.1155/2012/789623.

Conneely, O. M. (2001). Antiinflammatory activities of lactoferrin. J Am Coll Nutr, 20(5 Suppl), 389S-395S; discussion 396S-397S.

Corrales, R. M., Stern, M. E., De Paiva, C. S., Welch, J., Li, D. Q., & Pflugfelder, S. C. (2006). Desiccating stress stimulates expression of matrix metalloproteinases by the corneal epithelium. Invest Ophthalmol Vis Sci, 47(8), 3293-3302. doi: 10.1167/iovs.05-1382.

Dana, R. (2007). Comparison of topical interleukin-1 vs tumor necrosis factor-alpha blockade with corticosteroid therapy on murine corneal inflammation, neovascularization, and transplant survival (an American Ophthalmological Society thesis). Trans Am Ophthalmol Soc, 105, 330-343.

Dang, H., Geiser, A. G., Letterio, J. J., Nakabayashi, T., Kong, L., Fernandes, G., & Talal, N. (1995). SLE-like autoantibodies and Sjogren's syndrome-like lymphoproliferation in TGF-beta knockout mice. J Immunol, 155(6), 3205-3212.

Danjo, Y., Lee, M., Horimoto, K., & Hamano, T. (1994). Ocular surface damage and tear lactoferrin in dry eye syndrome. Acta Ophthalmol (Copenh), 72(4), 433-437.

De Paiva, C. S., Chotikavanich, S., Pangelinan, S. B., Pitcher, J. D., 3rd, Fang, B., Zheng, X., . . . Pflugfelder, S. C. (2009). IL-17 disrupts corneal barrier following desiccating stress. Mucosal Immunol, 2(3), 243-253. doi: 10.1038/mi.2009.5.

De Paiva, C. S., Corrales, R. M., Villarreal, A. L., Farley, W. J., Li, D.-Q., Stern, M. E., & Pflugfelder, S. C. (2006). Corticosteroid and doxycycline suppress MMP-9 and inflammatory cytokine expression, MAPK activation in the corneal epithelium in experimental dry eye. Experimental Eye Research, 83(3), 526-535. doi: http://dx.doi.org/10.1016/j.exer.2006.02.004.

De Paiva, C. S., Hwang, C. S., Pitcher, J. D., 3rd, Pangelinan, S. B., Rahimy, E., Chen, W., . . . Pflugfelder, S. C. (2010). Age-related T-cell cytokine profile parallels corneal disease severity in Sjogren's syndrome-like keratoconjunctivitis sicca in CD25KO mice. Rheumatology (Oxford), 49(2), 246-258. doi: 10.1093/rheumatology/kep357.

De Paiva, C. S., Pangelinan, S. B., Chang, E., Yoon, K. C., Farley, W. J., Li, D. Q., & Pflugfelder, S. C. (2009). Essential role for c-Jun N-terminal kinase 2 in corneal epithelial response to desiccating stress. ARCH OPHTHALMOL, 127(12), 1625-1631. doi: 10.1001/archophthalmol.2009.316.

De Paiva, C. S., Raince, J. K., McClellan, A. J., Shanmugam, K. P., Pangelinan, S. B., Volpe, E. A., . . . Pflugfelder, S. C. (2011). Homeostatic control of conjunctival mucosal goblet cells by NKT-derived IL-13. Mucosal Immunol, 4(4), 397-408. doi: 10.1038/mi.2010.82.

De Paiva, C. S., Volpe, E. A., Gandhi, N. B., Zhang, X., Zheng, X., Pitcher, J. D., 3rd, . . . Pflugfelder, S. C. (2011). Disruption of TGF-beta signaling improves ocular surface epithelial disease in experimental autoimmune keratoconjunctivitis sicca. PLoS One, 6(12), e29017. doi: 10.1371/journal.pone.0029017.

De Paiva, C. S., Volpe, E. A., Gandhi, N. B., Zhang, X., Zheng, X., Pitcher, J. D., III, . . . Pflugfelder, S. C. (2011). Disruption of TGF-β Signaling Improves Ocular Surface Epithelial Disease in Experimental Autoimmune Keratoconjunctivitis Sicca. PLoS One, 6(12), e29017. doi: 10.1371/journal.pone.0029017.

Dinarello, C. A. (2007). Historical insights into cytokines. Eur J Immunol, 37 Suppl 1, S34-45. doi: 10.1002/eji.200737772.

Dinarello, C. A. (2009). Interleukin-1β and the Autoinflammatory Diseases. New England Journal of Medicine, 360(23), 2467-2470. doi: doi:10.1056/NEJMe0811014.

Dinarello, C. A. (2011). Interleukin-1 in the pathogenesis and treatment of inflammatory diseases. Blood, 117(14), 3720-3732. doi: 10.1182/blood-2010-07-273417.

Dogru, M., Matsumoto, Y., Yamamoto, Y., Goto, E., Saiki, M., Shimazaki, J., . . . Tsubota, K. (2007). Lactoferrin in Sjogren's syndrome. Ophthalmology, 114(12), 2366-2367. doi: 10.1016/j.ophtha.2007.06.027.

Dohlman, T. H., Chauhan, S. K., Kodati, S., Hua, J., Chen, Y., Omoto, M., . . . Dana, R. (2013). The CCR6/CCL20 axis mediates Th17 cell migration to the ocular surface in dry eye disease. Invest Ophthalmol Vis Sci, 54(6), 4081-4091. doi: 10.1167/iovs.12-11216.

Dursun, D., Wang, M., Monroy, D., Li, D. Q., Lokeshwar, B. L., Stern, M. E., & Pflugfelder, S. C. (2002). A mouse model of keratoconjunctivitis sicca. Invest Ophthalmol Vis Sci, 43(3), 632-638.

Eckert, R. L., Broome, A. M., Ruse, M., Robinson, N., Ryan, D., & Lee, K. (2004). S100 proteins in the epidermis. J Invest Dermatol, 123(1), 23-33. doi: 10.1111/j.0022-202X.2004.22719.x

Ecoiffier, T., El Annan, J., Rashid, S., Schaumberg, D., & Dana, R. (2008). Modulation of integrin alpha4beta1 (VLA-4) in dry eye disease. ARCH OPHTHALMOL, 126(12), 1695-1699. doi: 10.1001/archopht.126.12.1695.

Ehrchen, J. M., Sunderkotter, C., Foell, D., Vogl, T., & Roth, J. (2009). The endogenous Toll-like receptor 4 agonist S100A8/S100A9 (calprotectin) as innate amplifier of infection, autoimmunity, and cancer. J Leukoc Biol, 86(3), 557-566. doi: 10.1189/jlb.1008647.

El Annan, J., Chauhan, S. K., Ecoiffier, T., Zhang, Q., Saban, D. R., & Dana, R. (2009). Characterization of effector T cells in dry eye disease. Invest Ophthalmol Vis Sci, 50(8), 3802-3807. doi: 10.1167/iovs.08-2417.

El Annan, J., Goyal, S., Zhang, Q., Freeman, G. J., Sharpe, A. H., & Dana, R. (2010). Regulation of T-cell chemotaxis by programmed death-ligand 1 (PD-L1) in dry eye-associated corneal inflammation. Invest Ophthalmol Vis Sci, 51(7), 3418-3423. doi: 10.1167/iovs.09-3684.

Erdinest, N., Shmueli, O., Grossman, Y., Ovadia, H., & Solomon, A. (2012). Anti-inflammatory effects of alpha linolenic acid on human corneal epithelial cells. Invest Ophthalmol Vis Sci, 53(8), 4396-4406. doi: 10.1167/iovs.12-9724.

Floyd, A. M., Zhou, X., Evans, C., Rompala, O. J., Zhu, L., Wang, M., & Chen, Y. (2012). Mucin deficiency causes functional and structural changes of the ocular surface. PLoS One, 7(12), e50704. doi: 10.1371/journal.pone.0050704.

Fujihara, T., Nagano, T., Nakamura, M., & Shirasawa, E. (1998). Lactoferrin suppresses loss of corneal epithelial integrity in a rabbit short-term dry eye model. J Ocul Pharmacol Ther, 14(2), 99-107.

Furuzawa-Carballeda, J., Vargas-Rojas, M. I., & Cabral, A. R. (2007). Autoimmune inflammation from the Th17 perspective. Autoimmunity Reviews, 6(3), 169-175.

Gamache, D. A., Dimitrijevich, S. D., Weimer, L. K., Lang, L. S., Spellman, J. M., Graff, G., & Yanni, J. M. (1997). Secretion of proinflammatory cytokines by human conjunctival epithelial cells. Ocul Immunol Inflamm, 5(2), 117-128.

Gandhi, N. B., Su, Z., Zhang, X., Volpe, E. A., Pelegrino, F. S., Rahman, S. A., . . . de Paiva, C. S. (2013). Dendritic cell-derived thrombospondin-1 is critical for the generation of the ocular surface Th17 response to desiccating stress. J Leukoc Biol. doi: 10.1189/jlb.1012524.

Gao, J., Morgan, G., Tieu, D., Schwalb, T. A., Luo, J. Y., Wheeler, L. A., & Stern, M. E. (2004). ICAM-1 expression predisposes ocular tissues to immune-based inflammation in dry eye patients and Sjogrens syndrome-like MRL/lpr mice. Exp Eye Res, 78(4), 823-835. doi: 10.1016/j.exer.2003.10.024.

Gerli, R., Agea, E., Muscat, C., Bertotto, A., Ercolani, R., Bistoni, O., . . . Venanzi, F. (1993). Functional characterization of T cells bearing the gamma/delta T-cell receptor in patients with primary Sjogren's syndrome. Clin Exp Rheumatol, 11(3), 295-299.

Gillette, T. E., & Allansmith, M. R. (1980). Lactoferrin in human ocular tissues. Am J Ophthalmol, 90(1), 30-37.

Goyal, S., Chauhan, S. K., & Dana, R. (2012). Blockade of prolymphangiogenic vascular endothelial growth factor C in dry eye disease. ARCH OPHTHALMOL, 130(1), 84-89. doi: 10.1001/archophthalmol.2011.266.

Goyal, S., Chauhan, S. K., El Annan, J., Nallasamy, N., Zhang, Q., & Dana, R. (2010). Evidence of corneal lymphangiogenesis in dry eye disease: a potential link to adaptive immunity? ARCH OPHTHALMOL, 128(7), 819-824. doi: 10.1001/archophthalmol.2010.124.

Goyal, S., Chauhan, S. K., Zhang, Q., & Dana, R. (2009). Amelioration of murine dry eye disease by topical antagonist to chemokine receptor 2. ARCH OPHTHALMOL, 127(7), 882-887. doi: 10.1001/archophthalmol.2009.125.

Gregorieff, A., Stange, D. E., Kujala, P., Begthel, H., van den Born, M., Korving, J., . . . Clevers, H. (2009). The ets-domain transcription factor Spdef promotes maturation of goblet and paneth cells in the intestinal epithelium. Gastroenterology, 137(4), 1333-1345 e1331-1333. doi: 10.1053/j.gastro.2009.06.044.

Hamrah, P., Liu, Y., Zhang, Q., & Dana, M. R. (2003). Alterations in corneal stromal dendritic cell phenotype and distribution in inflammation. ARCH OPHTHALMOL, 121(8), 1132-1140. doi: 10.1001/archopht.121.8.1132.

Harrington, L. E., Hatton, R. D., Mangan, P. R., Turner, H., Murphy, T. L., Murphy, K. M., & Weaver, C. T. (2005). Interleukin 17-producing CD4+ effector T cells develop via a lineage distinct from the T helper type 1 and 2 lineages. Nat Immunol, 6(11), 1123-1132. doi: 10.1038/ni1254.

Heur, M., Chaurasia, S. S., & Wilson, S. E. (2009). Expression of interleukin-1 receptor antagonist in human cornea. Exp Eye Res, 88(5), 992-994. doi: 10.1016/j.exer.2008.11.019.

Huang, J. F., Zhang, Y., Rittenhouse, K. D., Pickering, E. H., & McDowell, M. T. (2012). Evaluations of tear protein markers in dry eye disease: repeatability of measurement and correlation with disease. Invest Ophthalmol Vis Sci, 53(8), 4556-4564. doi: 10.1167/iovs.11-9054.

Huang, L. C., Jean, D., & McDermott, A. M. (2005). Effect of preservative-free artificial tears on the antimicrobial activity of human beta-defensin-2 and cathelicidin LL-37 in vitro. Eye Contact Lens, 31(1), 34-38.

Jabs, D. A., Lee, B., Burek, C. L., Saboori, A. M., & Prendergast, R. A. (1996). Cyclosporine therapy suppresses ocular and lacrimal gland disease in MRL/Mp-lpr/lpr mice. Invest Ophthalmol Vis Sci, 37(2), 377-383.

Jumblatt, M. M., McKenzie, R. W., & Jumblatt, J. E. (1999). MUC5AC mucin is a component of the human precorneal tear film. Invest Ophthalmol Vis Sci, 40(1), 43-49.

Kanyshkova, T. G., Buneva, V. N., & Nevinsky, G. A. (2001). Lactoferrin and its biological functions. Biochemistry (Mosc), 66(1), 1-7.

Kaufman, H. E. (2013). The practical detection of mmp-9 diagnoses ocular surface disease and may help prevent its complications. Cornea, 32(2), 211-216. doi: 10.1097/ICO.0b013e3182541e9a.

Kawashima, M., Kawakita, T., Inaba, T., Okada, N., Ito, M., Shimmura, S., . . . Tsubota, K. (2012). Dietary Lactoferrin Alleviates Age-Related Lacrimal Gland Dysfunction in Mice. PLoS One, 7(3), e33148. doi: 10.1371/journal.pone.0033148.

Keir, M. E., Liang, S. C., Guleria, I., Latchman, Y. E., Qipo, A., Albacker, L. A., . . . Sharpe, A. H. (2006). Tissue expression of PD-L1 mediates peripheral T cell tolerance. J Exp Med, 203(4), 883-895. doi: 10.1084/jem.20051776.

Kennedy, M. C., Rosenbaum, J. T., Brown, J., Planck, S. R., Huang, X., Armstrong, C. A., & Ansel, J. C. (1995). Novel production of interleukin-1 receptor antagonist peptides in normal human cornea. J Clin Invest, 95(1), 82-88. doi: 10.1172/jci117679.

Kim, H. S., Luo, L., Pflugfelder, S. C., & Li, D. Q. (2005). Doxycycline inhibits TGF-beta1-induced MMP-9 via Smad and MAPK pathways in human corneal epithelial cells. Invest Ophthalmol Vis Sci, 46(3), 840-848. doi: 10.1167/iovs.04-0929.

Kinoshita, S., Awamura, S., Oshiden, K., Nakamichi, N., Suzuki, H., & Yokoi, N. (2012). Rebamipide (OPC-12759) in the treatment of dry eye: a randomized, double-masked, multicenter, placebo-controlled phase II study. Ophthalmology, 119(12), 2471-2478. doi: 10.1016/j.ophtha.2012.06.052.

Knop, E., & Knop, N. (2005). Influence of the Eye-associated Lymphoid Tissue (EALT) on Inflammatory Ocular Surface Disease. The Ocular Surface, 3(4), S-180-S-186. doi: 10.1016/s1542-0124(12)70251-3.

Knop, N., & Knop, E. (2010). Regulation of the inflammatory component in chronic dry eye disease by the eye-associated lymphoid tissue (EALT). Dev Ophthalmol, 45, 23-39. doi: 10.1159/000315017.

Kovacs, L., Marczinovits, I., Gyorgy, A., Toth, G. K., Dorgai, L., Pal, J., . . . Pokorny, G. (2005). Clinical associations of autoantibodies to human muscarinic acetylcholine receptor 3(213-228) in primary Sjogren's syndrome. Rheumatology (Oxford), 44(8), 1021-1025. doi: 10.1093/rheumatology/keh672.

Kumar, S., & Jack, R. (2006). Invited review: Origin of monocytes and their differentiation to macrophages and dendritic cells. Journal of Endotoxin Research, 12(5), 278-284. doi: 10.1177/09680519060120050301.

Kunert, K. S., Tisdale, A. S., Stern, M. E., Smith, J. A., & Gipson, I. K. (2000). Analysis of topical cyclosporine treatment of patients with dry eye syndrome: effect on conjunctival lymphocytes. ARCH OPHTHALMOL, 118(11), 1489-1496.

Kymionis, G. D., Bouzoukis, D. I., Diakonis, V. F., & Siganos, C. (2008). Treatment of chronic dry eye: focus on cyclosporine. Clin Ophthalmol, 2(4), 829-836.

Lallemand, F., Daull, P., Benita, S., Buggage, R., & Garrigue, J. S. (2012). Successfully improving ocular drug delivery using the cationic nanoemulsion, novasorb. J Drug Deliv, 2012, 604204. doi: 10.1155/2012/604204.

Lam, H., Bleiden, L., de Paiva, C. S., Farley, W., Stern, M. E., & Pflugfelder, S. C. (2009). Tear cytokine profiles in dysfunctional tear syndrome. Am J Ophthalmol, 147(2), 198-205 e191. doi: 10.1016/j.ajo.2008.08.032.

Legrand, D., Elass, E., Carpentier, M., & Mazurier, J. (2005). Lactoferrin: a modulator of immune and inflammatory responses. Cell Mol Life Sci, 62(22), 2549-2559. doi: 10.1007/s00018-005-5370-2.

Li, C., Zhang, F., & Wang, Y. (2010). S100A proteins in the pathogenesis of experimental corneal neovascularization. Mol Vis, 16, 2225-2235.

Li, D. Q., Chen, Z., Song, X. J., Luo, L., & Pflugfelder, S. C. (2004). Stimulation of matrix metalloproteinases by hyperosmolarity via a JNK pathway in human corneal epithelial cells. Invest Ophthalmol Vis Sci, 45(12), 4302-4311. doi: 10.1167/iovs.04-0299.

Li, D. Q., Lokeshwar, B. L., Solomon, A., Monroy, D., Ji, Z., & Pflugfelder, S. C. (2001). Regulation of MMP-9 production by human corneal epithelial cells. Exp Eye Res, 73(4), 449-459. doi: 10.1006/exer.2001.1054.

Li, D. Q., Luo, L., Chen, Z., Kim, H. S., Song, X. J., & Pflugfelder, S. C. (2006). JNK and ERK MAP kinases mediate induction of IL-1beta, TNF-alpha and IL-8 following hyperosmolar stress in human limbal epithelial cells. Exp Eye Res, 82(4), 588-596. doi: 10.1016/j.exer.2005.08.019.

Li, N., He, J., Schwartz, C. E., Gjorstrup, P., & Bazan, H. E. (2010). Resolvin E1 improves tear production and decreases inflammation in a dry eye mouse model. J Ocul Pharmacol Ther, 26(5), 431-439. doi: 10.1089/jop.2010.0019.

Li, S., Li, B., Jiang, H., Wang, Y., Qu, M., Duan, H., . . . Shi, W. (2013). Macrophage Depletion Impairs Corneal Wound Healing after Autologous Transplantation in Mice. PLoS One, 8(4), e61799. doi: 10.1371/journal.pone.0061799.

Li, Z., Choi, W., Oh, H. J., & Yoon, K. C. (2012). Effectiveness of topical infliximab in a mouse model of experimental dry eye. Cornea, 31 Suppl 1, S25-31. doi: 10.1097/ICO.0b013e31826a80ea

Lindmark-Mansson, H., & Akesson, B. (2000). Antioxidative factors in milk. Br J Nutr, 84 Suppl 1, S103-110.

Liu, H., Begley, C., Chen, M., Bradley, A., Bonanno, J., McNamara, N. A., . . . Simpson, T. (2009). A Link between Tear Instability and Hyperosmolarity in Dry Eye. Invest Ophthalmol Vis Sci, 50(8), 3671-3679. doi: 10.1167/iovs.08-2689.

Lo, L.-H., Wu, P.-C., Wu, Y.-C., & Shiea, J. (2010). Characterization of human neutrophil peptides ([small alpha]-Defensins) in the tears of dry eye patients. Analytical Methods, 2(12), 1934-1940. doi: 10.1039/C0AY00243G.

Luo, L., Li, D. Q., Corrales, R. M., & Pflugfelder, S. C. (2005). Hyperosmolar saline is a proinflammatory stress on the mouse ocular surface. Eye Contact Lens, 31(5), 186-193.

Luo, L., Li, D. Q., Doshi, A., Farley, W., Corrales, R. M., & Pflugfelder, S. C. (2004). Experimental dry eye stimulates production of inflammatory cytokines and MMP-9 and activates MAPK signaling pathways on the ocular surface. Invest Ophthalmol Vis Sci, 45(12), 4293-4301. doi: 10.1167/iovs.03-1145.

Macri, A., Giuffrida, S., Amico, V., Iester, M., & Traverso, C. E. (2003). Effect of linoleic acid and gamma-linolenic acid on tear production, tear clearance and on the ocular surface after photorefractive keratectomy. Graefes Arch Clin Exp Ophthalmol, 241(7), 561-566. doi: 10.1007/s00417-003-0685-x

Maini, R. N., Taylor, P. C., Szechinski, J., Pavelka, K., Broll, J., Balint, G., . . . Kishimoto, T. (2006). Double-blind randomized controlled clinical trial of the interleukin-6 receptor antagonist, tocilizumab, in European patients with rheumatoid arthritis who had an incomplete response to methotrexate. Arthritis Rheum, 54(9), 2817-2829. doi: 10.1002/art.22033.

Management and Therapy of Dry Eye Disease: Report of the Management and Therapy Subcommittee of the International Dry Eye WorkShop (2007). (2007). The Ocular Surface, 5(2), 163-178.

Mannon, P. J., Fuss, I. J., Mayer, L., Elson, C. O., Sandborn, W. J., Present, D., . . . Strober, W. (2004). Anti-interleukin-12 antibody for active Crohn's disease. N Engl J Med, 351(20), 2069-2079. doi: 10.1056/NEJMoa033402.

Marko, C. K., Menon, B. B., Chen, G., Whitsett, J. A., Clevers, H., & Gipson, I. K. (2013). Spdef null mice lack conjunctival goblet cells and provide a model of dry eye. Am J Pathol, 183(1), 35-48. doi: 10.1016/j.ajpath.2013.03.017.

Marrazzo, G., Bellner, L., Halilovic, A., Li Volti, G., Drago, F., Dunn, M. W., & Schwartzman, M. L. (2011). The Role of Neutrophils in Corneal Wound Healing in HO-2 Null Mice. PLoS One, 6(6), e21180. doi: 10.1371/journal.pone.0021180.

Matthys, P., Vermeire, K., Mitera, T., Heremans, H., Huang, S., & Billiau, A. (1998). Anti-IL-12 antibody prevents the development and progression of collagen-induced arthritis in IFN-gamma receptor-deficient mice. Eur J Immunol, 28(7), 2143-2151. doi: 10.1002/(sici)1521-4141(199807)28:07<2143::aid-immu2143>3.0.co;2-c

McCallum, R. M., Cobo, L. M., & Haynes, B. F. (1993). Analysis of corneal and conjunctival microenvironments using monoclonal antibodies. Invest Ophthalmol Vis Sci, 34(5), 1793-1803.

McCartney-Francis, N. L., Mizel, D. E., Redman, R. S., Frazier-Jessen, M., Panek, R. B., Kulkarni, A. B., . . . Wahl, S. M. (1996). Autoimmune Sjogren's-like lesions in salivary glands of TGF-beta1-deficient mice are inhibited by adhesion-blocking peptides. J Immunol, 157(3), 1306-1312.

McDermott, A. M., Perez, V., Huang, A. J., Pflugfelder, S. C., Stern, M. E., Baudouin, C., . . . Kurie, E. (2005). Pathways of corneal and ocular surface inflammation: a perspective from the cullen symposium. Ocul Surf, 3(4 Suppl), S131-138.

Medina, E. (2009). Neutrophil extracellular traps: a strategic tactic to defeat pathogens with potential consequences for the host. J Innate Immun, 1(3), 176-180. doi: 10.1159/000203699.

Meijer, J. M., Meiners, P. M., Vissink, A., Spijkervet, F. K. L., Abdulahad, W., Kamminga, N., . . . Bootsma, H. (2010). Effectiveness of rituximab treatment in primary Sjögren's syndrome: A randomized, double-blind, placebo-controlled trial. Arthritis & Rheumatism, 62(4), 960-968. doi: 10.1002/art.27314.

Mircheff, A. K., Wang, Y., Jean Mde, S., Ding, C., Trousdale, M. D., Hamm-Alvarez, S. F., & Schechter, J. E. (2005). Mucosal immunity and self-tolerance in the ocular surface system. Ocul Surf, 3(4), 182-192.

Moscovici, B. K., Holzchuh, R., Chiacchio, B. B., Santo, R. M., Shimazaki, J., & Hida, R. Y. (2012). Clinical treatment of dry eye using 0.03% tacrolimus eye drops. Cornea, 31(8), 945-949. doi: 10.1097/ICO.0b013e31823f8c9b.

Moss, S. E., Klein, R., & Klein, B. E. (2000). Prevalence of and risk factors for dry eye syndrome. ARCH OPHTHALMOL, 118(9), 1264-1268.

Mott, K. R., Osorio, Y., Brown, D. J., Morishige, N., Wahlert, A., Jester, J. V., & Ghiasi, H. (2007). The corneas of naive mice contain both CD4+ and CD8+ T cells. Mol Vis, 13, 1802-1812.

Nacken, W., Roth, J., Sorg, C., & Kerkhoff, C. (2003). S100A9/S100A8: Myeloid representatives of the S100 protein family as prominent players in innate immunity. Microsc Res Tech, 60(6), 569-580. doi: 10.1002/jemt.10299.

Nakao, S., Hafezi-Moghadam, A., & Ishibashi, T. (2012). Lymphatics and lymphangiogenesis in the eye. J Ophthalmol, 2012, 783163. doi: 10.1155/2012/783163.

Narayanan, S., Corrales, R. M., Farley, W., McDermott, A. M., & Pflugfelder, S. C. (2008). Interleukin-1 receptor-1-deficient mice show attenuated production of ocular surface inflammatory cytokines in experimental dry eye. Cornea, 27(7), 811-817. doi: 10.1097/ICO.0b013e31816bf46c.

Narita, J., Kawamura, T., Miyaji, C., Watanabe, H., Honda, S., Koya, T., . . . Abo, T. (1999). Abundance of NKT cells in the salivary glands but absence thereof in the liver and thymus of aly/aly mice with Sjogren syndrome. Cell Immunol, 192(2), 149-158. doi: 10.1006/cimm.1998.1450.

Niederkorn, J. Y., Stern, M. E., Pflugfelder, S. C., De Paiva, C. S., Corrales, R. M., Gao, J., & Siemasko, K. (2006). Desiccating stress induces T cell-mediated Sjogren's Syndrome-like lacrimal keratoconjunctivitis. J Immunol, 176(7), 3950-3957.

Ogawa, Y., Kuwana, M., Yamazaki, K., Mashima, Y., Yamada, M., Mori, T., . . . Kawakami, Y. (2003). Periductal area as the primary site for T-cell activation in lacrimal gland chronic graft-versus-host disease. Invest Ophthalmol Vis Sci, 44(5), 1888-1896.

Ohashi, Y., Ishida, R., Kojima, T., Goto, E., Matsumoto, Y., Watanabe, K., . . . Tsubota, K. (2003). Abnormal protein profiles in tears with dry eye syndrome. Am J Ophthalmol, 136(2), 291-299.

Okanobo, A., Chauhan, S. K., Dastjerdi, M. H., Kodati, S., & Dana, R. (2012). Efficacy of topical blockade of interleukin-1 in experimental dry eye disease. Am J Ophthalmol, 154(1), 63-71. doi: 10.1016/j.ajo.2012.01.034.

Park, K.-S., Korfhagen, T. R., Bruno, M. D., Kitzmiller, J. A., Wan, H., Wert, S. E., . . . Whitsett, J. A. (2007). SPDEF regulates goblet cell hyperplasia in the airway epithelium. The Journal of Clinical Investigation, 117(4), 978-988. doi: 10.1172/JCI29176.

Pflugfelder, S. C., Farley, W., Luo, L., Chen, L. Z., de Paiva, C. S., Olmos, L. C., . . . Fini, M. E. (2005). Matrix metalloproteinase-9 knockout confers resistance to corneal epithelial barrier disruption in experimental dry eye. Am J Pathol, 166(1), 61-71. doi: 10.1016/s0002-9440(10)62232-8.

Pflugfelder, S. C., Jones, D., Ji, Z., Afonso, A., & Monroy, D. (1999). Altered cytokine balance in the tear fluid and conjunctiva of patients with Sjogren's syndrome keratoconjunctivitis sicca. Curr Eye Res, 19(3), 201-211.

Pisella, P. J., Brignole, F., Debbasch, C., Lozato, P. A., Creuzot-Garcher, C., Bara, J., . . . Baudouin, C. (2000). Flow cytometric analysis of conjunctival epithelium in ocular rosacea and keratoconjunctivitis sicca. Ophthalmology, 107(10), 1841-1849.

Postigo, A. A., Teixido, J., & Sanchez-Madrid, F. (1993). The alpha 4 beta 1/VCAM-1 adhesion pathway in physiology and disease. Res Immunol, 144(9), 723-735; discussion 754-762.

Rahimy, E., Pitcher, J. D., 3rd, Pangelinan, S. B., Chen, W., Farley, W. J., Niederkorn, J. Y., . . . De Paiva, C. S. (2010). Spontaneous autoimmune dacryoadenitis in aged CD25KO mice. Am J Pathol, 177(2), 744-753. doi: 10.2353/ajpath.2010.091116.

Ramamoorthy, P., & Nichols, J. J. (2008). Mucins in contact lens wear and dry eye conditions. Optom Vis Sci, 85(8), 631-642. doi: 10.1097/OPX.0b013e3181819f25.

Rashid, S., Jin, Y., Ecoiffier, T., Barabino, S., Schaumberg, D. A., & Dana, M. R. (2008). Topical omega-3 and omega-6 fatty acids for treatment of dry eye. ARCH OPHTHALMOL, 126(2), 219-225. doi: 10.1001/archophthalmol.2007.61.

Robinson, C. P., Brayer, J., Yamachika, S., Esch, T. R., Peck, A. B., Stewart, C. A., . . . Humphreys-Beher, M. G. (1998). Transfer of human serum IgG to nonobese diabetic Igmu null mice reveals a role for autoantibodies in the loss of secretory function of exocrine tissues in Sjogren's syndrome. Proceedings of the National Academy of Sciences of the United States of America, 95(13), 7538-7543.

Rolando, M., Barabino, S., Mingari, C., Moretti, S., Giuffrida, S., & Calabria, G. (2005). Distribution of conjunctival HLA-DR expression and the pathogenesis of damage in early dry eyes. Cornea, 24(8), 951-954.

Rose, C. M., Qian, L., Hakim, L., Wang, Y., Jerdeva, G. Y., Marchelletta, R., . . . Mircheff, A. K. (2005). Accumulation of catalytically active proteases in lacrimal gland acinar cell endosomes during chronic ex vivo muscarinic receptor stimulation. Scand J Immunol, 61(1), 36-50. doi: 10.1111/j.0300-9475.2005.01527.x

Sanz-Marco, E., Udaondo, P., Garcia-Delpech, S., Vazquez, A., & Diaz-Llopis, M. (2013). Treatment of Refractory Dry Eye Associated with Graft Versus Host Disease with 0.03% Tacrolimus Eyedrops. J Ocul Pharmacol Ther. doi: 10.1089/jop.2012.0265.

Schaumberg, D. A., Dana, R., Buring, J. E., & Sullivan, D. A. (2009). Prevalence of dry eye disease among US men: estimates from the Physicians' Health Studies. ARCH OPHTHALMOL, 127(6), 763-768. doi: 10.1001/archophthalmol.2009.103.

Schaumburg, C. S., Siemasko, K. F., De Paiva, C. S., Wheeler, L. A., Niederkorn, J. Y., Pflugfelder, S. C., & Stern, M. E. (2011). Ocular surface APCs are necessary for autoreactive T cell-mediated experimental autoimmune lacrimal keratoconjunctivitis. J Immunol, 187(7), 3653-3662. doi: 10.4049/jimmunol.1101442.

Schiffman, R. M., Walt, J. G., Jacobsen, G., Doyle, J. J., Lebovics, G., & Sumner, W. (2003). Utility assessment among patients with dry eye disease. Ophthalmology, 110(7), 1412-1419. doi: 10.1016/s0161-6420(03)00462-7.

Semba, C. P., Swearingen, D., Smith, V. L., Newman, M. S., O'Neill, C. A., Burnier, J. P., . . . Gadek, T. R. (2011). Safety and pharmacokinetics of a novel lymphocyte function-associated antigen-1 antagonist ophthalmic solution (SAR 1118) in healthy adults. J Ocul Pharmacol Ther, 27(1), 99-104. doi: 10.1089/jop.2009.0105.

Shatos, M. A., Rios, J. D., Horikawa, Y., Hodges, R. R., Chang, E. L., Bernardino, C. R., . . . Dartt, D. A. (2003). Isolation and characterization of cultured human conjunctival goblet cells. Invest Ophthalmol Vis Sci, 44(6), 2477-2486.

Shen, L., Jin, Y., Freeman, G. J., Sharpe, A. H., & Dana, M. R. (2007). The function of donor versus recipient programmed death-ligand 1 in corneal allograft survival. J Immunol, 179(6), 3672-3679.

Sheppard, J. D., Jr., Singh, R., McClellan, A. J., Weikert, M. P., Scoper, S. V., Joly, T. J., . . . Pflugfelder, S. C. (2013). Long-term Supplementation With n-6 and n-3 PUFAs Improves Moderate-to-Severe Keratoconjunctivitis Sicca: A Randomized Double-Blind Clinical Trial. Cornea. doi: 10.1097/ICO.0b013e318299549c

Shimmura, S., Shimazaki, J., & Tsubota, K. (1999). Results of a population-based questionnaire on the symptoms and lifestyles associated with dry eye. Cornea, 18(4), 408-411.

Shull, M. M., Ormsby, I., Kier, A. B., Pawlowski, S., Diebold, R. J., Yin, M., . . . et al. (1992). Targeted disruption of the mouse transforming growth factor-beta 1 gene results in multifocal inflammatory disease. Nature, 359(6397), 693-699. doi: 10.1038/359693a0

Siemasko, K. F., Gao, J., Calder, V. L., Hanna, R., Calonge, M., Pflugfelder, S. C., . . . Stern, M. E. (2008). *In vitro expanded CD4+CD25+Foxp3+ regulatory T cells maintain a normal phenotype and suppress immune-mediated ocular surface inflammation*. Invest Ophthalmol Vis Sci, 49(12), 5434-5440. doi: 10.1167/iovs.08-2075.

Sonawane, S., Khanolkar, V., Namavari, A., Chaudhary, S., Gandhi, S., Tibrewal, S., . . . Jain, S. (2012). *Ocular surface extracellular DNA and nuclease activity imbalance: a new paradigm for inflammation in dry eye disease*. Invest Ophthalmol Vis Sci, 53(13), 8253-8263. doi: 10.1167/iovs.12-10430.

Spadaro, A., Riccieri, V., Benfari, G., Scillone, M., & Taccari, E. (2001). *Soluble interleukin-2 receptor in Sjogren's syndrome: relation to main serum immunological and immunohistochemical parameters*. Clin Rheumatol, 20(5), 319-323.

Spurr-Michaud, S., Argueso, P., & Gipson, I. (2007). *Assay of mucins in human tear fluid*. Exp Eye Res, 84(5), 939-950. doi: 10.1016/j.exer.2007.01.018.

Stapleton, W. M., Chaurasia, S. S., Medeiros, F. W., Mohan, R. R., Sinha, S., & Wilson, S. E. (2008). *Topical interleukin-1 receptor antagonist inhibits inflammatory cell infiltration into the cornea*. Exp Eye Res, 86(5), 753-757. doi: 10.1016/j.exer.2008.02.001.

Stern, M. E., Gao, J., Schwalb, T. A., Ngo, M., Tieu, D. D., Chan, C. C., . . . Smith, J. A. (2002). *Conjunctival T-cell subpopulations in Sjogren's and non-Sjogren's patients with dry eye*. Invest Ophthalmol Vis Sci, 43(8), 2609-2614.

Stern, M. E., Schaumburg, C. S., & Pflugfelder, S. C. (2013). *Dry eye as a mucosal autoimmune disease*. Int Rev Immunol, 32(1), 19-41. doi: 10.3109/08830185.2012.748052.

Stern, M. E., Schaumburg, C. S., Siemasko, K. F., Gao, J., Wheeler, L. A., Grupe, D. A., . . . Pflugfelder, S. C. (2012). *Autoantibodies contribute to the immunopathogenesis of experimental dry eye disease*. Invest Ophthalmol Vis Sci, 53(4), 2062-2075. doi: 10.1167/iovs.11-9299.

Sun, Y., Zhang, R., Gadek, T. R., O'Neill, C. A., & Pearlman, E. (2013). *Corneal inflammation is inhibited by the LFA-1 antagonist, lifitegrast (SAR 1118)*. J Ocul Pharmacol Ther, 29(4), 395-402. doi: 10.1089/jop.2012.0102.

Takada, K., Takiguchi, M., Konno, A., & Inaba, M. (2005). *Autoimmunity against a tissue kallikrein in IQI/Jic Mice: a model for Sjogren's syndrome*. J Biol Chem, 280(5), 3982-3988. doi: 10.1074/jbc.M410157200.

Tong, L., Lan, W., Lim, R., & Chaurasia, S. S. (2013). *S100A Proteins as Molecular Targets in the Ocular Surface Inflammatory Diseases*. The Ocular Surface(0). doi: http://dx.doi.org/10.1016/j.jtos.2013.10.001

Tong, L., Zhou, L., Beuerman, R. W., Zhao, S. Z., & Li, X. R. (2011). *Association of tear proteins with Meibomian gland disease and dry eye symptoms*. Br J Ophthalmol, 95(6), 848-852. doi: 10.1136/bjo.2010.185256.

Tsubota, K., Fujihara, T., Saito, K., & Takeuchi, T. (1999). *Conjunctival epithelium expression of HLA-DR in dry eye patients*. Ophthalmologica, 213(1), 16-19.

Tsubota, K., Fujita, H., Tsuzaka, K., & Takeuchi, T. (2003). *Quantitative analysis of lacrimal gland function, apoptotic figures, Fas and Fas ligand expression of lacrimal glands in dry eye patients*. Exp Eye Res, 76(2), 233-240.

Tsubota, K., Kawashima, M., Inaba, T., Dogru, M., Matsumoto, Y., Ishida, R., . . . Kawakita, T. (2012). *The antiaging approach for the treatment of dry eye*. Cornea, 31 Suppl 1, S3-8. doi: 10.1097/ICO.0b013e31826a05a8.

Uchino, M., Schaumberg, D. A., Dogru, M., Uchino, Y., Fukagawa, K., Shimmura, S., . . . Tsubota, K. (2008). *Prevalence of dry eye disease among Japanese visual display terminal users*. Ophthalmology, 115(11), 1982-1988. doi: 10.1016/j.ophtha.2008.06.022.

Uchiyama, E., Aronowicz, J. D., Butovich, I. A., & McCulley, J. P. (2007). *Increased evaporative rates in laboratory testing conditions simulating airplane cabin relative humidity: an important factor for dry eye syndrome*. Eye Contact Lens, 33(4), 174-176. doi: 10.1097/01.icl.0000252881.04636.5e

Urashima, H., Okamoto, T., Takeji, Y., Shinohara, H., & Fujisawa, S. (2004). *Rebamipide increases the amount of mucin-like substances on the conjunctiva and cornea in the N-acetylcysteine-treated in vivo model*. Cornea, 23(6), 613-619.

Veldhoen, M., Hocking, R. J., Flavell, R. A., & Stockinger, B. (2006). *Signals mediated by transforming growth factor-beta initiate autoimmune encephalomyelitis, but chronic inflammation is needed to sustain disease*. Nat Immunol, 7(11), 1151-1156. doi: 10.1038/ni1391.

Versura, P., Nanni, P., Bavelloni, A., Blalock, W. L., Piazzi, M., Roda, A., & Campos, E. C. (2010). *Tear proteomics in evaporative dry eye disease*. Eye (Lond), 24(8), 1396-1402. doi: 10.1038/eye.2010.7

Versura, P., Profazio, V., Schiavi, C., & Campos, E. C. (2011). *Hyperosmolar stress upregulates HLA-DR expression in human conjunctival epithelium in dry eye patients and in vitro models. Invest Ophthalmol Vis Sci, 52(8), 5488-5496. doi: 10.1167/iovs.11-7215.*

Wan, Y. Y., & Flavell, R. A. (2007). *'Yin-Yang' functions of transforming growth factor-beta and T regulatory cells in immune regulation. Immunol Rev, 220, 199-213. doi: 10.1111/j.1600-065X.2007.00565.x*

Wartha, F., & Henriques-Normark, B. (2008). *ETosis: a novel cell death pathway. Sci Signal, 1(21), pe25. doi: 10.1126/stke.121pe25.*

Watanabe, H. (2002). *Significance of mucin on the ocular surface. Cornea, 21(2 Suppl 1), S17-22.*

Weng, J., He, C., Lai, P., Luo, C., Guo, R., Wu, S., . . . Du, X. (2012). *Mesenchymal stromal cells treatment attenuates dry eye in patients with chronic graft-versus-host disease. Mol Ther, 20(12), 2347-2354. doi: 10.1038/mt.2012.208.*

Whitcup, S. M., Chan, C. C., Kozhich, A. T., & Magone, M. T. (1999). *Blocking ICAM-1 (CD54) and LFA-1 (CD11a) inhibits experimental allergic conjunctivitis. Clin Immunol, 93(2), 107-113. doi: 10.1006/clim.1999.4775.*

Wildenberg, M. E., van Helden-Meeuwsen, C. G., van de Merwe, J. P., Drexhage, H. A., & Versnel, M. A. (2008). *Systemic increase in type I interferon activity in Sjogren's syndrome: a putative role for plasmacytoid dendritic cells. Eur J Immunol, 38(7), 2024-2033. doi: 10.1002/eji.200738008.*

Willoughby, D. A., Moore, A. R., Colville-Nash, P. R., & Gilroy, D. (2000). *Resolution of inflammation. International journal of immunopharmacology, 22(12), 1131-1135.*

Yang, W., Li, H., Chen, P. W., Alizadeh, H., He, Y., Hogan, R. N., & Niederkorn, J. Y. (2009). *PD-L1 expression on human ocular cells and its possible role in regulating immune-mediated ocular inflammation. Invest Ophthalmol Vis Sci, 50(1), 273-280. doi: 10.1167/iovs.08-2397.*

Yavuz, B., Bozdag Pehlivan, S., & Unlu, N. (2012). *An overview on dry eye treatment: approaches for cyclosporin a delivery. ScientificWorldJournal, 2012, 194848. doi: 10.1100/2012/194848.*

Yeh, S., Song, X. J., Farley, W., Li, D. Q., Stern, M. E., & Pflugfelder, S. C. (2003). *Apoptosis of ocular surface cells in experimentally induced dry eye. Invest Ophthalmol Vis Sci, 44(1), 124-129.*

Yoon, K. C., De Paiva, C. S., Qi, H., Chen, Z., Farley, W. J., Li, D. Q., & Pflugfelder, S. C. (2007). *Expression of Th-1 chemokines and chemokine receptors on the ocular surface of C57BL/6 mice: effects of desiccating stress. Invest Ophthalmol Vis Sci, 48(6), 2561-2569. doi: 10.1167/iovs.07-0002.*

Yoon, K. C., De Paiva, C. S., Qi, H., Chen, Z., Farley, W. J., Li, D. Q., . . . Pflugfelder, S. C. (2008). *Desiccating environmental stress exacerbates autoimmune lacrimal keratoconjunctivitis in non-obese diabetic mice. J Autoimmun, 30(4), 212-221. doi: 10.1016/j.jaut.2007.09.003.*

Yoon, K. C., Jeong, I. Y., Park, Y. G., & Yang, S. Y. (2007). *Interleukin-6 and tumor necrosis factor-alpha levels in tears of patients with dry eye syndrome. Cornea, 26(4), 431-437. doi: 10.1097/ICO.0b013e31803dcda2.*

Yoon, K. C., Park, C. S., You, I. C., Choi, H. J., Lee, K. H., Im, S. K., . . . Pflugfelder, S. C. (2010). *Expression of CXCL9, -10, -11, and CXCR3 in the tear film and ocular surface of patients with dry eye syndrome. Invest Ophthalmol Vis Sci, 51(2), 643-650. doi: 10.1167/iovs.09-3425.*

Yoshimura, T., Sonoda, K. H., Ohguro, N., Ohsugi, Y., Ishibashi, T., Cua, D. J., . . . Yoshimura, A. (2009). *Involvement of Th17 cells and the effect of anti-IL-6 therapy in autoimmune uveitis. Rheumatology (Oxford), 48(4), 347-354.*

Yusifov, T. N., Abduragimov, A. R., Narsinh, K., Gasymov, O. K., & Glasgow, B. J. (2008). *Tear lipocalin is the major endonuclease in tears. Mol Vis, 14, 180-188.*

Zhang, X., Schaumburg, C. S., Coursey, T. G., Siemasko, K. F., Volpe, E. A., Gandhi, N. B., . . . de Paiva, C. S. (2013). *CD8 cells regulate the T helper-17 response in an experimental murine model of Sjogren syndrome. Mucosal Immunol. doi: 10.1038/mi.2013.61.*

Zhang, X., Volpe, E. A., Gandhi, N. B., Schaumburg, C. S., Siemasko, K. F., Pangelinan, S. B., . . . De Paiva, C. S. (2012). *NK cells promote Th-17 mediated corneal barrier disruption in dry eye. PLoS One, 7(5), e36822. doi: 10.1371/journal.pone.0036822.*

Zheng, X., Bian, F., Ma, P., De Paiva, C. S., Stern, M., Pflugfelder, S. C., & Li, D. Q. (2010). *Induction of Th17 differentiation by corneal epithelial-derived cytokines. J Cell Physiol, 222(1), 95-102. doi: 10.1002/jcp.21926.*

Zheng, X., de Paiva, C. S., Li, D. Q., Farley, W. J., & Pflugfelder, S. C. (2010). *Desiccating stress promotion of Th17 differentiation by ocular surface tissues through a dendritic cell-mediated pathway.* Invest Ophthalmol Vis Sci, 51(6), 3083-3091. doi: 10.1167/iovs.09-3838.

Zheng, X., De Paiva, C. S., Rao, K., Li, D. Q., Farley, W. J., Stern, M., & Pflugfelder, S. C. (2010). *Evaluation of the transforming growth factor-beta activity in normal and dry eye human tears by CCL-185 cell bioassay.* Cornea, 29(9), 1048-1054. doi: 10.1097/ICO.0b013e3181cf98ff.

Zhou, D., Chen, Y. T., Chen, F., Gallup, M., Vijmasi, T., Bahrami, A. F., . . . McNamara, N. A. (2012). *Critical involvement of macrophage infiltration in the development of Sjogren's syndrome-associated dry eye.* Am J Pathol, 181(3), 753-760. doi: 10.1016/j.ajpath.2012.05.014.

Traditional Chinese Medicine in Dry Eye Disease

Pat Lim, Wanwen Lan, Wei Qi Ping, Louis Tong

1 Introduction

Dry eye disease is a lacrimal film abnormality caused by decreased lacrimal secretions, or hyperactive lacrimal evaporation (DEWS, 2007). The condition is presented with symptoms of discomfort in the eye which may accompany other ocular surface diseases. If patients present only isolated symptoms of dry eyes, they may recover with rest or short-term use of artificial tears (Johnson ME & Murphy PJ, 2004). If there are no ocular surface damage and/or any other local or systemic causes present, it is termed 'simple dry eye'. If patients present both symptoms and clinical signs of dry eyes, it is termed 'dry eye disease'. With the increased usage of the computer and other IT gadgets in modern lifestyle, the incidence of dry eyes has gradually increased while the average age of onset is much lower than before. Dry eye disease imposes a significant direct health care burden and even more so indirectly (Waduthantri S *et al.*, 2012). Dry eye disease affects millions of people around the world with prevalence rates estimated to be as high as 35% in the general population (McCarty CA *et al.*, 1998).

Traditional Chinese Medicine (TCM) is a holistic system of healthcare developed by the Chinese and has been practiced for thousands of years. The first record of TCM is dated back to 2000 years ago in the Yellow Emperor's Cannon of Internal Medicine (*Huang-di nei jing*). Over the years, Chinese medicine is developed from the foundations laid in the Yellow Emperor's Cannon of Internal Medicine, however the core values of TCM never deviated from it, that is, (1) holistic treatment: to look at a disease holistically and treat from the disease roots, while addressing the symptoms; (2) strengthening the body's resistance (*zheng qi*) and dispelling pathogenic factors (*xie qi*), and (3) personalization of treatment based on environmental factors and individual constitution.

There are various modalities of treatment in TCM, including acupuncture, herbal remedies, massage (tui *na*), cupping, moxibustion, ear acupuncture and scraping (*gua sha*). The most commonly employed methods today are acupuncture, herbal remedies and massage, although massage is mostly used for relaxation than its healing functions today. Acupuncture is the insertion of needles into the skin or even the tongues and mucosal layer, based on the system of meridians and its connectivity to the various organs deep in the human body. A modification to the ancient technique of acupuncture is the development of electro stimulation, where needles are connected to weak pulses of electricity for increased stimulation of the acupoints. Herbal remedies are usually prescribed in the form of decoctions, although pills, pastes and baths are also available. Herbal remedies could be based on a single herb or a combination of a few or many, depending on the individual constitution, and modification of the remedies is commonly done. The principle of all modalities of treatment would be to eliminate pathogenic forces, while restoring the body's balance and strengthening it.

In Chinese medicine, the disease pertains to *bai se zheng* (白涩症，white dry eyes), or *shen shui jiang ku* (神水将枯，impending desiccation of spirit water), belonging to the category of *zao zheng* (燥症，dryness pattern) (Ping WQ). The causes are mostly attributed to lung *yin* deficiency or liver and kidney *yin* deficiency, which lead to nutritional deficiency of the eyes.

2   Clinical Manifestation of Dry Eye Disease

Common ocular symptoms include asthenopia (eye strain), sensation of foreign bodies in the eyes, dryness, burning sensation, swelling, ophthalmalgia (pain in eye), photophobia, redness, etc. If these symptoms are presented, patients should be asked in detail on their history of dry eyes sensation in order to find the underlying causes. For patients who present with severe dry eyes, the clinician should check if their condition is accompanied by dry mouth or joint pain, as the dry eye symptoms could be an indication of Sjörgren's Disease and require prompt treatment. Clinical signs of dry eye include vasodilatation, edema, folding of bulbar conjunctiva, shortened tear meniscus height (TMH), and occasional mucopurulent discharge in the lower fornix and punctuate staining in corneal epithelium in the palpebral fissure area. When dry eye disease is suspected, relevant objective tests may be considered, including Schirmer's test and tear break up time (TBUT) test.(Tong L *et al.*, 2012) Dry eyes may affect visual acuity in early stages, and further develop into filamentary keratitis. At later stages, if left untreated, dry eye disease may lead to corneal thinning, ulcers, and perforation, or in some cases, a secondary bacterial infection.

2.1   Types of Dry Eye Patterns in TCM

In most patients presenting with dry eye, their disease condition could be attributed to one or a combination of five main categories of 'disease pattern'. These disease patterns are identified as pathologies stemming from the 'organs', or the root of the disease, and usually present overlapping symptoms apart from dry eye. These patterns include deficiency of lung *yin*, deficiency of liver and kidney *yin*, and dry eye initiated by heat in various organs. These will be described in the sections below:

2.1.1   Deficiency of Lung Yin

Patients in this category often present with the following characteristics: Dry eyes that result in inability to see clearly over a long period, mild conjunctiva hyperemia, point lesions of the superficial corneal layer, relapses with poor recovery, dry cough with little phlegm, dry pharynx, constipation, reddish tongue with dry mouth and a thready rapid pulse.

   The treatment in this case is to enrich yin and moisten the lung meridian. A representative formula is the Yang Yin Qing Fei Tang (养阴清肺汤, yin-nourishing lung-clearing decoction). (Wei Q-P *et al.*, 2011) Refer to Table 1 for the prescription. Please note that this prescription is often modified in 3 scenarios:

- For cases with pronounced dry throat and mouth, add *bei sha shen* (北沙参, *Glehmia littoralis Fr. Schmidt ex Miq.*) 15g, *Shi Hu* (石斛, *Dendrobium loddigesii Rolfe.*) 10g to boost the *qi* and nourish the *yin*.

- For cases with constipation, add *jue ming zi* (决明子, *Cassisa obtusifolia L.*) 15g to moisten the intestines and allow the stool to move down the rectum.

- For cases with point lesions of the cornea, add *chan tui* (蝉蜕, *Cryptotympana pustulata Fabricius*) 6g, *ju hua* (菊花, *Chrysanthemum morifolium Ramat.*) 12g, *mi meng hua* (密蒙花, *Buddleja officinalis Maxim.*) 10g to clear the heat, and brighten the eyes.

Herb	Chinese character	Latin name	Amount
Mu dan pi	牡丹皮	*Paeonia suffruticosa Andr.*	10 g
Bai shao	白芍	*Paeonia lactiflora Pall.*	10 g
Sheng gan cao	生甘草	*Glycyrrhiza uralensis Fisch*	10 g
Sheng di	生地	*Rehmannia glutinosa Libosch.*	10 g
Bo he	薄荷	*Metha haplocalyz Briq.*	6 g
Xuan shen	玄参	*Scrophularia ningpoensis Hemsl.*	10 g
Mai dong	麦冬	*Ophiopogon japonicus (L.f.) Ker-Gawl.*	15 g
Bei mu	贝母	*Fritillaria thunbergii Miq.*	10 g
Tai zi shen	太子参	*Pseudostellaria heterophylla (Miq.)*	15 g
Wu wei zi	五味子	*Schisandrae chinensis (Turez.) Baill.*	10 g

Table 1: Prescription for *Yang Yin Qing Fei Tang* (yin-nourishing lung-clearing decoction)

2.1.2 Liver and Kidney Yin Deficiency

In this syndrome, dry eye is accompanied with symptoms of ocular discomfort, photophobia, and dry mouth with scant saliva, lumbago, weak and/or painful knees, dizziness, tinnitus, insomnia with profuse dreams, red tongue with thin coating and a thready pulse.

The treatment principle is to nourish the liver and kidney meridians, and a representative formula is the Modified Qi Ju Di Huang Wan (杞菊地黄丸, lycium berry, chrysanthemum and rehmannia pill) (Table 2).

Herb	Chinese character	Latin name	Amount
Gou qi zi	枸杞子	*Lycium barbarum L.*	15 g
Ju hua	菊花	*Chrysanthemum morifolium Ramat.*	10 g
Shu di	熟地	*Rehmannia glutinosa Libosch.*	10 g
Shan zhu yu	山茱萸	*Cornus officinalis Sieb.et Zucc.*	10 g
Shan yao	山药	*Dioscrorea opposite Thunb.*	10 g
Ze xie	泽泻	*Alisma orientalis (Sam.) Juzep.*	10 g
Fu ling	茯苓	*Poria cocos (Schw.) Wolf*	10 g
Mu dan pi	牡丹皮	*Paeonia suffruticasa Andr.*	10 g

Table 2: Prescription for Modified Qi Ju Di Huang Wan.

In certain scenarios, this formulation can be modified:

- For cases with dry mouth, with scanty saliva, add mai dong (麦冬, *Ophiopogon japonicus (L.f.)Ker-Gawl.*) 10g, xuan shen (玄参, *Scrophularia ningpoensis Hemsl*) 10g to nourish the yin and engender the fluid.

- For cases with obvious conjunctival hyperaemia, add sang bai pi (桑白皮, *Morus alba L.*) 9g, di gu pi (地骨皮, *Lycium chinensis Mill.*) 10g to clear the heat and reduce congestion.

2.1.3   Dry Eye Initiated by Wind and Heat

This type of dry eye is caused by wind and heat, including xerosis conjunctiva, fulminant red eye with acute mebula and conjunctival edema. The principle of treatment is to 'scatter' the wind and clear the heat. The representative formula is *Sang Ju Ying* (桑菊饮，Mulberry leaf and chrysanthemum beverage (Table 3).

Herb	Chinese character	Latin name	Amount
Sang ye	桑叶	*Morus alba L.*	9 g
Ju hua	菊花	*Chrysanthemum morifolium Ramat.*	9 g
Lian qiao	连翘	*Forsythia suspense (Thunb.)Vahl.*	9 g
Ju geng	桔梗	*Platycodon grandiflorum (Jaoq.)A.DC.*	9 g
Xing ren	杏仁	*Prunus armeniaca L.var.ansu Maxim.*	9 g
Ze xie	泽泻	*Alisma orientalis (Sam.) Juzep.*	6 g
Gan cao	甘草	*Glycyirrhiza uralensis Fisch*	3 g
Lu gen	芦根	*Phragmites communis (L.) Trin.*	15 g

Table 3: Formulation for Mulberry Leaf and Chrysanthemum Beverage.

2.1.4   Dry Eye Initiated by Heart–heat

This is dry eye initiated by overwork from prolonged use of computers, insufficient sleep or stress-induced insomnia, and usually presents with photophobia, eye strain, eye sore or pain, with red tongue tip and rapid pulse. In this scenario, the treatment principle is to clear the heart-heat from the heart meridian by promoting urination. A representative formulation to address this is found in Table 4.

Herb	Chinese character	Latin name	Amount
Sheng di	生地	*Rehmannia glutinosa Libosch.*	18 g
Mu tong	木通	*Aristolochia manshuriensis Kom.*	9 g
Dan zhu ye	淡竹叶	*Lophatherum gracile Brongn.*	12 g
Shan zhi zi	山栀子	*Gardenia jasminoides Ellis*	12 g
Huang bai	黄柏	*Phellodendron amurense Rupr.*	9 g
Zhi mu	知母	*Anemarhena asphodeloides Bge.*	9 g
Deng xin cao	灯芯草	*Juncus effuses L.*	6 g
Gan cao	甘草	*Glycyirrhiza uralensis Fisch*	6 g

Table 4: Treatment to reduce heat in the heart – formulation of dao chi san.

2.1.5   Dry Eye Initiated by Liver- heat

Heat can also be initiated by the liver. In this syndrome, dry eye is initiated by prolonged visual tasks, and the patients in this category are stressed and easily agitated or frustrated with dry eye with headache. He also suffers from pain in the side abdomens at times, has red tongue with white coat and a rapid thready pulse.

Here, the physician aims to clear the liver heat and dampness from the lower part of the body meridians. A formulation such as that in Table 5 can be employed.

Herb	Chinese character	Latin name	Amount
Long dan cao	龙胆草	*Gentiana scabra Bge.*	12 g
Sheng di	生地	*Rehmannia glutinosa Libosch.*	18 g
Dang gui	当归	*Angelica sinensis (Oliv.)*	6 g
Chai hu	柴胡	*Bupleurum chinensis DC.*	6 g
Mu tong	木通	*Aristolochia manshuriensis Kom.*	9 g
Ze xie	泽泻	*Alisma orientalis (Sam.) Juzep.*	9 g
Che qian zi	车前子	*Plantago asiatica L.*	9 g
Shan zhi Zi	山栀子	*Gardenia jasminoides Ellis*	9 g
Huang qin	黄芩	*Scuttellaria baicalensis Georgi.*	9 g
Gan cao	甘草	*Glycyrrhiza uralensis Fisch*	5 g

Table 5: Formulation for treatment of liver heat – long dan xie gan tang.

3   TCM Treatments of Dry Eye

3.1   Acupuncture Treatment for Dry Eye

The history of using acupuncture treatment for dry eye is dated back to the Ancient Times – Northern and Southern Dynasties (581A.D). The Yellow Emperor's Inner Classic (*Huang Di Nei Jing*, 黄帝内经) had records of the anatomy and physiology of the eyes, as well as the etiology, pathology, clinical manifestation, and acupuncture strategies for eye disorders (Wei Q-P *et al.*, 2011). More than 30 eye diseases were recorded in this book. In each typical treatment session, 4 – 6 acupoints were selected, needles retained for 20 – 30 minutes, and treatment was performed once every day. Ten treatments constitute one course of treatment(Wei Q-P *et al.*, 2011) (Table 6). Most studies conducted previously did not have proper control groups. Recently, investigators in Korea have conducted randomized controlled studies in acupuncture compared to sham acupuncture.(Shin MS *et al.*, 2010) The results show that compared to patients on sham acupuncture, the acupuncture patients have improved tear break up time, Schirmer's tests and corneal fluorescein staining at 3 weeks after treatment.

ST1 (*cheng qi*)	承泣	太阳（*tai yang*）	GB20 (*feng chi*)	风池
BL2 (*cuan zhu*)	攒竹	鱼腰 (*yu yao*)	SJ 23 (*si zhu kong*)	丝竹空
ST2 (*si bai*)	四白	LV3 (*tai chong*) 太冲	GB37 (*guang ming*)	光明
SP6 (*san yin jiao*) 三阴交		LI4 (*he gu*) 合谷	DU23 (*shang xing*)	上星
DU20 (*bai hui*)	百会			

Table 6: Acupuncture points for treatment of dry eye.

Commonly used Acupoints in Dry Eye Syndrome are shown in the above table. Their locations and applications are as follows:

Acupoints around the eye (6 acupoints):

1. ST1 (cheng qi, 承泣): Between the infraorbital ridge and the eye ball, 0.7 cun (ancient Chinese measurement in inches) directly below the pupil when the eyes are looking straight ahead. Puncture perpendicularly 0.5 – 1.5 cun along the infraorbital ridge.

2. BL2 (cuan zhu, 攒竹): In the depression over the medial end of the eyebrow. Oblique puncture downward to a depth of 0.3 – 0.5 cun.

3. ST2 (si bai, 四白): 1 cun directly below the pupil, in the depression over the infraorbital foramen. Perpendicularly puncture for 0.2 – 0.3 cun.

4. Tai yang 太阳: In the depression about 1 cun behind the midpoint between the lateral end of the eyebrow and the outer canthus. Perpendicularly or obliquely puncture for 0.3 – 0.5 cun.

5. Yu yao 鱼腰: At the midpoint of the eyebrow, directly above the pupil. Horizontally puncture towards medial or lateral side for 0.5 cun.

6. SJ23 (si zhu kong, 丝竹空): In the depression over the tip of eyebrow. Horizontally puncture to 0.3 – 0.5 cun.

Relative body acupoints (7 acupoints):

1. SP6 (san yin jiao, 三阴交): On the medial side of the leg, 3 cun above the tip of the medial malleolus, posterior to the medial border of the tibia. Perpendicularly puncture to a depth of 0.5 – 1 cun. Moxibustion is applicable.

2. DU20 (bai hui, 百会): 7 cun directly above the midpoint of the posterior hairline. Horizontally puncture to a depth of 0.5 – 0.8 cun.

3. LV3 (tai chong, 太冲): On the dorsum of the foot between the 1st and 2nd toes, in the depression 1.5 cun to LR2. Perpendicularly puncture to a depth of 0.5 – 0.8 cun. Moxibustion is applicable.

4. LI4 (he gu, 合谷): In the depression between the first and second metacarpophalangeal joint. Perpendicularly puncture to a depth of 0.5 – 0.8 cun.

5. GB20 (feng chi, 风池): In the depression between the upper ends of the sternocleidomastoid and trapezius muscles, at the level of DU 16 (feng fu). Obliquely puncture 1 – 2 cun towards the fellow eye. Moxibustion is applicable.

6. GB37 (guang ming, 光明): 5 cun above the tip of the external malleolus, on the anterior boarder of the fibula. Perpendicularly puncture to a depth of 0.5 – 1 cun. Moxibustion is applicable.

7. DU23 (shang xing, 上星): 1 cun directly above the midpoint of the anterior hairline. Horizontally puncture to a depth of 0.5 – 0.8 cun. Moxibustion is applicable.

The principle of selecting acupoints in the practice of TCM ophthalmic acupuncture is based on diagnosis and pattern differentiations, usually using whole-body pattern differentiation combined with local acupoints to obtain the goal of supporting healthy qi, dispelling pathogens, relieving sickness by dredging the channels and collaterals, regulating zang-fu organs, and relating qi and blood. The essence of the five zang and six fu flow upward to the eyes. Therefore, all the pathological conditions of the zang, fu, qi, blood, channels and collaterals should be taken into consideration when making a pattern differentiation.

In TCM theory, all the vessels are related to the eyes. The eyes are abundant with channels; collaterals, qi and blood, and thus they may become vulnerable to disease. Therefore, needling the local acupoints around the eye can have a direct and rapid impact on relieving the symptoms. In clinical practice, we commonly select local acupoints around the eyes in combination with body acupoints to promote a whole treatment process.

Therefore for the dry eye syndrome, besides the local acupoints, different acupoints from different meridians – Spleen meridian (SP), Stomach meridian(ST), Liver meridian(LV), Gallbladder meridian (GB) will be selected accordingly, in completing the points selection.

3.2   Chinese Patent Medicines

In western or clinical medicine, patients with dry eye may be given lubricants such as 1% sodium hyaluronate or carboxymethylcellulose eyedrops used frequently daily. Patients with more severe or uncontrolled symptoms may seek advice or treatment from an Ophthalmologist, who may initiate immunosuppressive, anti-inflammatory treatment, or punctum occlusion methods.

In contrast, TCM advocates the use of simple remedies comprising core herbs such as ju hua (菊花, *Chrysanthemum morifolium Ramat.*), mai dong (麦冬, *O.japonicus(L.f)Ker-Gawl*) gou qi zi (枸杞子, *Lycium barbarum L.*), mu hu die (木蝴蝶, *Oroxylum indicum (L.) Kurz*) which possess yin-nourishing properties. Depending on the condition and constitution of the patients, a selection of herbs are added (10g each) into a prescription and wrapped as a tea drink. Alternatively, they are brewed in a teapot with boiling water, and consumed 6 – 9 times in small amounts daily, Chinese physicians may choose one of these more standard therapies:

1. Qi Ju Di Huang Wan (杞菊地黄丸, lycium berry, chrysanthemum and rehmannia pill) 6 pills, twice daily; applicable to liver-kidney yin deficiency

2. Zhi Bai Di Huang Wan (知柏地黄丸, Lycium berry, chrysanthemum and redmannia pill)6 pills, twice daily; applicable to liver-kidney yin deficiency or effulgent yin-deficiency

3. Yang Yin Qing Fei Kou Fu Ye (养阴清肺口服液, yin-nourishing lung-clearing oral liquid) 10ml, twice daily, applicable to deficiency of lung-yin deficiency

3.3   Dietary Therapy and Preventive Management

Like in all types of medicine, Chinese medicine recognizes that environmental and dietary factors contribute to disease. Therefore, preventive measures and ways to adjust the environment that one is exposed to maybe just as helpful as therapeutic medications.(Wei Q-P *et al.*, 2011) Some of these measures include:

- Avoiding prolonged and excessive visual tasks. Patients are counseled that TV, computers and other IT gadgets should be placed in a position below eye level.

- Avoidance of air conditioning and dust, and measures to maintain a certain degree of humidity in the room

- Adopting a positive attitude to life and have a happy outlook, paying particular attention to balanced and sufficient dietary components and maintaining a healthy eating habit including the consumption of fresh vegetables and fruits, while increasing vitamins A, B, C and E intake. The patients should be advised against over-consumption of spicy, greasy-fried, or fatty and processed food.

- Regulation of the internal emotions and working on cultivating an optimistic mood; maintaining a proper balance between work and relaxation.

4   Clinical Trials in Dry Eye

Sometimes, Tradition Chinese Medicine physicians employ a mixture of acupuncture and oral therapies. Recently, randomized controlled studies in the use of TCM in dry eye have been published, with data that suggest TCM is useful in improving the disease condition (Chang YH et al., 2005; Gronlund MA et al., 2004; Lee MS et al., 2011; Nepp J, 2005; Nepp J et al., 1998; Shin MS et al., 2010; Tseng KL et al., 2006). In a randomized placebo-controlled study, the group receiving *Chi-Ju-Di-Huang-Wan* medication had a significantly improved Rose-Bengal and fluorescein TBUT compared to placebo group at 2 and 4 weeks respectively (Chang Y-H et al., 2005). A Korean study showed that in TBUT in an acupuncture group had improved TBUT (p not statistically significant) after 3 weeks (Lan W & Tong L, 2011; Shin MS et al., 2010). Finally, in one meta-analysis of 6 randomized controlled trials, the authors found that acupuncture significantly improved TBUT ($p < 0.0001$), Schirmer's test ($p < 0.00001$) and cornea fluorescein staining ($p = 0.0001$) (Lee MS et al., 2011).

We have recently conducted a clinical research study involving qi ju gan lu yin and qi ju gan lu yin with acupuncture on the treatment of lung and kidney yin deficiency type of dry eye (Lim P) at Singapore Chung Hwa Medical Institution.

In the study, we aimed to evaluate the efficacy of TCM herbal medicine "qi ju gan lu yin" in treating dry eye, compared to the same "qi ju gan lu yin with acupuncture" and a total of 89 age- and gender-matched subjects were recruited. This included 44 in Group 1, the TCM Herbal Medicine Group, and 45 in Group 2, the TCM Combined Methods Group. All participants had dry eyes as their main complaint and were aged 40-70 years old. All subjects had good general health, no ocular disease, non-smoking and were non-contact lens wearer. The inclusion criteria of dry eye subjects were a positive score in the SPEED Questionnaire (Standard Patient Evaluation for Eye Dryness Questionnaire). The study group (Group 1, TCM Herbal Medicine Group) of 44 patients were given qi ju gan lu yin orally and the control group (Group 2, TCM Combined Methods Group) of 45 patients were given qi ju gan lu yin combined with acupuncture twice a week. Both groups were treated for 30 days. Pre- and post-treatment measurements of Schirmer's and TBUT test were obtained for the TCM Herbal Medicine Group (Group 1) and TCM Combined Methods Group (Group 2). We used the Right eye as the main observation eye and for Schirmer's I test (mm/5 min) result in Group 1, $p = 0.04$.

In Group 2, p = 0.668. For Tear Break-Up Time (TBUT), the values were p = 0.001 in Group 1 and p = 0.099 Group 2.

No significant differences were found in Schirmer's test readings between the two groups Z = –1.441 p = 0.150 Significant differences were obtained for the TBUT between Group 1 and Group 2 at the post treatment visit. Group 1 performed better than Group 2, where Z = –7.013 p = 0.001 for Group 1; and Z = –1.650, p = 0.099 in Group 2.The total efficacy or % in improvement in SPEED was 54.4% for Group 1 and similar in Group 2 (53.3%). The SPEED improvement in group 1 was 3.58 ± 5.40 and Group 2 was 4.40 ± 7.82. There was no significant difference between the two groups (t = 0.520, p = 0.604). The percentage improvement in the SANDE(Schaumberg DA et al., 2007) or Visual Analogue Score (VAS) in Group 1 and 2 was 61% and 55.5% respectively. VAS (Visual Analogue Score) improvement for Group 1 was 24.01 ± 23.99 and Group 2 was 22.70 ± 24.33. The improvement between the 2 groups was not significantly different (t = − 0.252, p = 0.802).

In addition we found that the TCM lung and kidney yin deficiency score aggregates for Group 1 was 68.18% and for Group 2 was 71.11%.The TCM lung and kidney yin deficiency improvement in Group 1 was 3.76 ± 6.04 and Group 2 was 4.50 ± 5.81. These were not significantly different between the two groups (t = –0.205, p = 0.838).

The findings demonstrate the usefulness of TCM treatment in treating the commonly seen dry eye disease in Singapore. In this study, acupuncture does not demonstrate any additional therapeutic effect over and above herbal medication alone. In fact, for TBUT, Group 1 (TCM Herbal Medicine alone) has in fact shown a better result than the combined TCM methods. The result findings suggest that TCM herbal medicine may be used as an alternative medicine to treat dry eyes in Singapore.

In addition, we performed a review of other clinical trials investigating the efficacy of TCM in the treatment of dry eye disease (Table 7).

5   Conclusions

A previous study in Singapore has evaluated the knowledge, attitude and practice of TCM practitioners in treatment of dry eye (Lan W et al., 2012). This study shows that at least in institutional practice, the registered Chinese physicians were keened to participate in the treatment of dry eye. Although there has been randomized controlled studies in TCM in dry eye, the results are often controversial (Lan W & Tong L, 2011) and much larger studies are being planned and conducted (Kim TH et al., 2010; Kim TH et al., 2009). Use of combined modalities of TCM may not necessarily be advantageous over a single modality, although the specific nature of the modality used may determine the outcome.

It seems that in Asian countries, the use of TCM is widespread and prevalent increasingly, health care workers have realized the holistic nature of dry eye. As TCM deals holistically with patients' conditions, many dry eye patients are willing to be treated with TCM. In any case, the coordination of care of dry eye between TCM and western practitioners may be advantageous for many patients. We eagerly await the outcome of the major trials being conducted in this area.

Author, year	Sample size	Type of treatment	Duration of follow-up	Randomization	Control group	Outcome	Language
(Chang YH et al., 2005)	80	Chi-Ju-Di-Huang-Wan	4 weeks	-	Yes	Symt,TBUT, ST, St	English
(Shi JL & Miao WH, 2012)	65	Acupuncture	3 weeks	Yes	Yes	TBUT, ST	Chinese
(Kim TH et al., 2012)	150	Acupuncture	4 weeks	Yes	Yes	Symt,TBUT,ST	English
(Xu XH & Fang XL, 2012)	30	Acupuncture	2 sessions	Yes	Yes	Symt	Chinese
(Chen LQ, 2008)	70	moxibustion	-	Yes	Yes	Symt,TBUT, St	Chinese
(Qiu X et al., 2011)	10 rabbits	Acupuncture	10 sessions	-	-	Tear proteins	English
(Jeon JH et al., 2010)	36	Acupuncture	4 weeks	-	-	Symt,TBUT, ST	English
(Kim TH et al., 2010)	150	Acupuncture	4weeks	Yes	Yes	Symt,TBUT,ST	English
(Shin MS et al., 2010)	42	Acupuncture	3weeks	Yes	Yes	Symt,TBUT,ST	English
(Wei LX et al., 2010)	80	Acupuncture	-	Yes	Yes	Symt,TBUT,ST	Chinese
(Gong L et al., 2010)	44	Acupuncture	3 weeks	No	No	Symt	English
(Gao WP et al., 2010)	56	Acupuncture	-	No	No	Symt, TBUT,St	Chinese
(Gong L & Sun X, 2007)	Rabbits	Acupuncture	-	No	No	ST	English
(Zhang Y & Yang W, 2007)	61	Acupuncture, moxibustion	-	Yes	Yes	Symt,TBUT,ST	English
(Bai H et al., 2007)	57	Electroacupuncture	2 months	No	No	Symt	Chinese
(Tseng KL et al., 2006)	43	Acupuncture, SSP	4 weeks	Yes	Yes	Symt,TBUT,ST	English
(Gronlund MA et al., 2004)	25	Acupuncture	10 sessions	Yes	Yes	Symt,	English
(Blom M & Lundeberg T, 2000)	70	Acupuncture	6 months	-	-	SFR	English
(Nepp J et al., 1999)	102	Acupuncture	10 sessions	Yes	Yes	TBUT,ST	German
(Blom M et al., 1999)	32	Acupuncture	1 month	No	No	SFR	English
(List T et al., 1998)	21	Acupuncture	10 weeks	-	Yes	SS	English
(Nepp J et al., 1998)	-	Acupuncture	-	Yes	Yes	-	English
(Blom M et al., 1993)	21	Acupuncture	-	No	No	SFR	English

Table 7: Clinical trials on use of TCM in dry eye management.

Authors

Pat Lim
Singapore Chung Hwa Medical Institution, Singapore
Beijing University of Chinese Medicine, China

Wanwen Lan
Singapore Eye Research Institute, Singapore
Yong Loo Lin School of Medicine, National University of Singapore, Singapore

Wei Qi Ping
Beijing University of Chinese Medicine, China

Louis Tong
Singapore Eye Research Institute, Singapore
Singapore National Eye Center, Singapore
Duke-National University of Singapore Graduate Medical School, National University of Singapore, Singapore

References

Bai, H., Yu, P., & Yu, M. (2007). [Effect of electroacununcture on sex hormone levels in patients with Sjogren's syndrome]. *Zhen Ci Yan Jiu, 32(3)*, 203-206.

Blom, M., Kopp, S., & Lundeberg, T. (1999). Prognostic value of the pilocarpine test to identify patients who may obtain long-term relief from xerostomia by acupuncture treatment. *Arch Otolaryngol Head Neck Surg, 125(5)*, 561-566.

Blom, M., & Lundeberg, T. (2000). Long-term follow-up of patients treated with acupuncture for xerostomia and the influence of additional treatment. *Oral Dis, 6(1)*, 15-24.

Blom, M., Lundeberg, T., Dawidson, I., & Angmar-Mansson, B. (1993). Effects on local blood flux of acupuncture stimulation used to treat xerostomia in patients suffering from Sjogren's syndrome. *J Oral Rehabil, 20(5)*, 541-548.

Chang, Y.-H., Lin, H.-J., & Li, W.-C. (2005). Clinical evaluation of the traditional chinese prescription Chi-Ju-Di-Huang-Wan for Dry Eye.

Chang, Y. H., Lin, H. J., & Li, W. C. (2005). Clinical evaluation of the traditional chinese prescription Chi-Ju-Di-Huang-Wan for dry eye. *Phytother Res, 19(4)*, 349-354.

Chen, L. Q. (2008). [Observation on therapeutic effect of moxibustion with thunder-fire herbal moxa stick on xerophthalmia of oligodacrya]. *Zhongguo Zhen Jiu, 28(8)*, 585-588.

DEWS. (2007). The definition and classification of dry eye disease: report of the Definition and Classification Subcommittee of the International Dry Eye WorkShop (2007). *Ocul Surf, 5(2)*, 75-92.

Gao, W. P., Liu, M., & Zhang, Y. B. (2010). [Observation on therapeutic effect of dry eye syndrome treated with acupuncture on the acupoints around the eyes]. *Zhongguo Zhen Jiu, 30(6)*, 478-480.

Gong, L., & Sun, X. (2007). Treatment of intractable dry eyes: tear secretion increase and morphological changes of the lacrimal gland of rabbit after acupuncture. *Acupunct Electrother Res, 32(3-4)*, 223-233.

Gong, L., Sun, X., & Chapin, W. J. (2010). Clinical curative effect of acupuncture therapy on xerophthalmia. *Am J Chin Med, 38(4)*, 651-659.

Gronlund, M. A., Stenevi, U., & Lundeberg, T. (2004). Acupuncture treatment in patients with keratoconjunctivitis sicca: a pilot study. *Acta Ophthalmol Scand, 82(3 Pt 1)*, 283-290.

Jeon, J. H., Shin, M. S., Lee, M. S., Jeong, S. Y., Kang, K. W., Kim, Y. I., et al. (2010). Acupuncture reduces symptoms of dry eye syndrome: a preliminary observational study. *J Altern Complement Med, 16(12)*, 1291-1294.

Johnson, M. E., & Murphy, P. J. (2004). Changes in the tear film and ocular surface from dry eye syndrome. Prog Retin Eye Res, 23(4), 449-474.

Kim, T. H., Kang, J. W., Kim, K. H., Kang, K. W., Shin, M. S., Jung, S. Y., et al. (2012). Acupuncture for the treatment of dry eye: a multicenter randomised controlled trial with active comparison intervention (artificial teardrops). PLoS One, 7(5), e36638.

Kim, T. H., Kang, J. W., Kim, K. H., Kang, K. W., Shin, M. S., Jung, S. Y., et al. (2010). Acupuncture for dry eye: a multicentre randomised controlled trial with active comparison intervention (artificial tear drop) using a mixed method approach protocol. Trials, 11, 107.

Kim, T. H., Kim, J. I., Shin, M. S., Lee, M. S., Choi, J. Y., Jung, S. Y., et al. (2009). Acupuncture for dry eye: a randomised controlled trial protocol. Trials, 10, 112.

Lan, W., Lee, S. Y., Lee, M. X., & Tong, L. (2012). Knowledge, attitude, and practice of dry eye treatment by institutional Chinese physicians in Singapore. ScientificWorldJournal, 2012, 923059.

Lan, W., & Tong, L. (2011). Comments: acupuncture for treating dry eye: a randomized placebo-controlled trial. Acta Ophthalmol, 89(4), e371-372; author reply e372.

Lee, M. S., Shin, B. C., Choi, T. Y., & Ernst, E. (2011). Acupuncture for treating dry eye: a systematic review. Acta Ophthalmol, 89(2), 101-106.

Lim, P. Unpublished data. Beijing, PRC.

List, T., Lundeberg, T., Lundstrom, I., Lindstrom, F., & Ravald, N. (1998). The effect of acupuncture in the treatment of patients with primary Sjogren's syndrome. A controlled study. Acta Odontol Scand, 56(2), 95-99.

McCarty, C. A., Bansal, A. K., Livingston, P. M., Stanislavsky, Y. L., & Taylor, H. R. (1998). The epidemiology of dry eye in Melbourne, Australia. Ophthalmology, 105(6), 1114-1119.

Nepp, J. (2005). Acupuncture in dry eye syndromes. Arch Soc Esp Oftalmol, 80(5), 267-270.

Nepp, J., Derbolav, A., Haslinger-Akramian, J., Mudrich, C., Schauersberger, J., & Wedrich, A. (1999). [Effect of acupuncture in keratoconjunctivitis sicca]. Klin Monbl Augenheilkd, 215(4), 228-232.

Nepp, J., Wedrich, A., Akramian, J., Derbolav, A., Mudrich, C., Ries, E., et al. (1998). Dry eye treatment with acupuncture. A prospective, randomized, double-masked study. Adv Exp Med Biol, 438, 1011-1016.

Ping, W. Q. Impending Dessication of Spirit Water (Shen Shui Jiang Ku Zheng), Previous Classic on Ophthalmology (Shen Shi Yao Han).

Qiu, X., Gong, L., Sun, X., Guo, J., & Chodara, A. M. (2011). Efficacy of acupuncture and identification of tear protein expression changes using iTRAQ quantitative proteomics in rabbits. Curr Eye Res, 36(10), 886-894.

Schaumberg, D. A., Gulati, A., Mathers, W. D., Clinch, T., Lemp, M. A., Nelson, J. D., et al. (2007). Development and validation of a short global dry eye symptom index. Ocul Surf, 5(1), 50-57.

Shi, J. L., & Miao, W. H. (2012). [Effects of acupuncture on lactoferrin content in tears and tear secretion in patients suffering from dry eyes: a randomized controlled trial]. Zhong Xi Yi Jie He Xue Bao, 10(9), 1003-1008.

Shin, M. S., Kim, J. I., Lee, M. S., Kim, K. H., Choi, J. Y., Kang, K. W., et al. (2010). Acupuncture for treating dry eye: a randomized placebo-controlled trial. Acta Ophthalmol, 88(8), e328-333.

Tong, L., Tan, J., Thumboo, J., & Seow, G. (2012). Dry eye. BMJ, 345, e7533.

Tseng, K. L., Liu, H. J., Tso, K. Y., Woung, L. C., Su, Y. C., & Lin, J. G. (2006). A clinical study of acupuncture and SSP (silver spike point) electro-therapy for dry eye syndrome. Am J Chin Med, 34(2), 197-206.

Waduthantri, S., Yong, S. S., Tan, C. H., Shen, L., Lee, M. X., Nagarajan, S., et al. (2012). Cost of dry eye treatment in an Asian clinic setting. PLoS One, 7(6), e37711.

Wei, L. X., Yang, W., Wang, H. C., Zhang, O., Ding, R. Q., & Liu, Z. H. (2010). [Efficacy assessment of acupuncture and moxibustion on tear secretion in xerophthalmia]. Zhongguo Zhen Jiu, 30(9), 709-712.

Wei, Q.-P., Rosenfarb, A., & Liang, L.-n. (2011). Ophthalmology in Chinese Medicine.): People's Medical Publishing House Co, LTD.

Xu, X. H., & Fang, X. L. (2012). [Efficacy observation of xerophthalmia treated with acupuncture of warming-promotion needling technique]. Zhongguo Zhen Jiu, 32(3), 233-236.

Zhang, Y., & Yang, W. (2007). Effects of acupuncture and moxibustion on tear-film of the patients with xerophthalmia. J Tradit Chin Med, 27(4), 258-260.

Mechanisms of Goji Berry and Its Taurine Component in the Prevention and Management of Diabetic Retinopathy

Min Kyong Song, Basil D. Roufogalis and Tom Hsun-Wei Huang

1 Diabetic Retinopathy

Diabetic retinopathy (DR) is one of the most prevalent diabetic eye diseases. It is a vision-threatening disease presenting neurodegenerative features associated with extensive vascular changes (Fong *et al.*, 2004b; Silva *et al.*, 2009). The prevalence of DR increases with the duration of diabetes, and nearly all patients with type I diabetes and more than 60 % with type II diabetes have some degree of retinopathy after 20 years (Fong *et al.*, 2003; Fong *et al.*, 2004a; Williams *et al.*, 2004a). Therefore, early detection and prevention are the current management strategies (Ciulla *et al.*, 2003). Chronic hyperglycemia is believed to be the primary pathogenic factor for inducing damage to retinal cells (Hammes, 2005; Knudsen *et al.*, 2002; Yanagi, 2008). However, the mechanisms that lead to DR are not fully understood (West *et al.*, 2006). DR is characterised by increased vascular permeability, due to a breakdown in the blood retinal barrier (BRB), which causes macular edema, followed later by the development of vascular microaneurysms, hemorrhages, hard exudates and intraocular pathological neovascularization (Cunha-Vaz *et al.*, 1975; Fong *et al.*, 2004a). Moreover, degenerative changes, including increased apoptosis, glial cell activation, microglial activation, and altered glutamate metabolism, occur beyond the vascular cells of the retina (Barber, 2003). Laser photocoagulation therapy is the most common treatment modality for DR. However, this therapy may damage neural tissue, resulting in the deterioration of vision (Bloomgarden, 2007). Therefore, development of new therapeutic strategies for the treatment of excessive retinal vasopermeability, angiogenic changes and apoptosis of neurons are the basis for further research focus (Barber, 2003; Garcia *et al.*, 2008).

Diabetes damages all the major cells of the retina, vascular cells (endothelial cells and pericytes) (Hammes *et al.*, 1995; Mizutani *et al.*, 1996), pigment epithelial cells (Decanini *et al.*, 2008), retinal microglial cells and retinal ganglion cells (Aoun *et al.*, 2003; Ibrahim *et al.*, 2011). Basement membrane thickening, pericyte drop out and retinal capillary non-perfusion occur prior to the damage, which changes the production pattern of a number of mediators, such as growth factors, vasoactive agents, coagulation factors and adhesion molecules. These result in increased blood flow and capillary diameter, proliferation of the extracellular matrix and thickening of basal membranes, altered cell turnover (apoptosis, proliferation, hypertrophy) and procoagulant/proaggregant patterns, and finally angiogenesis with tissue remodeling.

These pathological changes cause increased retinal vasopermeability and breakdown of the BRB, resulting in retinal hemorrhage, swelling, exudates, and retinal detachment (Ciulla *et al.*, 2003; Gardner *et al.*, 2000; Yam *et al.*, 2007). DR has many elements that suggest chronic neurodegeneration, including neural apoptosis, loss of ganglion cell bodies, reduction in thickness of the inner retina, glial reactivity, neurofilament abnormality, slowing of optic nerve retrograde transport, changes in electrophysiological activity, and resultant deficits in perception (Villarroel *et al.*, 2010). Moreover, neuoretinal degeneration initiates and/or activates several metabolic and signaling pathways as well as in the disruption of the BRB (Tretiach *et al.*, 2005).

The underlying pathophysiological mechanisms associated with hyperglycemia-induced diabetic retinopathy are through excessive formation of advanced glycation end products (AGEs) and production of excessive oxidative stress (Abu El-Asrar *et al.*, 2009; Ciulla *et al.*, 2003). Moreover, these biochemical mechanisms lead to a cascade of events, such as promotion of apoptosis, inflammation, neurodegeneration and angiogenesis, which induce damage to diabetic retina, leading to DR (Abu El-Asrar *et al.*, 2009; Barber, 2003; Ciulla *et al.*, 2003) (Figure 1).

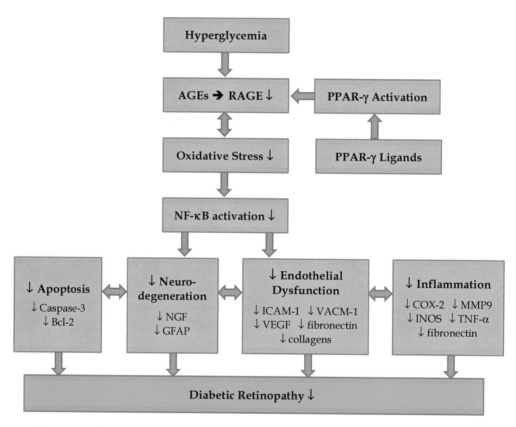

Figure 1: Schematic representation showing the role of PPAR-γ and its receptor system in the progression of diabetic retinopathy. Black arrows indicate pathway, red arrows indicate increase or decrease in activity following PPAR-γ activation (adapted from Yamagishi *et al.* 2009).

1.1   AGEs in Diabetic Retinopathy

AGEs are associated with modification of proteins or lipids that are generated from intermediate glycation products by non-enzymatic reaction of glucose with protein side chains (Goh *et al.*, 2008; Schmidt *et al.*, 1994). These intermediate glycation products undergo further condensation, dehydration or rearrangement, leading to eventual irreversible AGEs formation (Chu *et al.*, 2008).

AGEs formation occurs normally over time whereas an accelerated rate of AGE formation is accompanied by hyperglycemia (Munch *et al.*, 1998). The accumulated AGEs products are detected in the neural retina and vascular cells of diabetic animals, responsible for mediating the pathological angiogenesis and hyper-permeability in retina (Hammes *et al.*, 1999; Stitt *et al.*, 1997).

Several bodies of evidence suggest that the interaction between AGEs and their receptor (RAGE) activates nicotinamide adenine dinucleotide phosphate (NADPH) oxidase and enhances the formation of oxygen radicals, with subsequent activation and translocation of Nuclear Factor-KappaB (NF-κB), followed by release of pro-inflammatory cytokines and growth factors (Abu El-Asrar *et al.*, 2009). Moreover, AGEs can provide the early molecular pathogenesis mechanisms responsible for neuronal apoptosis and neuro-glial reaction (Lecleire-Collet *et al.*, 2005). In addition, AGEs enhance apoptosis in retinal pericytes, corneal endothelial cells and neuronal cells through increased oxidative stress or via induced expression of pro-apoptotic cytokines (Denis *et al.*, 2002; Kaji *et al.*, 2003; Kasper *et al.*, 2000). Indeed, AGEs induce apoptosis, angiogenesis, breakdown of the BRB, and leukocyte adhesion in the retina. Thus, AGEs are detrimental to the retinal vasculature and contribute to the pathogenesis of DR (Sato *et al.*, 2006; Stitt, 2001).

1.2 Oxidative Stress in Diabetic Retinopathy

Oxidative stress appears when there is a serious imbalance between generation of reactive oxygen species (ROS) and its clearance by anti-oxidant defenses (Brownlee, 2005; Ceriello *et al.*, 2001). Activation of RAGE results in production of oxidative stress (conversely, glycation itself is promoted by oxidative stress), and subsequent activation of NF-κB transcription factor in micro-vascular endothelial cells that are considered to be linked to endothelial dysfunction (Moore *et al.*, 2003; Vincent *et al.*, 2007). Retina, a tissue rich in polyunsaturated fatty acid, uses more oxygen and glucose oxidation than any other tissue in the body, and is very susceptible to damage (Schmidt *et al.*, 2003). Diabetic induced-oxidative stress, followed by activation of NF-κB in the retina, are early events in the pathogenesis of DR (Kowluru, 2005; Kowluru *et al.*, 1996; Kowluru *et al.*, 2001b; Obrosova *et al.*, 2005). Moreover, oxidative stress has been linked to the accelerated apoptosis of retinal ganglion cells, retinal capillary cells and micro-vascular abnormalities in DR (Allen *et al.*, 2005; Kern *et al.*, 2008).

1.3 NF-κB in Diabetic Retinopathy

NF-κB is a multi-protein complex which can activate many kinds of genes involved in cellular functions. Pathogenic stimuli allow NF-κB to enter the nucleus and to bind to DNA recognition sites in regulatory regions of target genes (Baeuerle *et al.*, 1994; Boileau *et al.*, 2003; Schreck *et al.*, 1992). NF-κB is required for maximal transcription of many pro-inflammatory molecules thought to be important in the generation of inflammation, including cell interaction molecules (eg intracellular adhesion molecule 1), critical enzymes (eg inducible nitric oxidase synthase, cyclooxygenase-2), and a number of cytokines (eg interleukin-1β, tumor necrosis factor-α, IL-6) (Blackwell *et al.*, 1997; Siebenlist *et al.*, 1994). The activation of NF-κB is considered a key signaling pathway by which high glucose induces apoptosis in endothelial cells (Du *et al.*, 1999). In the retina, NF-κB is localised in sub-retinal membranes and in micro-vessels

(Hammes *et al.*, 1999) and its activation is considered responsible for the accelerated loss of pericytes observed in DR (Romeo *et al.*, 2002). Moreover, the study has shown that diabetes-induced capillary degeneration, observed in DR, is at least closely associated with NF-κB activation in both vascular and neural compartments of retina and subsequent inflammatory response (Zheng *et al.*, 2007).

1.4 Inflammation in Diabetic Retinopathy

In recent years inflammation has been linked to vascular leakage in DR, at least in part (Adamis, 2002; Joussen *et al.*, 2002). Hyperglycemia is a contributing risk factor for the development of vascular dysfunction and production of inflammatory markers (Haubner *et al.*, 2007; Tawfik *et al.*, 2009). Indeed, pro-inflammatory cytokines, chemokines and other inflammatory mediators play an important role in the pathogenesis of DR. These lead to persistent low-grade inflammation, which in turn leads to neuronal cell death, the adhesion of leukocytes to the retinal vasculature (leukostasis), breakdown of BRB and tissue ischemia (Ali *et al.*, 2008; El-Remessy *et al.*, 2006; Joussen *et al.*, 2004; Kern, 2007). Several inflammatory molecules are involved in the pathogenesis of DR, including tumor necrotic factor (TNF-α, fibronectin, cyclo-oxygenase-2 (COX-2), intercellular cell adhesion molecule-1 (ICAM-1), vascular cell adhesion molecule-1 (VCAM-1) and matrix metalloproteinase-9 (MMP-9) (Joussen *et al.*, 2004; Miyamoto *et al.*, 1999; Yuuki *et al.*, 2001).

1.5 Angiogenesis in Diabetic Retinopathy

Angiogenesis is defined as the growth of new vessels from pre-existing capillaries, which is a complex process comprising endothelial cell proliferation, migration, extracellular proteolysis, tube formation and vessel remodeling (Beck *et al.*, 1997). In retina, vascular endothelial growth factor (VEGF) is the major angiogenic factor for neovascularization and vascular leakage via the mitogen-activated protein kinase (MAPK) pathway (De Luca *et al.*, 2008; Kliffen *et al.*, 1997; Miller *et al.*, 1994). Additional pro-angiogenic factors, including MMP-9, are also required for the process of ocular neovascularization through either synergistic effect with angiogenic factor or as a stimulant for the secretion of angiogenic factors (Hollborn *et al.*, 2007). In addition, MMP-9 expression acts as a factor in increasing vascular permeability in ocular neovascularization (Herzlich *et al.*, 2008). Neurotrophic factor, such as nerve growth factor (NGF), alone or in combination with other biological active endogenous molecules, have been found to exert angiogenic activity *in vitro* and *in vivo* (Calza *et al.*, 2001; Cantarella *et al.*, 2002). Moreover, NGF has been shown to induce neuronal-driven angiogenesis, leading to pathologic retinopathy (Liu *et al.*, 2010).

1.6 Apoptosis in Diabetic Retinopathy

Apoptosis is programmed cell death and is characterised by chromatin condensation, fragmentation, and formation of apoptotic bodies that can be triggered by various signals (Leal *et al.*, 2009; Li *et al.*, 1998; Nagata, 1997). Retinal microvascular cells are lost selectively via apoptosis before other histopathology is detectable in diabetes (Kern *et al.*, 2000; Kowluru *et al.*, 2004; Mizutani *et al.*, 1996). As oxidative stress is closely linked to apoptosis in diabetes, oxidative stress-induced apoptotic episodes have been demonstrated by retinal abnormalities, potential visual changes and the onset of the first neural and vascular change (El-Remessy *et al.*,

2006; Kowluru, 2005; Lopes de Faria *et al.*, 2001). Moreover, apoptotic cell death in retinal regions is a probable stimulus for the increased expression of molecules that enhance the breakdown of the BRB and lead to vascular proliferation (Henkind, 1978; Patz, 1982). Several studies have shown that retinal pigment epithelial cells, Glial cells (Zeng *et al.*, 2009), retinal ganglion cells (Abu El-Asrar *et al.*, 2004) and retinal pericytes (Leal *et al.*, 2009; Zeng *et al.*, 2010) undergo high glucose induced-apoptosis. The studies have shown that diabetes causes a chronic loss of neurons from the inner retina by increasing the frequency of apoptosis (de Faria *et al.*, 2002; Zhang *et al.*, 2000). Moreover, it has been well established that apoptosis represents a final common pathway of cell loss and hence vision loss (Doonan *et al.*, 2009). In addition, high glucose causes activation of several proteins involved in apoptotic cell death, including members of the caspase and Bcl-2 family (Allen *et al.*, 2005). Therefore, apoptosis plays an important role in the progression and pathogenesis of DR (Allen *et al.*, 2005; Leal *et al.*, 2009).

1.7 Neurodegeneration in Diabetic Retinopathy

Neurodegeneration is recognised as a pivotal feature of many diseases of the central nervous system. Although much of the research effort has focused on vascular changes, it is becoming apparent that the degenerative changes occur beyond the vascular cells of the retina. These include apoptosis, glial cell reactivity, microglial activation, and altered glutamate metabolism (Barber, 2003). Moreover, early neuronal and glial alterations are also evident in diabetes, including decrease in components of the electroretinogram (Sakai *et al.*, 1995) and increased apoptosis of retinal neurons (Barber *et al.*, 1998). Indeed, current evidences has shown that neurodegeneration of the retina is a critical component of DR (Barber, 2003). In addition, early in the course of DR, Müller cells markedly up-regulate their expression of glial fibrillary acidic protein (GFAP) (Barber *et al.*, 2000). Retinal ganglion cells are the earliest cells affected and have the highest rate of apoptosis. Moreover, neuroretinal degeneration initiates and/or activates several metabolic and signaling pathways which participate in the microangiographic process as well as the disruption of the BRB (Tretiach *et al.*, 2005). Elevated levels of glutamate, the major excitatory neurotransmitter in the retina, have been found in experimental models of diabetes (Pulido *et al.*, 2007).

1.8 Pathogenesis of Microglial Cells in Diabetic Retinopathy

Retinal glial cells, including macroglia (Müller cells and astrocytes) and microglia, are considered channels of communication between retinal blood vessels and neurons owing to their special spatial arrangement and regulatory functions. Under normal conditions, microglia are characterised by a down-regulated phenotype when compared to other macrophage populations of peripheral tissues (Malchiodi-Albedi *et al.*, 2008). The maintenance of microglia in the "inhibited" state is crucial for the maintaining tissue homeostasis and preventing the destructive potential of inflammatory response (Zeng *et al.*, 2008). Moreover, microglial activation appears early in the course of DR, before the onset of overt neuronal cell death (Krady *et al.*, 2005). In diabetes, retinal microglial cells are activated to release inflammatory cytokines, such as IL-1β, TNF-α, NO, MMPs and VEGF, and excitatory amino acids, such as glutamate that initiate neuronal loss and BRB breakdown seen in DR (Ibrahim *et al.*, 2011; Langmann, 2007). The study has shown that in STZ-induced diabetic rats treated with minocycline, a semi-synthetic tetracycline that counteracts microglial activation, as well as decreasing the expression of pro-inflammatory cytokines, caspase-3 levels are also decreased, suggesting a potential neuroprotective anti-apoptotic effect of inhibition of microglial activation (Krady *et al.*, 2005; Malchiodi-Albedi *et al.*, 2008). Moreover, in mice with alloxan-induced diabetes, changes in microglial cell morphology were the first detectable cellular modifications, apparently preceding ganglion cell apoptosis and increase in BRB permeability (Gaucher *et al.*, 2007).

1.9 Pathogenesis of Ganglion Cells in Diabetic Retinopathy

Although the clinically demonstrable changes to the retinal vasculature in diabetes have led to the general assumption that the retinopathy is solely a microvascular disease, diabetes also damages non-vascular cells of the retina, resulting in loss of ganglion cells (Kern *et al.*, 2008). Numerous studies have suggested that exposure to AGEs, inflammation or oxidative stress might contribute to retinal ganglion cell apoptosis (Kern *et al.*, 2008). Moreover, the diabetes-induced degeneration of retinal ganglion has been shown to involve inhibiting the activation of the pro-inflammatory NF-κB (Zheng *et al.*, 2007). Another potential cause of retinal ganglion cell loss is excitotoxicity due to excessive synaptic glutamate activity (Kowluru *et al.*, 2001a). Immunohistochemical studies of cross-sections of human retinas demonstrated an increase in expression of Bax, caspase-3 and caspase-9 in retinal ganglion cells from diabetic patients, suggesting at least some retinal ganglion cells might die via apoptosis (Oshitari *et al.*, 2008). Moreover, activated microglial cells in hypoxic neonatal retina produce increased amounts of pro-inflammatory cytokines, including TNF-α and IL-1β that could induce retinal ganglion cell death (Sivakumar *et al.*, 2011).

1.10 Pathogenesis of Retinal Pigment Epithelium in Diabetic Retinopathy

The retinal pigment epithelial (RPE) cells form a monolayer between the neuroretina and the choriocapillaris which are the essential components of the outer BRB that maintain physiological and structural balance within the retina (Bok, 1993; Rizzolo, 1997). The main characteristics of RPE cells are the presence of tight junctions at the apical side of their lateral molecules, which limit access of blood components to the retina. Moreover, RPE and photoreceptors are particularly susceptible to oxidative stress because of high oxygen consumption by photoreceptors (Beatty *et al.*, 2000). In response to damage caused by the hyperglycemic condition, RPE cells migrate and proliferate, leading to a break-down in adhesion between the RPE and the choroidal capillaries, followed by BRB breakdown compromising blood flow within the RPE layer and leading to eventual retinal edema (Kennedy *et al.*, 1995). These cascade episodes trigger the serum components and inflammatory cells to enter the vitreous cavity and sub-retinal space, exposing the RPE cells to a variety of cytokines, pro-inflammatory mediators, extracellular matrix proteins and growth factors, causing DR (Kimoto *et al.*, 2004). Several studies have shown that the expression of angiogenic cytokines, growth factors (e.g. VEGF) and metalloproteinases (e.g. MMP-9) are produced by RPE (Grossniklaus *et al.*, 2002). Moreover, the combined effects from chronic sustained inflammation and ROS generation promotes the development of RPE damage (de Jong, 2006; SanGiovanni *et al.*, 2005; Winkler *et al.*, 1999).

1.11 PPAR-γ and Diabetic Retinopathy

PPAR-γ is heterogeneously expressed in the mammalian eye, prominently present in the retinal pigmented epithelium, photoreceptor outer segments, choriocapillaries, and retinal ganglion cells (Aoun *et al.*, 2003; Herzlich *et al.*, 2008; Murata *et al.*, 2000). Recent studies have shown that retinal expression of PPAR-γ was suppressed in experimental models of diabetes and in endothelial cells treated with high glucose (Tawfik *et al.*, 2009). Moreover, PPAR-γ ligands are potent inhibitors of corneal angiogenesis and neovascularization (Muranaka *et al.*, 2006; Xin *et al.*, 1999). Administration of 15d-PGJ$_2$ has shown to inhibit VEGF-stimulated angiogenesis in rat cornea (Xin *et al.*, 1999). Similarly, choroidal neovascularization was markedly reduced by intravitreous injection of troglitazone. Laser photocoagulation-induced lesions in rat and monkey eyes showed significantly less leakage in troglitazone-treated animals (Murata *et al.*, 2000). In neonatal mice, intravitreous injection of rosiglitazone or troglitazone inhibited development of new retinal vessels. In the same study, TZDs have been found to inhibit retinal endothelial cell proliferation, migration, and tube formation in response to VEGF treatment (Touyz *et al.*, 2006). In addition, rosiglitazone inhibits both the retinal leukostasis and retinal leakage observed in experimental diabetic rats, which leads to the aggravation of retinal leukostasis, and retinal leakage in diabetic mice (Muranaka *et al.*, 2006). Moreover, rosiglitazone has been shown to delay the onset of DR (Shen *et al.*, 2008).

As inflammation plays a role in several neurodegenerative diseases, numerous research has been conducted on the role of PPAR-γ in inflammation-induced neurodegeneration (Arimoto *et al.*, 2003; Banati *et al.*, 1993; Heneka *et al.*, 2000). Moreover, it has more recently become appreciated that PPAR-γ agonists act on neurons and microglia to inhibit neurotoxic inflammation and subsequently neurodegeneration, partially through the abilities of agonist bound PPAR-RXR heterodimers to antagonise NFκ-B mediated gene transcription of several inflammatory mediators such as COX-2 and inducible nitric oxide synthase (iNOS) *in vitro* and *in vivo* (Bernardo *et al.*, 2000; Braissant *et al.*, 1996; Kim *et al.*, 2002; Luna-Medina *et al.*, 2005; Storer *et al.*, 2005). Troglitazone has been shown to prevent neuronal death induced by glutamate toxicity *in vitro* (Uryu *et al.*, 2002). Similarly, retinal ganglion cells were rescued from death by troglitazone (Aoun *et al.*, 2003). Therefore, the anti-inflammatory, anti-oxidative stress properties of PPAR-γ activation may allow the neuroprotection seen with PPAR-γ agonism (Hunter *et al.*, 2007). These findings suggest that PPAR-γ is involved in the pathogenesis of DR (Figure 1).

1.12 PPAR-γ and AGEs

PPAR-γ ligands have a significant role in prevention of AGEs-induced micro-vascular complications, including DR (Dolhofer-Bliesener *et al.*, 1996; Watson *et al.*, 2005). Indeed, PPAR-γ ligands have shown to inhibit the formation of AGEs (Rahbar *et al.*, 2000; Sobal *et al.*, 2005). The inhibitory action of PPAR-γ ligands on AGE formation may be ascribed to their anti-oxidative properties (Gerry *et al.*, 2008; Giaginis *et al.*, 2008; Sulistio *et al.*, 2008; Yamagishi *et al.*, 2007). The study has shown that rosiglitazone inhibits extracellular matrix accumulation, fibronectin and type IV collagen in AGE-injected rats, and also inhibits the AGE-induced proliferation and NO production in cardiac fibroblasts (Li *et al.*, 2008; Yu *et al.*, 2007b). Moreover, activation of PPAR-γ by rosiglitazone inhibits AGE-induced inducible NO synthase expression, nitrite release, fibronectin and type IV collagen production (Chang *et al.*, 2004b; Yu *et al.*, 2007b).

1.13 PPAR-γ in NF-κB, Inflammatory Mediators and Angiogenesis

PPAR-γ plays an important role in a variety of biological processes, including inflammation and angiogenesis, mediated through the inhibition of NF-κB (Kim *et al.*, 2007; Lee *et al.*, 2006; Rosen *et al.*, 2001; Sung *et al.*, 2006). Rosiglitazone was shown to inhibit both retinal leukostasis and retinal leakage by the inhibition of NF-κB activation, with consequent suppression of ICAM-1 expression (Muranaka *et al.*, 2006). In addition, recent evidence has shown that the suppression of PPAR-γ in diabetic retina is associated with the activation of NF-κB target gene expression (Remels *et al.*, 2009; Tawfik *et al.*, 2009). Stimulation of a pro-inflammatory response in microglia *in vitro* and the resulting production of neurotoxic inflammatory mediators were found to be suppressed by administration of a number structurally distinct PPAR-γ agonists (Luna-Medina *et al.*, 2005; Storer *et al.*, 2005). In addition, TZDs have been shown to attenuate lipopolysaccharide-induced neuroinflammation by PPAR-γ activation in neural cells (Luna-Medina *et al.*, 2005).

The activation of PPAR-γ inhibits the pro-inflammatory pathways, including cytokine secretion (Uchimura *et al.*, 2001; Wong *et al.*, 2001) and iNOS expression (Petrova *et al.*, 1999; Reilly *et al.*, 2001) in a variety of cell lines. Indeed, PPAR-γ agonists have been shown to suppress cytokine evoked neuronal iNOS expression, thereby preventing NO-mediated cell death of neurons (Heneka *et al.*, 1999). Inhibition of ICAM-1 expression and retinal vascular leakage in experimental diabetes has been shown by rosiglitazone, and the increase in the same parameters by depletion of the gene encoding PPAR-γ (Muranaka *et al.*, 2006). PPAR-γ ligands have also been shown to inhibit the expression of VEGF receptors and the subsequent activation of downstream signaling pathways (Murata *et al.*, 2001; Xin *et al.*, 1999). Moreover, rosiglitazone has been shown to inhibit retinal neovascularization in OIR by a mechanism downstream from VEGF-induced angiogenesis (Murata *et al.*, 2001). In addition, it has been suggested that ICAM-1 is involved in VEGF-induced leukocyte-endothelial cell interactions and subsequent (BRB) breakdown in the diabetic retina (Miyahara *et al.*, 2004). Furthermore, PPAR-γ activation inhibits VEGF-mediated angiogenesis through the modulation of the stimulated COX-2 expression and activity (Scoditti *et al.*, 2009).

1.14 PPAR-γ and Apoptosis

Apoptosis is a complex process, involving a multitude of signaling pathways that regulate the activities of pro- and anti-apoptotic members of the Bcl-2 family of proteins which play an important role in various cell types (Bonne, 2005; Fehlberg *et al.*, 2003; Fuenzalida *et al.*, 2007b). Oxidative stress can induce mitochondrial dysfunction, followed by cytochrome c release and subsequent activation of caspases, a group of enzymes that execute apoptosis (Danial *et al.*, 2004; Lin *et al.*, 2006). A recent study has shown that rosiglitazone protects against oxidative stress-induced apoptosis through up-regulation of anti-apoptotic Bcl-2 family proteins (Ren *et al.*, 2009). Moreover, rosiglitazone and PPAR-γ over-expression protect against apoptosis induced by oxygen and glucose deprivation followed by re-oxygenation and up-regulation of Bcl-2 (Wu *et al.*, 2009). In contrast, down-regulation of NF-κB activation by PPAR-γ ligands protects the cells from destruction via the apoptotic pathways (Baker *et al.*, 2001; Grey *et al.*, 1999). A screen of FDA-approved compounds identified rosiglitazone as a novel anti-apoptotic agent in retinal cells both *in vivo* and *in vitro* (Doonan *et al.*, 2009). Troglitazone has shown cytoprotective activity in apoptotic-induced ARPE-19 cells (Rodrigues *et al.*, 2010). One further study has indicated that 15d-PGJ$_2$ helps RPE cells to maintain mitochondrial integrity by prevention of cytochrome c release and subsequent activation of the apoptosis pathway (Chang *et al.*, 2008b; Garg *et al.*, 2004). Moreover, rosiglitazone has been shown to protect hippocampal and dorsal root ganglion neurons against Aβ-induced mitochondrial damage and NGF deprivation-induced apoptosis (Fuenzalida *et al.*, 2007a).

1.15 PPAR-γ in Retinal Microglia and Retinal Ganglion Cells

The beneficial effects of PPAR-γ ligands on the ocular system have been supported by various reports. Troglitazone and 15d-PGJ$_2$ have been shown to protect retinal ganglion cells, RGC-5, from glutamate-induced apoptosis (Aoun *et al.*, 2003). Microglial cells have shown to express PPAR-γ and that such basal expression is increased by its specific agonists, while it is reduced in the presence of microglial activators such as lipopolysaccharide (LPS) and interferon-γ (IFN-γ) (Forman *et al.*, 1995). Moreover, 15d-PGJ$_2$ has been shown to prevent LPS-induced iNOS expression and TNF-α production in primary microglial cultures, by mechanisms involving PPAR-γ activation and reduced activation of NFκ-B, which is known to mediate LPS and IFN-γ signaling (Bernardo *et al.*, 2000). Similarly, PPAR-γ agonists have been shown to modulate LPS-induced neuronal death in mixed cortical neurons, suggesting a PPAR-γ mediated mechanism of neuroprotection (Kim *et al.*, 2002).

1.16 PPAR-γ and RPE Cells

A number of studies have shown that RPE might be the prime target for oxidative stress and PPAR-γ ligands modulate cellular defense against the oxidative stress (Chang *et al.*, 2008a). 15-dPGJ$_2$ protects RPE cells from oxidative stress by elevating GSH and enhancing MAPK activation through a PPAR-γ independent pathway (Qin *et al.*, 2006). In addition, 15-dPGJ$_2$, independent of its PPAR-γ activity, protects RPE cells from oxidative injury by raising intracellular GSH levels and extending hydrogen peroxide-induced activation of JNK and p38, suggesting the possible application of the agents in preventing ocular diseases from oxidative stress (Garg *et al.*, 2003; Qin *et al.*, 2006).

2 Lycium Barbarum - a Traditional Chinese Medicine (TCM)

2.1 Botanical Description

The fruit from *Lycium barbarum* L. (LB) in the family Solanaceae is a well-known traditional Chinese medicine. The earliest Chinese medicinal monograph documented medicinal use of LB around 2300 years ago (Luo *et al.*, 2004) (Figure 2).

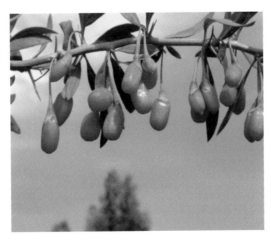

Figure 2: *Lycium barbarum.*

"Wolfberry' is the common English name for the plant, while the name "Goji berry" is in common use in the health food market for berries from this plant (J Helmer, 2006; Marchuck, 2005). LB is deciduous woody shrub with thorny branches up to 10 feet in length and bright red edible berries which are the source of the Chinese medicine "gou qi" or "gou qi zi". The number of seeds in each berry varies widely based on cultivar and fruit sizes, containing any-where between 10-60 tiny yellow seeds that are compressed with a curved embryo. The berries ripen from July to October in the northern hemisphere (Chiu *et al.*, 2009; Flint, 1997). LB is sim-ilar in texture and size to a raisin, and is widely consumed in China for its pleasant flavor. The dried berries can be chewed and eaten without further processing, or added in teas, soups and stews (Cheng *et al.*, 2005).

2.2 Traditional Use

According to the traditional Chinese medicine literature, LB has been known for balancing "Yin" and "Yang" in the body, nourishing the liver, kidney and improving visual acuity for more than 2500 years (Chang *et al.*, 2008b; Gao *et al.*, 2000). LB has been regarded as an upper class traditional Chinese medicine in several ancient Chinese pharmacopoeias since the Tang Dynasty, indicating that LB is one of the ingredients in Chinese medicinal products (Chang *et al.*, 2008b). According to Chinese literature, LB contains several valuable and important prop-erties and useful for various treatments and health supplements. These include nourishing the blood, enriching the yin, tonifying the kidney and liver, and moistening the lungs. It is applied in the treatment of early-onset diabetes, tuberculosis, dizziness, blurred vision, diminished visual acuity and chronic cough (Yu *et al.*, 2005). Moreover, LB has been used in various oph-thalmic conditions, including glaucoma, cataract and retinitis pigmentosa (Tu, 1992).

2.3 Lycium *Barbarum* in Diabetic Retinopathy

DR is a frequent complication in the eye of individuals with long-term diabetes and remains the leading cause of vision loss in working-age adults throughout the world (Ciulla *et al.*, 2003). Control of metabolic abnormalities of diabetes has been shown to effectively prevent the development and progression of DR (Aiello *et al.*, 2001). However, many patients fail to achieve or maintain optimal levels of metabolic control. Therefore, early detection and timely treatment of DR remains standard management (Ciulla *et al.*, 2003). Laser photocoagulation therapy and vitrectomy have proven effective for reducing DR progression and sight-saving interventions. However, these treatments are invasive, associated with destructive side effects, and only treat the late stages of disease and cause significant financial burden (Ciulla *et al.*, 2003; Lewis *et al.*, 1992). Therefore, emerging treatments, possibly in combination with stand-ard therapy, may provide a superior efficacy and safety profile, targeting the underlying bio-chemical mechanisms for the treatment or prevention of DR. LB has been widely used as nu-tritional food product with a large variety of beneficial effects, such as reducing blood glucose and serum lipids, anti-oxidant, immune-modulation, neuroprotection, and anti-inflammatory activity (Cao *et al.*, 1993; Peng *et al.*, 2001; Wang *et al.*, 2002). There is a growing body of evi-dence indicating that LB intake increases the fasting plasma zeaxanthin levels, beneficial for maintaining macular pigment density in age-related macular degeneration (Cheng *et al.*, 2005). LB has been shown to be effective in the treatment of glaucoma and modulating immunity in retinal ganglion cells in a rat hypertension model (Chan *et al.*, 2007; Chiu *et al.*, 2009). Moreo-ver, LB polysaccharides has been shown to improve insulin resistance by increasing the cell-surface level of glucose transporter 4 (GLUT4), improving GLUT4 trafficking and intracellular insulin signaling in streptozotocin-induced diabetic rats (Zhao *et al.*, 2005).

Even though there is a significant and growing body of *in vitro* and animal research on the efficacy of LB in various medical fields in recent years, there is limited high-quality research available on its efficacy and possible mechanisms for vision enhancement or prevention of vision disorders. Moreover, given the body of traditional knowledge on the effect of LB in eye pathophysiology further research is warranted on the active constituents of LB and their investigation for maximum therapeutic potential for treatment of DR.

2.4 Taurine Content in *Lycium Barbarum* (Goji Berry)

LB has been widely used as nutritional food product with a large variety of beneficial effects, such as reducing blood glucose and serum lipids, anti-oxidant, immune-modulation, neuro-protection, and anti-inflammatory activity (Cao *et al.*, 1993; Peng *et al.*, 2001; Wang *et al.*, 2002). Taurine is one of the chemical components abundantly present in LB. The chromatographic methods have been reported for the identification and quantification of taurine content from LB extracts (Cao *et al.*, 2003; Song *et al.*, 2011c; Xie *et al.*, 1997).

2.5 Taurine in Diabetic Retinopathy

LB contains a high content of taurine which crosses the blood-retinal barrier (Cao *et al.*, 2003; Tomi *et al.*, 2007; Xie *et al.*, 1997). A dietary source of taurine is essential for those animals (e.g. cat and humans) which cannot synthesise sufficient taurine and where greater consumption of taurine is required, such as in diabetes (Kawasaki, 1998). Moreover, the concentration of taurine in photoreceptors, RPE cells and retina is estimated to be around 60 to 80 mM, which corresponds to about 40-75% of the total free amino acid content considered necessary to maintain physiological functions, including membrane stabilisation, neuromodulation and integrity of retina (Hayes *et al.*, 1975; Pasantes-Morales *et al.*, 1972; Vilchis *et al.*, 1996). Several previous articles have reported that taurine potentiates the effect of insulin (Donadio *et al.*, 1964; Lampson *et al.*, 1983) and possibly modulates the insulin receptor (Kulakowski *et al.*, 1990; Maturo *et al.*, 1988). Moreover, it has been shown that taurine inhibits the activation of caspase-3 in ischaemic cardiomyocytes (Takatani *et al.*, 2004). Taurine has also been found to prevent high-glucose-mediated endothelial cell apoptosis through its antioxidant property (Wu *et al.*, 1999).

Taurine has been recommended as a complementary therapeutic agent for the prevention of diabetic complications in type II diabetes (McCarty, 1997; Yu *et al.*, 2008). Taurine (Figure 3) is a sulfur-containing amino acid that is found in high intracellular concentrations in most animal tissues (Hansen, 2001). Although the main function of taurine is the formation of bile salts, other functions have been reported, including effects on retinal development, antioxidation, neuroinhibition, maintenance of excitatory activity in muscle, inhibitory action of inflammatory cytokines in the brain, osmotic regulation of cell volume and formation of *N*-chlorotaurine in leukocytes as part of the host defense (Chang *et al.*, 2001; Hansen, 2001). A glucose lowering effect of taurine was first reported in the 1930s and repeated in later studies (Dokshina *et al.*, 1976; Hansen, 2001; Kulakowski *et al.*, 1984; Silaeva *et al.*, 1976). Several papers have reported that taurine potentiates the effect of insulin (Donadio *et al.*, 1964; Lampson *et al.*, 1983) and possibly affects the insulin receptor (Kulakowski *et al.*, 1990; Maturo *et al.*, 1988). In addition, one recent study has stated that high concentrations of taurine are capable of en

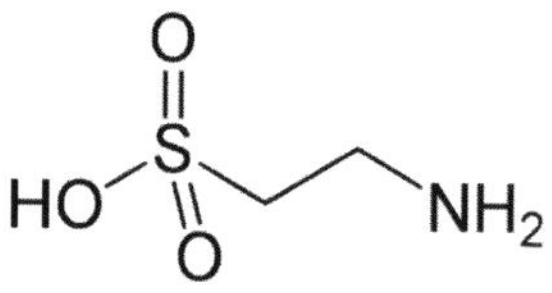

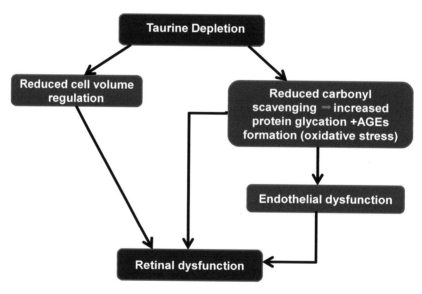

Figure 3: Chemical Structure of Taurine.

hancing the phosphatidylinositide 3 (PI3)-kinase/Akt signaling pathway responsible for insulin-mediated stimulation of GLUT4 activity and glucose uptake (Takatani *et al.*, 2004).

Several clinical trials have found that poorly controlled diabetes or ketoacidosis is associated with high urinary taurine excretion (Martensson *et al.*, 1984; Szabo *et al.*, 1991). A dietary source of taurine is essential for those animals (cat and humans) which cannot synthesize sufficient taurine and in conditions where more consumption of taurine is required, such as diabetes (Kawasaki, 1998). Alteration of taurine metabolism and the development of cellular dysfunction have been observed in diabetes (Figure 4) (Hansen, 2001). Moreover, it has been recommended that taurine be used as a complementary therapeutic agent for the prevention of diabetic complications in type II diabetes (McCarty, 1997).

Figure 4: Scheme illustrating the possible consequences of depletion of taurine for the endothelium and retinal function. The loss of cellular volume regulation and decreased scavenging of reactive carbonyl compounds induce dysfunctions of several cell types (adapted from Hansen *et al.* 2001).

The concentration of taurine in photoreceptors, retinal pigment epithelial (RPE) cells is estimated to be around 60 to 80 mM, which corresponds to about 40-75% of the total free amino acid content required to maintain the structure and functional integrity of retina (Hayes *et al.*, 1975; Pasantes-Morales *et al.*, 1972; Vilchis *et al.*, 1996). Moreover, taurine is actively transported by Na$^+$-dependent taurine transporter protein into the retina and RPE through the blood-retinal barrier (Heller-Stilb *et al.*, 2002). Down-regulation of the taurine transporter activity has been observed in retinal epithelial cells by glucose-induced protein kinase C activation (Stevens *et al.*, 1999).

Taurine is known to reduce high glucose-induced AGEs formation through the glycation scavenger function (Devamanoharan *et al.*, 1997; Hansen, 2001; Nandhini *et al.*, 2004). Taurine has been reported to protect against retinal damage produced by photochemical stress via antioxidant and anti-apoptotic mechanisms in rats (Yu *et al.*, 2007a). Moreover, taurine has been shown to diminish the expression of the angiotensin AT_2 receptor in the diabetic cardiomyocyte (Li *et al.*, 2005), an action that provides a direct link between the beneficial effects of taurine and modulation of ROS generation by angiotensin II (Gurujeyalakshmi *et al.*, 2000; Ricci *et al.*, 2008). The taurine-taurinechloramine system is reported to down-regulate NF-κB activity (Barua *et al.*, 2001; Kim *et al.*, 2005; Kontny *et al.*, 2000), nitric oxide synthase 2, TNF-α, COX-2 (Liu *et al.*, 1998; Park *et al.*, 2002) and inflammatory cytokines (Kontny *et al.*, 1999; Park *et al.*, 1993). One other study has shown that taurine down-regulates VEGF in diabetic retina (Zeng *et al.*, 2009). Interestingly, taurine administration decreases the levels of glutamate and GABA in diabetic retinas, so as to effectively protect against DR via anti-excitotoxicity of glutamate (Yu *et al.*, 2008).

Even though, a significant number of studies have been carried out on the efficacy of taurine on DR, a more comprehensive understanding of underlying mechanisms is needed for better elucidation of the relationship between taurine and DR.

3 Current Research on *Lycium barbarum*

LB has been widely used as a functional food, with promotion of a large variety of beneficial effects, such as serum lipids, anti-oxidant, anti-aging, immune-modulating, neuroprotection, anti-cancer, anti-fatigue, and anti-inflammatory (Cao *et al.*, 1993; Peng *et al.*, 2001; Wang *et al.*, 2002). The most abundant and well-researched chemical components to date are the polysaccharides, the caroteinoids (lutein and zeaxanthin) (Huang *et al.*, 2001; Luo *et al.*, 2006; Peng *et al.*, 2005).

There is a growing body of evidence to support the efficacy of LB and its related mechanisms in various biological systems. LB polysaccharides (LBP) has been shown to antagonize glutamate excitotoxicity in rat cortical neurons (Ho *et al.*, 2009). Feeding mice with LBP at 100 mg/kg daily has shown to reduce serum AGEs levels in erythrocytes (Deng *et al.*, 2003). Interestingly, LBP shows an inhibitory effect on apoptosis and anti-inflammatory action in cultured seminiferous epithelium (Wang *et al.*, 2002). Indeed, LBP appears to reduce the expression of VEGF and transforming growth factor-β1 (TGF-β1) in H~2~2-bearing mice (Yanli, 2005). LBP has also been shown to activate NF-κB and activator protein 1 (AP-1), and to induce TNF-α, interleukin 1β (IL-1β) mRNA expression in RWA264.7 macrophage cells (Chen *et al.*, 2009). Moreover, one LBP fraction showed up-regulation of NF-κB and AP-1 expression and stimulated proliferation of isolated splenocytes and B-lymphocytes (Peng *et al.*, 2001). A recent study has shown that mice drinking LB juice are protected from UV radiation-induced skin damage through anti-oxidant pathways by up-regulation of haem oxygenase-1 and metallothionein l (Reeve *et al.*, 2010).

LB is also considered to benefit vision because of its high antioxidant content (Bucheli *et al.*, 2011). One human supplementation trial showed that LB intake increased the fasting plasma zeaxathin levels, beneficial for maintaining macular pigment density in age-related macular degeneration (Cheng *et al.*, 2005). LBPs have also been shown to increase anti-apoptotic protein Bcl-2 levels in epithelial cells of the whole lens incubated in culture medium and exposed to hydrogen peroxide (Wang *et al.*, 2002). LBP has been shown to be neuroprotective in retinal ganglion cells against ocular hypertension (Chiu *et al.*, 2009). LB has been shown to be effective in glaucoma and in modulating immune functions in retinal ganglion cells in a rat hypertension model (Chan *et al.*, 2007). Moreover, LBP has been shown to reduce neuronal damage, blood retinal barrier disruption and oxidative stress in retinal ischemia/reperfusion injury (Li *et al.*, 2011).

3.1 Lycium Barbarum (Goji Berry) Extracts and its Taurine Component Inhibit PPAR-gamma-dependent Gene Transcription in Human Retinal Pigment Epithelial Cells: Possible Implications for Diabetic Retinopathy Treatment (*Biochemical Pharmacology*, 2011, 82(9): 1209-1218)

The study by Song *et al* investigated the mechanism of action of an extract from LB on a model of DR, the retinal ARPE-19 cell line, and identified the receptor function of taurine, an active component of LB extract, which is potentially responsible for the protective effect on DR (Song *et al.*, 2011c). Through bioassay and TLC analytical screening methods, we demonstrated that taurine present in methanol LB extract appears to be the active component responsible for the PPAR-γ activation. The range of taurine concentrations in the LB extract used in the experiments, 0.086 – 0.86 mM, falls within the range of pure taurine concentrations (0.001- 1.00 mM) used. The study has demonstrated for the first time that LB and its taurine component dose-dependently enhance PPAR-γ luciferase activity in HEK293 cell line transfected with PPAR-γ reporter gene. This activity was significantly decreased by a selective PPAR-γ antagonist GW9662. Moreover, LB extract and taurine dose-dependently enhanced the expression of PPAR-γ mRNA and protein. In an inflammation model, where ARPE-19 cells were exposed to high glucose, LB extract and taurine down-regulated the mRNA of pro-inflammatory mediators encoding MMP-9, fibronectin and the protein expression of COX-2 and iNOS proteins. The predicted binding mode of taurine in the PPAR-γ ligand binding site was found to mimic key electrostatic interactions seen with known PPAR-γ agonists. Therefore, PPAR-γ activation by LB extract is mimicked by taurine, which may explain at least in part its use in diabetic retinopathy progression.

The agonist-receptor binding affinity of LB extract and its taurine component as PPAR-γ activators could further be explored using ligand binding assay to determine whether the activators directly or indirectly bind to the receptor and allow binding affinity profiles to be established. Moreover, more *in vitro* studies can be further carried out to confirm *in vivo* observations and the proposed consequences of these interactions to the nuclear receptor and its biological effects. In order to determine the key chemical interactions responsible for PPAR-γ activity, the molecular structure of taurine was simulated in the binding site of the PPAR-γ crystal structure via computational analysis. An induced-fit docking approach was used as it accounts for side-chain rearrangements induced by ligand binding in (Song *et al.*, 2011c). However, further work would be required to elucidate a truly accurate conformation of the taurine-PPAR-γ complex, which would require exhaustive computational approaches (e.g. molecular dynamics) or other experimental techniques (e.g. x-ray crystallography). The ensemble of 10 IFD poses presented here serves as an efficient guide into the plausible binding modes of taurine. Although it is highly plausible that taurine activates PPAR-γ directly, taurine has shown weak binding affinity overall (Song *et al.*, 2011c). This is presumably a consequence of stronger desolvation penalty caused by its zwitterionic state, its smaller size and the lack of hydrophobic functional groups seen in more potent agonists. Therefore, further studies could be focused on finding taurine-like compound(s) from LB with high binding affinity by virtual high throughput screening using computer-generated models. Moreover, multiple rigid-receptor dockings and IFD have been shown to support the identification of novel hit compounds and to enable a detailed ligand-receptor binding complex proposal (Salam *et al.*, 2008).

3.2 Modulation of RAGE and the Downstream Targets of RAGE Signaling Cascades by Taurine in Lycium Barbarum (Goji Berry): Protection of Human Retinal Pigment Epithelial Barrier Function and Its Potential Benefit in Diabetic Retinopathy (*Journal Of Diabetes & Metabolism*, 2011, 2(9): 162)

RPE barrier disruption is an early event in DR. One of the underlying pathophysological mechanisms associated with hyperglycaemia-induced DR is excessive formation of AGEs and subsequent interaction with their receptor advanced glycation end products (RAGE) (Stitt, 2003). Activation of RAGE results in oxidative stress, and the subsequent activation of NF-κB transcription factor is considered to be linked to epithelial dysfunction (Ma *et al.*, 2007). These cascade episodes trigger serum components and inflammatory cells to enter the vitreous cavity and sub-retinal space, exposing the RPE cells to pro-inflammatory mediators, including ICAM-1 and VEGF, causing BRB breakdown and vascular leakage, leading to further progression of DR (Kimoto *et al.*, 2004; Wang *et al.*, 2011). A body of evidence has shown that PPAR-γ ligands inhibit the formation of AGEs (Rahbar *et al.*, 2000; Sobal *et al.*, 2005). Moreover, rosiglitazone has been shown to inhibit both retinal leukostasis and retinal leakage by inhibition of NF-κB activation, with consequent suppression of ICAM-1 expression (Muranaka *et al.*, 2006). Study by Song *et al.* investigated the effect of pure taurine and an extract of LB extract rich in taurine on a model of DR, the ARPE-19 cell line treated with high glucose, and whether their effects on RPE barrier disruption by glucose may contribute to protection against DR (Song *et al.*, 2011b). Both taurine and the extract of LB rich in taurine dose-dependently down-regulate the increased levels of RAGE, NF-κB, VEGF and ICAM-1 in the ARPE-19 cell line exposed to 33.3 mM glucose. This reversal was associated with attenuation of high glucose-induced RPE barrier disruption, which was shown by increased TER, reduced FITC-dextran permeability, characteristic morphological staining and dose-dependent modulation of claudin-1 and connexin 43 protein expression. Pure taurine and LB extract protect against barrier disruption following exposure of ARPE-19 cells to high glucose (Song *et al.*, 2011b). These effects are associated with altered NF-κB, ICAM-1 activity and VEGF secretion. Taurine and LB extract decrease RAGE (Song *et al.*, 2011b) . As they are known to activate PPAR-γ we proposed that their effects on barrier disruption may occur through their effects on RAGE and the downstream targets of RAGE signaling cascades. This pathway provides a rationale for the potential of taurine and the LB extract for protection against progression of DR.

3.3 Reversal of the Caspase-Dependent Apoptotic Cytotoxicity Pathway by Taurine from Lycium Barbarum (Goji Berry) in Human Retinal Pigment Epithelial Cells: Potential Benefit in Diabetic Retinopathy (*Evidence-Based Complementary And Alternative Medicine*, 2012, 2012:323784)

Apoptosis is important in the progression and pathogenesis of DR (Song *et al.*, 2012b). Research has suggested that apoptotic episodes in retinal cells during the initial stage of diabetes play an integral role in the early stage of vision loss (Barber *et al.*, 2011). Retinal pigment epithelial cell apoptosis is an early event in DR. Moreover, recent studies have suggested that ligand-activated PPAR-γ modulates apoptosis, contributing to tissue protection (Wu *et al.*, 2009). Song et al., 2012 investigated the cytoprotective effect of pure taurine and an extract of LB rich in taurine on a model of DR, the retinal ARPE-19 cell line exposed to high glucose (Song *et al.*, 2012b). In the study it was demonstrated for the first time that LB extract and the active ligand, taurine, dose-dependently enhance cell viability following high glucose-treatment in the ARPE-19 retinal epithelial cell line. This cytoprotective effect was associated with the attenuation of high glucose-induced apoptosis, which was shown by characteristic morphological staining and the dose-dependent decrease in the number of apoptotic cells, determined by flow cytometry. Moreover, LB extract and taurine have been shown to dose-dependently down-regulate caspase-3 protein expression and the enzymatic activity of caspase-3 (Song *et al.*, 2012b). Therefore, taurine, has a cytoprotective effect against glucose exposure in the human retinal epithelial cell line, and may provide useful approaches to delaying DR progression.

3.4 Final Thoughts

Overall LB extract and its taurine component may be involved at least in part in delaying the progression of DR through activation of PPAR-γ. However, future effort will focus on research to further demonstrate the effectiveness of LB extract and its taurine component in the prevention of DR. Synthetic PPAR-γ agonists, including rosiglitazone have beneficial effects on diabetes, a trail of evidence indicates that long term intake of these agents may increase the risk of cardiovascular-related disease, such as myocardial infarction (Barnett *et al.*, 2003; Khanderia *et al.*, 2008; Rendell *et al.*, 2004; Roehr, 2010). This issue has prompted the search for safe and novel compounds (of non-thiazolidione-related types) to manage diabetic complications, with herbal and natural products being an important source (Ceylan-Isik *et al.*, 2008; Song *et al.*, 2011a). Taurine is endogenously produced by the human body, and often exogenously supplemented when there is deficiency to maintain the structural and functional integrity of retina (Bouckenooghe *et al.*, 2006; Chang *et al.*, 2004a; Franconi *et al.*, 2004; Yu *et al.*, 2005). Moreover, several studies have suggested that taurine has strong cardiovascular protective effects (Ahn, 2009; Oudit *et al.*, 2004). Therefore, more conclusive studies on the mechanism of action of taurine and its relation to its long term safety and efficacy in DR are warranted.

Although much of the research effort has focused on vascular changes, it is becoming apparent that the degenerative changes occur beyond the vascular cells of the retina. These include apoptosis, glial cell reactivity, microglial activation, and altered glutamate metabolism (Barber, 2003). Early neuronal and glial alterations are also evident in diabetes. These changes include decreases in components of the electroretinogram, an objective method of evaluating retinal function (Sakai *et al.*, 1995), and increased apoptosis of retinal neurons (Barber *et al.*, 1998). Indeed, current evidence has shown that neurodegeneration of the retina is a critical component of DR (Barber, 2003). Moreover, it has more recently become appreciated that PPAR-γ agonists act on neurons and microglia to inhibit neurotoxic inflammation and subsequently neurodegeneration, partially through the abilities of agonist bound PPAR-RXR heterodimers to antagonise NFκ-B mediated gene transcription of several inflammatory mediators such as COX-2 and iNOS *in vitro* and *in vivo* (Bernardo *et al.*, 2000; Braissant *et al.*, 1996; Kim *et al.*, 2002; Luna-Medina *et al.*, 2005; Storer *et al.*, 2005). Therefore, further investigations into their specific mechanisms in various retinal cells are warranted to confirm the modulating effect of LB and its taurine component in the progression of DR through the PPAR-γ activation.

Taurine levels in physiological fluids have been a useful tool for both pathological diagnostic purpose and establishing disease therapy management (Schuller-Levis *et al.*, 2006). Taurine has been measured in animal models of disease as well as a variety of human conditions (Gamagedara *et al.*, 2012; Timbrell *et al.*, 1995). However, it remains unclear how taurine could be used as a reliable prognostic or diagnostic biomarker for DR. Therefore, future studies could be focused on conclusive *in vivo* and clinical validation of the biomarker using appropriate parameters.

4   Conclusion

Diabetic retinopathy remains one of the major risk factors and a leading cause of preventable blindness worldwide. There is a strong body of evidence on the prevalence of the variety of anti-angiogenic agents, anti-inflammatory agents, anti-oxidants, anti-fibrogenesis and neuroprotective agents present in the retinal regions for slowing down the progression of DR (Song *et al.*, 2012c). Moreover, the increasing importance of understanding the specific molecular and biochemical changes in DR leads to the requirement for development of novel therapeutic interventions. Although it is an important cause of blindness, initially DR presents few visual or ophthalmic symptoms until complete visual loss occurs (Fong *et al.*, 2004a). Current treatments of DR rarely improve visual function and are limited to surgical options in an advanced stage, with excessive side effects and significant financial burden. Hence, emerging treatments, possibly in combination with standard therapy, may provide superior efficacy and safety profile for the treatment or prevention of DR. Moreover, the new strategies move a paradigm in treating the early stages of DR. The recent advancements in the knowledge of the pathogenic alterations driving ocular damage and vision loss in DR strongly focus on PPAR-γ as a valuable target to control high glucose-induced inflammation, apoptosis and angiogenesis (Song *et al.*, 2012a). PPAR-γ functions as a transcription factor and thereby controlling cellular processes at the level of gene expression, through modulation by its nuclear receptor activity of selective downstream gene expression (Huang *et al.*, 2005). Moreover, PPAR-γ is an attractive and relatively unexploited target for herbal-derived medicines in DR (Song *et al.*, 2012a). This chapter confirms that the traditional Chinese medicine LB and its taurine component enhance PPAR-γ activity. At the same time both LB extract and pure taurine inhibited a variety of PPAR-γ dependent downstream pro-inflammatory mediators in the retinal cells. Moreover, LB is cytoprotective against high glucose cytotoxicity in ARPE-19 cells, at least in part by regulating apoptosis as a result of caspase-3 modulation, possibly through PPAR-γ activation. The effects of the extract are mimicked by taurine at concentrations present in the extracts. Finally, LB and its taurine component have been shown to protect against barrier permeability disruption following exposure of ARPE-19 cells to high glucose. These effects are associated with altered NF-κB, ICAM-1 activity and VEGF secretion. Taurine and LB decrease RAGE. As they have been shown to activate PPAR-γ, their effects on barrier disruption may occur through their effects on RAGE and the downstream targets of RAGE signaling cascades. These pathways provide a rationale for the potential of taurine and the LB extract for protection against progression of DR. Delineation of the similar effects of LB extract and taurine provides a rationale for the therapeutic use of this valuable medicinal herb and its taurine component. In combination with standard therapy it may provide superior efficacy and safety profile for the treatment or prevention of DR. However, further investigation into their exact mechanism is warranted and required to gather proof of efficacy and safety of LB for possible protection against DR-related pathophysiology and disease progression.

Authors

Min Kyong Song
Faculty of Pharmacy, The University of Sydney, Australia

Basil D. Roufogalis
Faculty of Pharmacy and Discipline of Pharmacology, School of Medical Sciences, The University of Sydney, Australia

Tom Hsun-Wei Huang
Faculty of Pharmacy, The University of Sydney, Australia

References

Abu El-Asrar AM, Al-Mezaine HS, Ola MS (2009). *Pathophysiology and management of diabetic retinopathy. Expert Rev Ophthalmol 4(6): 627-647.*

Abu El-Asrar AM, Dralands L, Missotten L, Al-Jadaan I, Geboes K (2004). *Expression of apoptosis markers in the retinas of human subjects with diabetes. Investigative Ophthalmology & Visual Science 45(8): 2760-2766.*

Adamis AP (2002). *Is diabetic retinopathy an inflammatory disease? Br J Ophthalmol 86(4): 363-365.*

Ahn CS (2009). *Effect of taurine supplementation on plasma homocysteine levels of the middle-aged Korean women. Adv Exp Med Biol 643: 415-422.*

Aiello LP, Cahill MT, Wong JS (2001). *Systemic considerations in the management of diabetic retinopathy. Am J Ophthalmol 132(5): 760-776.*

Ali TK, Matragoon S, Pillai BA, Liou GI, El-Remessy AB (2008). *Peroxynitrite mediates retinal neurodegeneration by inhibiting nerve growth factor survival signaling in experimental and human diabetes. Diabetes 57(4): 889-898.*

Allen DA, Yaqoob MM, Harwood SM (2005). *Mechanisms of high glucose-induced apoptosis and its relationship to diabetic complications. J Nutr Biochem 16(12): 705-713.*

Aoun P, Simpkins JW, Agarwal N (2003). *Role of PPAR-gamma ligands in neuroprotection against glutamate-induced cytotoxicity in retinal ganglion cells. Invest Ophthalmol Vis Sci 44(7): 2999-3004.*

Arimoto T, Bing GY (2003). *Up-regulation of inducible nitric oxide synthase in the substantia nigra by lipopolysaccharide causes microglial activation and neurodegeneration. Neurobiology of Disease 12(1): 35-45.*

Baeuerle PA, Henkel T (1994). *Function and activation of NF-kappa B in the immune system. Annu Rev Immunol 12: 141-179.*

Baker MS, Chen X, Cao XC, Kaufman DB (2001). *Expression of a dominant negative inhibitor of NF-kappaB protects MIN6 beta-cells from cytokine-induced apoptosis. J Surg Res 97(2): 117-122.*

Banati RB, Gehrmann J, Schubert P, Kreutzberg GW (1993). *Cytotoxicity of microglia. Glia 7(1): 111-118.*

Barber AJ (2003). *A new view of diabetic retinopathy: a neurodegenerative disease of the eye. Prog Neuropsychopharmacol Biol Psychiatry 27(2): 283-290.*

Barber AJ, Antonetti DA, Gardner TW (2000). *Altered expression of retinal occludin and glial fibrillary acidic protein in experimental diabetes. The Penn State Retina Research Group. Invest Ophthalmol Vis Sci 41(11): 3561-3568.*

Barber AJ, Gardner TW, Abcouwer SF (2011). *The significance of vascular and neural apoptosis to the pathology of diabetic retinopathy. Invest Ophthalmol Vis Sci 52(2): 1156-1163.*

Barber AJ, Lieth E, Khin SA, Antonetti DA, Buchanan AG, Gardner TW (1998). *Neural apoptosis in the retina during experimental and human diabetes. Early onset and effect of insulin. J Clin Invest 102(4): 783-791.*

Barnett AH, Grant PJ, Hitman GA, Mather H, Pawa M, Robertson L, et al. (2003). *Rosiglitazone in Type 2 diabetes mellitus: an evaluation in British Indo-Asian patients. Diabet Med 20(5): 387-393.*

Barua M, Liu Y, Quinn MR (2001). *Taurine chloramine inhibits inducible nitric oxide synthase and TNF-alpha gene expression in activated alveolar macrophages: decreased NF-kappaB activation and IkappaB kinase activity. J Immunol 167(4): 2275-2281.*

Beatty S, Koh H, Phil M, Henson D, Boulton M (2000). *The role of oxidative stress in the pathogenesis of age-related macular degeneration. Surv Ophthalmol 45(2): 115-134.*

Beck L, Jr., D'Amore PA (1997). *Vascular development: cellular and molecular regulation. FASEB J 11(5): 365-373.*

Bernardo A, Levi G, Minghetti L (2000). *Role of the peroxisome proliferator-activated receptor-gamma (PPAR-gamma) and its natural ligand 15-deoxy-Delta(12,14)-prostaglandin J(2) in the regulation of microglial functions. Eur J Neurosci 12(7): 2215-2223.*

Blackwell TS, Christman JW (1997). *The role of nuclear factor-kappa B in cytokine gene regulation. Am J Respir Cell Mol Biol 17(1): 3-9.*

Bloomgarden ZT (2007). *Screening for and managing diabetic retinopathy: current approaches. Am J Health Syst Pharm 64(17 Suppl 12): S8-14.*

Boileau TW, Bray TM, Bomser JA (2003). *Ultraviolet radiation modulates nuclear factor kappa B activation in human lens epithelial cells. J Biochem Mol Toxicol 17(2): 108-113.*

Bok D (1993). *The retinal pigment epithelium: a versatile partner in vision. J Cell Sci Suppl 17: 189-195.*

Bonne C (2005). *[PPAR gamma: a novel pharmacological target against retinal and choroidal neovascularization]. J Fr Ophtalmol 28(3): 326-330.*

Bouckenooghe T, Remacle C, Reusens B (2006). *Is taurine a functional nutrient? Curr Opin Clin Nutr Metab Care 9(6): 728-733.*

Braissant O, Foufelle F, Scotto C, Dauca M, Wahli W (1996). *Differential expression of peroxisome proliferator-activated receptors (PPARs): Tissue distribution of PPAR-alpha, -beta, and -gamma in the adult rat. Endocrinology 137(1): 354-366.*

Brownlee M (2005). *The pathobiology of diabetic complications: a unifying mechanism. Diabetes 54(6): 1615-1625.*

Bucheli P, Vidal K, Shen L, Gu Z, Zhang C, Miller LE, et al. (2011). *Goji berry effects on macular characteristics and plasma antioxidant levels. Optom Vis Sci 88(2): 257-262.*

Calza L, Giardino L, Giuliani A, Aloe L, Levi-Montalcini R (2001). *Nerve growth factor control of neuronal expression of angiogenetic and vasoactive factors. Proc Natl Acad Sci U S A 98(7): 4160-4165.*

Cantarella G, Lempereur L, Presta M, Ribatti D, Lombardo G, Lazarovici P, et al. (2002). *Nerve growth factor-endothelial cell interaction leads to angiogenesis in vitro and in vivo. Faseb Journal 16(8): 1307-+.*

Cao G, Alessio HM, Cutler RG (1993). *Oxygen-radical absorbance capacity assay for antioxidants. Free Radical Biol Med 14(3): 303-311.*

Cao Y, Zhang X, Chu Q, Fang Y, Ye J (2003). *Determination of Taurine in Lycium Barbarum L. and Other Foods by Capillary Electrophoresis with Electrochemical Detection. Electroanalysis 15(10): 898-902.*

Ceriello A, Mercuri F, Quagliaro L, Assaloni R, Motz E, Tonutti L, et al. (2001). *Detection of nitrotyrosine in the diabetic plasma: evidence of oxidative stress. Diabetologia 44(7): 834-838.*

Ceylan-Isik AF, Fliethman RM, Wold LE, Ren J (2008). *Herbal and traditional Chinese medicine for the treatment of cardiovascular complications in diabetes mellitus. Curr Diabetes Rev 4(4): 320-328.*

Chan HC, Chang RC, Koon-Ching Ip A, Chiu K, Yuen WH, Zee SY, et al. (2007). *Neuroprotective effects of Lycium barbarum Lynn on protecting retinal ganglion cells in an ocular hypertension model of glaucoma. Exp Neurol 203(1): 269-273.*

Chang JY, Bora PS, Bora NS (2008a). *Prevention of Oxidative Stress-Induced Retinal Pigment Epithelial Cell Death by the PPARgamma Agonists, 15-Deoxy-Delta 12, 14-Prostaglandin J(2). PPAR Res 2008: 720163.*

Chang L, Zhao J, Xu J, Jiang W, Tang CS, Qi YF (2004a). *Effects of taurine and homocysteine on calcium homeostasis and hydrogen peroxide and superoxide anions in rat myocardial mitochondria. Clin Exp Pharmacol Physiol 31(4): 237-243.*

Chang PC, Chen TH, Chang CJ, Hou CC, Chan P, Lee HM (2004b). *Advanced glycosylation end products induce inducible nitric oxide synthase (iNOS) expression via a p38 MAPK-dependent pathway. Kidney Int 65(5): 1664-1675.*

Chang RC, So KF (2008b). *Use of anti-aging herbal medicine, Lycium barbarum, against aging-associated diseases. What do we know so far? Cell Mol Neurobiol 28(5): 643-652.*

Chang RC, Stadlin A, Tsang D (2001). *Effects of tumor necrosis factor alpha on taurine uptake in cultured rat astrocytes. Neurochem Int 38(3): 249-254.*

Chen Z, Soo MY, Srinivasan N, Tan BK, Chan SH (2009). *Activation of macrophages by polysaccharide-protein complex from Lycium barbarum L. Phytother Res 23(8): 1116-1122.*

Cheng CY, Chung WY, Szeto YT, Benzie IF (2005). *Fasting plasma zeaxanthin response to Fructus barbarum L. (wolfberry; Kei Tze) in a food-based human supplementation trial. Br J Nutr 93(1): 123-130.*

Chiu K, Chan HC, Yeung SC, Yuen WH, Zee SY, Chang RC, et al. (2009). *Modulation of microglia by Wolfberry on the survival of retinal ganglion cells in a rat ocular hypertension model. J Ocul Biol Dis Infor 2(2): 47-56.*

Chu J, Ali Y (2008). *Diabetic Retinopathy: A Review. Drug Development Research 69: 1-14.*

Ciulla TA, Amador AG, Zinman B (2003). *Diabetic retinopathy and diabetic macular edema: pathophysiology, screening, and novel therapies. Diabetes Care 26(9): 2653-2664.*

Cunha-Vaz J, Faria de Abreu JR, Campos AJ (1975). *Early breakdown of the blood-retinal barrier in diabetes. The British journal of ophthalmology 59(11): 649-656.*

Danial NN, Korsmeyer SJ (2004). *Cell death: critical control points. Cell 116(2): 205-219.*

de Faria JML, Russ H, Costa VP (2002). *Retinal nerve fibre layer loss in patients with type 1 diabetes mellitus without retinopathy. British Journal of Ophthalmology 86(7): 725-728.*

de Jong PT (2006). *Age-related macular degeneration. N Engl J Med 355(14): 1474-1485.*

De Luca A, Carotenuto A, Rachiglio A, Gallo M, Maiello MR, Aldinucci D, et al. (2008). *The role of the EGFR signaling in tumor microenvironment. J Cell Physiol 214(3): 559-567.*

Decanini A, Karunadharma PR, Nordgaard CL, Feng X, Olsen TW, Ferrington DA (2008). *Human retinal pigment epithelium proteome changes in early diabetes. Diabetologia 51(6): 1051-1061.*

Deng HB, Cui DP, Jiang JM, Feng YC, Cai NS, Li DD (2003). *Inhibiting effects of Achyranthes bidentata polysaccharide and Lycium barbarum polysaccharide on nonenzyme glycation in D-galactose induced mouse aging model. Biomed Environ Sci 16(3): 267-275.*

Denis U, Lecomte M, Paget C, Ruggiero D, Wiernsperger N, Lagarde M (2002). *Advanced glycation end-products induce apoptosis of bovine retinal pericytes in culture: involvement of diacylglycerol/ceramide production and oxidative stress induction. Free Radic Biol Med 33(2): 236-247.*

Devamanoharan PS, Ali AH, Varma SD (1997). *Prevention of lens protein glycation by taurine. Mol Cell Biochem 177(1-2): 245-250.*

Dokshina GA, Silaeva T, Lartsev EI (1976). *[Insulin-like effects of taurine]. Vopr Med Khim 22(4): 503-507.*

Dolhofer-Bliesener R, Lechner B, Gerbitz KD (1996). *Possible significance of advanced glycation end products in serum in end-stage renal disease and in late complications of diabetes. Eur J Clin Chem Clin Biochem 34(4): 355-361.*

Donadio G, Fromageot P (1964). *[Influence Exerted by Taurine on the Utilization of Glucose by the Rat.]. Bull Soc Chim Biol (Paris) 46: 293-302.*

Doonan F, Wallace DM, O'Driscoll C, Cotter TG (2009). *Rosiglitazone acts as a neuroprotectant in retinal cells via up-regulation of sestrin-1 and SOD-2. J Neurochem 109(2): 631-643.*

Du X, Stocklauser-Farber K, Rosen P (1999). *Generation of reactive oxygen intermediates, activation of NF-kappaB, and induction of apoptosis in human endothelial cells by glucose: role of nitric oxide synthase? Free Radic Biol Med 27(7-8): 752-763.*

El-Remessy AB, Al-Shabrawey M, Khalifa Y, Tsai NT, Caldwell RB, Liou GI (2006). *Neuroprotective and blood-retinal barrier-preserving effects of cannabidiol in experimental diabetes.* American Journal of Pathology 168(1): 235-244.

Fehlberg S, Gregel CM, Goke A, Goke R (2003). *Bisphenol A diglycidyl ether-induced apoptosis involves Bax/Bid-dependent mitochondrial release of apoptosis-inducing factor (AIF), cytochrome c and Smac/DIABLO.* Br J Pharmacol 139(3): 495-500.

Flint HL (1997). *"Lycium barbarum". Landscape plants for Eastern North Ameria: exclusive of Florida and the immediate Gulf Coast.* edn. Chichester: John Wiley & Sons.

Fong DS, Aiello L, Gardner TW, King GL, Blankenship G, Cavallerano JD, et al. (2003). *Diabetic retinopathy.* Diabetes Care 26(1): 226-229.

Fong DS, Aiello L, Gardner TW, King GL, Blankenship G, Cavallerano JD, et al. (2004a). *Retinopathy in diabetes.* Diabetes Care 27 Suppl 1: S84-87.

Fong DS, Aiello LP, Ferris FL, 3rd, Klein R (2004b). *Diabetic retinopathy.* Diabetes Care 27(10): 2540-2553.

Forman BM, Tontonoz P, Chen J, Brun RP, Spiegelman BM, Evans RM (1995). *15-Deoxy-delta 12, 14-prostaglandin J2 is a ligand for the adipocyte determination factor PPAR gamma.* Cell 83(5): 803-812.

Franconi F, Di Leo MA, Bennardini F, Ghirlanda G (2004). *Is taurine beneficial in reducing risk factors for diabetes mellitus?* Neurochem Res 29(1): 143-150.

Fuenzalida K, Quintanilla R, Ramos P, Piderit D, Fuentealba RA, Martinez G, et al. (2007a). *Peroxisome proliferator-activated receptor gamma up-regulates the Bcl-2 anti-apoptotic protein in neurons and induces mitochondrial stabilization and protection against oxidative stress and apoptosis.* Journal of Biological Chemistry 282(51): 37006-37015.

Fuenzalida K, Quintanilla R, Ramos P, Piderit D, Fuentealba RA, Martinez G, et al. (2007b). *Peroxisome proliferator-activated receptor gamma up-regulates the Bcl-2 anti-apoptotic protein in neurons and induces mitochondrial stabilization and protection against oxidative stress and apoptosis.* J Biol Chem 282(51): 37006-37015.

Gamagedara S, Shi H, Ma Y (2012). *Quantitative determination of taurine and related biomarkers in urine by liquid chromatography-tandem mass spectrometry.* Anal Bioanal Chem 402(2): 763-770.

Gao XM, Xu ZM, Li ZW (2000). *Traditional Chinese Medicine.* edn. People's Health Publishing House: Beijing.

Garcia C, Aranda J, Arnold E, Thebault S, Macotela Y, Lopez-Casillas F, et al. (2008). *Vasoinhibins prevent retinal vasopermeability associated with diabetic retinopathy in rats via protein phosphatase 2A-dependent eNOS inactivation.* J Clin Invest 118(6): 2291-2300.

Gardner TW, Antonetti DA, Barber AJ, LaNoue KF, Nakamura M (2000). *New insights into the pathophysiology of diabetic retinopathy: potential cell-specific therapeutic targets.* Diabetes Technol Ther 2(4): 601-608.

Garg TK, Chang JY (2004). *15-deoxy-delta 12, 14-Prostaglandin J2 prevents reactive oxygen species generation and mitochondrial membrane depolarization induced by oxidative stress.* BMC Pharmacol 4: 6.

Garg TK, Chang JY (2003). *Oxidative stress causes ERK phosphorylation and cell death in cultured retinal pigment epithelium: prevention of cell death by AG126 and 15-deoxy-delta 12, 14-PGJ2.* BMC Ophthalmol 3: 5.

Gaucher D, Chiappore JA, Paques M, Simonutti M, Boitard C, Sahel JA, et al. (2007). *Microglial changes occur without neural cell death in diabetic retinopathy.* Vision research 47(5): 612-623.

Gerry JM, Pascual G (2008). *Narrowing in on cardiovascular disease: the atheroprotective role of peroxisome proliferator-activated receptor gamma.* Trends Cardiovasc Med 18(2): 39-44.

Giaginis C, Tsourouflis G, Theocharis S (2008). *Peroxisome proliferator-activated receptor-gamma (PPAR-gamma) ligands: novel pharmacological agents in the treatment of ischemia reperfusion injury.* Curr Mol Med 8(6): 562-579.

Goh SY, Cooper ME (2008). *Clinical review: The role of advanced glycation end products in progression and complications of diabetes.* J Clin Endocrinol Metab 93(4): 1143-1152.

Grey ST, Arvelo MB, Hasenkamp W, Bach FH, Ferran C (1999). *A20 inhibits cytokine-induced apoptosis and nuclear factor kappaB-dependent gene activation in islets.* J Exp Med 190(8): 1135-1146.

Grossniklaus HE, Ling JX, Wallace TM, Dithmar S, Lawson DH, Cohen C, et al. (2002). *Macrophage and retinal pigment epithelium expression of angiogenic cytokines in choroidal neovascularization.* Mol Vis 8: 119-126.

Gurujeyalakshmi G, Wang Y, Giri SN (2000). *Suppression of bleomycin-induced nitric oxide production in mice by taurine and niacin.* Nitric Oxide 4(4): 399-411.

Hammes HP (2005). Pericytes and the pathogenesis of diabetic retinopathy. Horm Metab Res 37 Suppl 1: 39-43.

Hammes HP, Hoerauf H, Alt A, Schleicher E, Clausen JT, Bretzel RG, et al. (1999). N(epsilon)(carboxymethyl)lysin and the AGE receptor RAGE colocalize in age-related macular degeneration. Invest Ophthalmol Vis Sci 40(8): 1855-1859.

Hammes HP, Strodter D, Weiss A, Bretzel RG, Federlin K, Brownlee M (1995). Secondary intervention with aminoguanidine retards the progression of diabetic retinopathy in the rat model. Diabetologia 38(6): 656-660.

Hansen SH (2001). The role of taurine in diabetes and the development of diabetic complications. Diabetes Metab Res Rev 17(5): 330-346.

Haubner F, Lehle K, Munzel D, Schmid C, Birnbaum DE, Preuner JG (2007). Hyperglycemia increases the levels of vascular cellular adhesion molecule-1 and monocyte-chemoattractant-protein-1 in the diabetic endothelial cell. Biochem Biophys Res Commun 360(3): 560-565.

Hayes KC, Carey RE, Schmidt SY (1975). Retinal degeneration associated with taurine deficiency in the cat. Science 188(4191): 949-951.

Heller-Stilb B, van Roeyen C, Rascher K, Hartwig HG, Huth A, Seeliger MW, et al. (2002). Disruption of the taurine transporter gene (taut) leads to retinal degeneration in mice. FASEB J 16(2): 231-233.

Heneka MT, Feinstein DL, Galea E, Gleichmann M, Wullner U, Klockgether T (1999). Peroxisome proliferator-activated receptor gamma agonists protect cerebellar granule cells from cytokine-induced apoptotic cell death by inhibition of inducible nitric oxide synthase. Journal of Neuroimmunology 100(1-2): 156-168.

Heneka MT, Klockgether T, Feinstein DL (2000). Peroxisome proliferator-activated receptor-gamma ligands reduce neuronal inducible nitric oxide synthase expression and cell death in vivo. Journal of Neuroscience 20(18): 6862-6867.

Henkind P (1978). Ocular neovascularization. The Krill memorial lecture. Am J Ophthalmol 85(3): 287-301.

Herzlich AA, Tuo J, Chan CC (2008). Peroxisome proliferator-activated receptor and age-related macular degeneration. PPAR Res 2008: 389507.

Ho YS, Yu MS, Yang XF, So KF, Yuen WH, Chang RC (2009). Neuroprotective Effects of Polysaccharides from Wolfberry, the Fruits of Lycium barbarum, Against Homocysteine-induced Toxicity in Rat Cortical Neurons. J Alzheimers Dis 19: 813-827.

Hollborn M, Stathopoulos C, Steffen A, Wiedemann P, Kohen L, Bringmann A (2007). Positive feedback regulation between MMP-9 and VEGF in human RPE cells. Invest Ophthalmol Vis Sci 48(9): 4360-4367.

Huang LJ, Tian GY, Wang ZF, Dong JB, Wu MP (2001). [Studies on the glycoconjugates and glycans from Lycium barbarum L in inhibiting low density lipoprotein (LDL) peroxidation]. Yao Xue Xue Bao 36(2): 108-111.

Huang TH, Kota BP, Razmovski V, Roufogalis BD (2005). Herbal or natural medicines as modulators of peroxisome proliferator-activated receptors and related nuclear receptors for therapy of metabolic syndrome. Basic Clin Pharmacol Toxicol 96(1): 3-14.

Hunter RL, Bing GY (2007). Agonism of peroxisome proliferator receptor-gamma may have therapeutic potential for neuroinflammation and Parkinson's disease. Current Neuropharmacology 5(1): 35-46.

Ibrahim AS, El-Remessy AB, Matragoon S, Zhang W, Patel Y, Khan S, et al. (2011). Retinal microglial activation and inflammation induced by amadori-glycated albumin in a rat model of diabetes. Diabetes 60(4): 1122-1133.

J Helmer (2006). Goji Berries. Better Nutrition 68: 18-18.

Joussen AM, Poulaki V, Le ML, Koizumi K, Esser C, Janicki H, et al. (2004). A central role for inflammation in the pathogenesis of diabetic retinopathy. FASEB J 18(12): 1450-1452.

Joussen AM, Poulaki V, Mitsiades N, Kirchhof B, Koizumi K, Dohmen S, et al. (2002). Nonsteroidal anti-inflammatory drugs prevent early diabetic retinopathy via TNF-alpha suppression. FASEB J 16(3): 438-440.

Kaji Y, Amano S, Usui T, Oshika T, Yamashiro K, Ishida S, et al. (2003). Expression and function of receptors for advanced glycation end products in bovine corneal endothelial cells. Invest Ophthalmol Vis Sci 44(2): 521-528.

Kasper M, Roehlecke C, Witt M, Fehrenbach H, Hofer A, Miyata T, et al. (2000). Induction of apoptosis by glyoxal in human embryonic lung epithelial cell line L132. Am J Respir Cell Mol Biol 23(4): 485-491.

Kawasaki K (1998). [Preretinopathic changes in the oscillatory potential in diabetic retina: interpretation and significance]. Nippon Ganka Gakkai Zasshi 102(12): 813-836.

Kennedy CJ, Rakoczy PE, Constable IJ (1995). Lipofuscin of the retinal pigment epithelium: a review. Eye (Lond) 9 (Pt 6): 763-771.

Kern TS (2007). Contributions of inflammatory processes to the development of the early stages of diabetic retinopathy. Exp Diabetes Res 2007: 95103.

Kern TS, Barber AJ (2008). Retinal ganglion cells in diabetes. J Physiol 586(Pt 18): 4401-4408.

Kern TS, Tang J, Mizutani M, Kowluru RA, Nagaraj RH, Romeo G, et al. (2000). Response of capillary cell death to aminoguanidine predicts the development of retinopathy: comparison of diabetes and galactosemia. Invest Ophthalmol Vis Sci 41(12): 3972-3978.

Khanderia U, Pop-Busui R, Eagle KA (2008). Thiazolidinediones in type 2 diabetes: a cardiology perspective. Ann Pharmacother 42(10): 1466-1474.

Kim EJ, Kwon KJ, Park JY, Lee SH, Moon CH, Baik EJ (2002). Effects of peroxisome proliferator-activated receptor agonists on LPS-induced neuronal death in mixed cortical neurons: associated with iNOS and COX-2. Brain Research 941(1-2): 1-10.

Kim EK, Kwon KB, Koo BS, Han MJ, Song MY, Song EK, et al. (2007). Activation of peroxisome proliferator-activated receptor-gamma protects pancreatic beta-cells from cytokine-induced cytotoxicity via NF kappaB pathway. Int J Biochem Cell Biol 39(6): 1260-1275.

Kim JW, Kim C (2005). Inhibition of LPS-induced NO production by taurine chloramine in macrophages is mediated though Ras-ERK-NF-kappaB. Biochem Pharmacol 70(9): 1352-1360.

Kimoto K, Nakatsuka K, Matsuo N, Yoshioka H (2004). p38 MAPK mediates the expression of type I collagen induced by TGF-beta 2 in human retinal pigment epithelial cells ARPE-19. Invest Ophthalmol Vis Sci 45(7): 2431-2437.

Kliffen M, Sharma HS, Mooy CM, Kerkvliet S, de Jong PT (1997). Increased expression of angiogenic growth factors in age-related maculopathy. Br J Ophthalmol 81(2): 154-162.

Knudsen ST, Bek T, Poulsen PL, Hove MN, Rehling M, Mogensen CE (2002). Macular edema reflects generalized vascular hyperpermeability in type 2 diabetic patients with retinopathy. Diabetes Care 25(12): 2328-2334.

Kontny E, Grabowska A, Kowalczewski J, Kurowska M, Janicka I, Marcinkiewicz J, et al. (1999). Taurine chloramine inhibition of cell proliferation and cytokine production by rheumatoid arthritis fibroblast-like synoviocytes. Arthritis Rheum 42(12): 2552-2560.

Kontny E, Szczepanska K, Kowalczewski J, Kurowska M, Janicka I, Marcinkiewicz J, et al. (2000). The mechanism of taurine chloramine inhibition of cytokine (interleukin-6, interleukin-8) production by rheumatoid arthritis fibroblast-like synoviocytes. Arthritis Rheum 43(10): 2169-2177.

Kowluru RA (2005). Diabetic retinopathy: mitochondrial dysfunction and retinal capillary cell death. Antioxid Redox Signal 7(11-12): 1581-1587.

Kowluru RA, Engerman RL, Case GL, Kern TS (2001a). Retinal glutamate in diabetes and effect of antioxidants. Neurochem Int 38(5): 385-390.

Kowluru RA, Kern TS, Engerman RL, Armstrong D (1996). Abnormalities of retinal metabolism in diabetes or experimental galactosemia. III. Effects of antioxidants. Diabetes 45(9): 1233-1237.

Kowluru RA, Odenbach S (2004). Effect of long-term administration of alpha-lipoic acid on retinal capillary cell death and the development of retinopathy in diabetic rats. Diabetes 53(12): 3233-3238.

Kowluru RA, Tang J, Kern TS (2001b). Abnormalities of retinal metabolism in diabetes and experimental galactosemia. VII. Effect of long-term administration of antioxidants on the development of retinopathy. Diabetes 50(8): 1938-1942.

Krady JK, Basu A, Allen CM, Xu Y, LaNoue KF, Gardner TW, et al. (2005). Minocycline reduces proinflammatory cytokine expression, microglial activation, and caspase-3 activation in a rodent model of diabetic retinopathy. Diabetes 54(5): 1559-1565.

Kulakowski EC, Maturo J (1990). Does taurine bind to the insulin binding site of the insulin receptor? Prog Clin Biol Res 351: 95-102.

Kulakowski EC, Maturo J (1984). Hypoglycemic properties of taurine: not mediated by enhanced insulin release. Biochem Pharmacol 33(18): 2835-2838.

Lampson WG, Kramer JH, Schaffer SW (1983). Potentiation of the actions of insulin by taurine. Can J Physiol Pharmacol 61(5): 457-463.

Langmann T (2007). Microglia activation in retinal degeneration. J Leukoc Biol 81(6): 1345-1351.

Leal EC, Aveleira CA, Castilho AF, Serra AM, Baptista FI, Hosoya K, et al. (2009). High glucose and oxidative/nitrosative stress conditions induce apoptosis in retinal endothelial cells by a caspase-independent pathway. Exp Eye Res 88(5): 983-991.

Lecleire-Collet A, Tessier LH, Massin P, Forster V, Brasseur G, Sahel JA, et al. (2005). Advanced glycation end products can induce glial reaction and neuronal degeneration in retinal explants. Br J Ophthalmol 89(12): 1631-1633.

Lee KS, Kim SR, Park SJ, Park HS, Min KH, Jin SM, et al. (2006). Peroxisome proliferator activated receptor-gamma modulates reactive oxygen species generation and activation of nuclear factor-kappaB and hypoxia-inducible factor 1alpha in allergic airway disease of mice. J Allergy Clin Immunol 118(1): 120-127.

Lewis H, Abrams GW, Blumenkranz MS, Campo RV (1992). Vitrectomy for diabetic macular traction and edema associated with posterior hyaloidal traction. Ophthalmology 99(5): 753-759.

Li C, Cao L, Zeng Q, Liu X, Zhang Y, Dai T, et al. (2005). Taurine may prevent diabetic rats from developing cardiomyopathy also by downregulating angiotensin II type2 receptor expression. Cardiovasc Drugs Ther 19(2): 105-112.

Li H, Zhu H, Xu CJ, Yuan J (1998). Cleavage of BID by caspase 8 mediates the mitochondrial damage in the Fas pathway of apoptosis. Cell 94(4): 491-501.

Li J, Liu NF, Wei Q (2008). Effect of rosiglitazone on cardiac fibroblast proliferation, nitric oxide production and connective tissue growth factor expression induced by advanced glycation end-products. J Int Med Res 36(2): 329-335.

Li SY, Yang D, Yeung CM, Yu WY, Chang RC, So KF, et al. (2011). Lycium barbarum polysaccharides reduce neuronal damage, blood-retinal barrier disruption and oxidative stress in retinal ischemia/reperfusion injury. PLoS One 6(1): e16380.

Lin MT, Beal MF (2006). Mitochondrial dysfunction and oxidative stress in neurodegenerative diseases. Nature 443(7113): 787-795.

Liu XL, Wang DD, Liu YZ, Luo Y, Ma W, Xiao W, et al. (2010). Neuronal-Driven Angiogenesis: Role of NGF in Retinal Neovascularization in an Oxygen-Induced Retinopathy Model. Investigative Ophthalmology & Visual Science 51(7): 3749-3757.

Liu Y, Tonna-DeMasi M, Park E, Schuller-Levis G, Quinn MR (1998). Taurine chloramine inhibits production of nitric oxide and prostaglandin E2 in activated C6 glioma cells by suppressing inducible nitric oxide synthase and cyclooxygenase-2 expression. Brain Res Mol Brain Res 59(2): 189-195.

Lopes de Faria JM, Katsumi O, Cagliero E, Nathan D, Hirose T (2001). Neurovisual abnormalities preceding the retinopathy in patients with long-term type 1 diabetes mellitus. Graefes Arch Clin Exp Ophthalmol 239(9): 643-648.

Luna-Medina R, Cortes-Canteli M, Alonso M, Santos A, Martinez A, Perez-Castillo A (2005). Regulation of inflammatory response in neural cells in vitro by thiadiazolidinones derivatives through peroxisome proliferator-activated receptor gamma activation. J Biol Chem 280(22): 21453-21462.

Luo Q, Cai Y, Yan J, Sun M, Corke H (2004). Hypoglycemic and hypolipidemic effects and antioxidant activity of fruit extracts from Lycium barbarum. Life Sci 76(2): 137-149.

Luo Q, Li Z, Huang X, Yan J, Zhang S, Cai YZ (2006). Lycium barbarum polysaccharides: Protective effects against heat-induced damage of rat testes and H2O2-induced DNA damage in mouse testicular cells and beneficial effect on sexual behavior and reproductive function of hemicastrated rats. Life Sci 79(7): 613-621.

Ma W, Lee SE, Guo J, Qu W, Hudson BI, Schmidt AM, et al. (2007). RAGE ligand upregulation of VEGF secretion in ARPE-19 cells. Invest Ophthalmol Vis Sci 48(3): 1355-1361.

Malchiodi-Albedi F, Matteucci A, Bernardo A, Minghetti L (2008). PPAR-gamma, Microglial Cells, and Ocular Inflammation: New Venues for Potential Therapeutic Approaches. PPAR Res 2008: 295784.

Marchuck M (2005). Goji Berry-Ancient Herb, New Discovery. New Life Journal: Carolina Edition 6: 37-37.

Martensson J, Hermansson G (1984). Sulfur amino acid metabolism in juvenile-onset nonketotic and ketotic diabetic patients. Metabolism 33(5): 425-428.

Maturo J, Kulakowski EC (1988). Taurine binding to the purified insulin receptor. Biochem Pharmacol 37(19): 3755-3760.

McCarty MF (1997). Exploiting complementary therapeutic strategies for the treatment of type II diabetes and prevention of its complications. Med Hypotheses 49(2): 143-152.

Miller JW, Adamis AP, Shima DT, D'Amore PA, Moulton RS, O'Reilly MS, et al. (1994). *Vascular endothelial growth factor/vascular permeability factor is temporally and spatially correlated with ocular angiogenesis in a primate model. Am J Pathol 145(3): 574-584.*

Miyahara S, Kiryu J, Yamashiro K, Miyamoto K, Hirose F, Tamura H, et al. (2004). *Simvastatin inhibits leukocyte accumulation and vascular permeability in the retinas of rats with streptozotocin-induced diabetes. Am J Pathol 164(5): 1697-1706.*

Miyamoto K, Ogura Y (1999). *Pathogenetic potential of leukocytes in diabetic retinopathy. Semin Ophthalmol 14(4): 233-239.*

Mizutani M, Kern TS, Lorenzi M (1996). *Accelerated death of retinal microvascular cells in human and experimental diabetic retinopathy. J Clin Invest 97(12): 2883-2890.*

Moore TC, Moore JE, Kaji Y, Frizzell N, Usui T, Poulaki V, et al. (2003). *The role of advanced glycation end products in retinal microvascular leukostasis. Invest Ophthalmol Vis Sci 44(10): 4457-4464.*

Munch G, Schinzel R, Loske C, Wong A, Durany N, Li JJ, et al. (1998). *Alzheimer's disease--synergistic effects of glucose deficit, oxidative stress and advanced glycation endproducts. J Neural Transm 105(4-5): 439-461.*

Muranaka K, Yanagi Y, Tamaki Y, Usui T, Kubota N, Iriyama A, et al. (2006). *Effects of peroxisome proliferator-activated receptor gamma and its ligand on blood-retinal barrier in a streptozotocin-induced diabetic model. Invest Ophthalmol Vis Sci 47(10): 4547-4552.*

Murata T, Hata Y, Ishibashi T, Kim S, Hsueh WA, Law RE, et al. (2001). *Response of experimental retinal neovascularization to thiazolidinediones. Arch Ophthalmol 119(5): 709-717.*

Murata T, He S, Hangai M, Ishibashi T, Xi XP, Kim S, et al. (2000). *Peroxisome proliferator-activated receptor-gamma ligands inhibit choroidal neovascularization. Invest Ophthalmol Vis Sci 41(8): 2309-2317.*

Nagata S (1997). *Apoptosis by death factor. Cell 88(3): 355-365.*

Nandhini AT, Thirunavukkarasu V, Anuradha CV (2004). *Stimulation of glucose utilization and inhibition of protein glycation and AGE products by taurine. Acta Physiol Scand 181(3): 297-303.*

Obrosova IG, Julius UA (2005). *Role for poly(ADP-ribose) polymerase activation in diabetic nephropathy, neuropathy and retinopathy. Curr Vasc Pharmacol 3(3): 267-283.*

Oshitari T, Yamamoto S, Hata N, Roy S (2008). *Mitochondria- and caspase-dependent cell death pathway involved in neuronal degeneration in diabetic retinopathy. Br J Ophthalmol 92(4): 552-556.*

Oudit GY, Trivieri MG, Khaper N, Husain T, Wilson GJ, Liu P, et al. (2004). *Taurine supplementation reduces oxidative stress and improves cardiovascular function in an iron-overload murine model. Circulation 109(15): 1877-1885.*

Park E, Jia J, Quinn MR, Schuller-Levis G (2002). *Taurine chloramine inhibits lymphocyte proliferation and decreases cytokine production in activated human leukocytes. Clin Immunol 102(2): 179-184.*

Park E, Quinn MR, Wright CE, Schuller-Levis G (1993). *Taurine chloramine inhibits the synthesis of nitric oxide and the release of tumor necrosis factor in activated RAW 264.7 cells. J Leukoc Biol 54(2): 119-124.*

Pasantes-Morales H, Klethi J, Ledig M, Mandel P (1972). *Free amino acids of chicken and rat retina. Brain Res 41(2): 494-497.*

Patz A (1982). *Clinical and experimental studies on retinal neovascularization. XXXIX Edward Jackson Memorial Lecture. Am J Ophthalmol 94(6): 715-743.*

Peng X, Tian G (2001). *Structural characterization of the glycan part of glycoconjugate LbGp2 from Lycium barbarum L. Carbohydr Res 331(1): 95-99.*

Peng Y, Ma C, Li Y, Leung KS, Jiang ZH, Zhao Z (2005). *Quantification of zeaxanthin dipalmitate and total carotenoids in Lycium fruits (Fructus Lycii). Plant Foods Hum Nutr 60(4): 161-164.*

Petrova TV, Akama KT, Van Eldik LJ (1999). *Cyclopentenone prostaglandins suppress activation of microglia: down-regulation of inducible nitric-oxide synthase by 15-deoxy-Delta12,14-prostaglandin J2. Proc Natl Acad Sci U S A 96(8): 4668-4673.*

Pulido JE, Pulido JS, Erie JC, Arroyo J, Bertram K, Lu MJ, et al. (2007). *A role for excitatory amino acids in diabetic eye disease. Exp Diabetes Res 2007: 36150.*

Qin S, McLaughlin AP, De Vries GW (2006). *Protection of RPE cells from oxidative injury by 15-deoxy-delta12,14-prostaglandin J2 by augmenting GSH and activating MAPK. Invest Ophthalmol Vis Sci 47(11): 5098-5105.*

Rahbar S, Natarajan R, Yerneni K, Scott S, Gonzales N, Nadler JL (2000). *Evidence that pioglitazone, metformin and pentoxifylline are inhibitors of glycation. Clin Chim Acta 301(1-2): 65-77.*

Reeve VE, Allanson M, Arun SJ, Domanski D, Painter N (2010). *Mice drinking goji berry juice (Lycium barbarum) are protected from UV radiation-induced skin damage via antioxidant pathways.* Photochem Photobiol Sci 9(4): 601-607.

Reilly CM, Oates JC, Sudian J, Crosby MB, Halushka PV, Gilkeson GS (2001). *Prostaglandin J(2) inhibition of mesangial cell iNOS expression.* Clin Immunol 98(3): 337-345.

Remels AH, Langen RC, Gosker HR, Russell AP, Spaapen F, Voncken JW, et al. (2009). *PPARgamma inhibits NF-kappaB-dependent transcriptional activation in skeletal muscle.* Am J Physiol Endocrinol Metab 297(1): E174-183.

Ren Y, Sun C, Sun Y, Tan H, Wu Y, Cui B, et al. (2009). *PPAR gamma protects cardiomyocytes against oxidative stress and apoptosis via Bcl-2 upregulation.* Vascul Pharmacol 51(2-3): 169-174.

Rendell M, Lundberg GD (2004). *Advances in diabetes for the millennium: an e-symposium.* MedGenMed 6(3 Suppl): 15.

Ricci C, Pastukh V, Leonard J, Turrens J, Wilson G, Schaffer D, et al. (2008). *Mitochondrial DNA damage triggers mitochondrial-superoxide generation and apoptosis.* Am J Physiol Cell Physiol 294(2): C413-422.

Rizzolo LJ (1997). *Polarity and the development of the outer blood-retinal barrier.* Histol Histopathol 12(4): 1057-1067.

Rodrigues GA, Maurier-Mahe F, Shurland DL, McLaughlin AP, Luhrs K, Throo E, et al. (2010). *Differential effects of PPARgamma ligands on oxidative stress-induced death of retinal pigmented epithelial cells.* Invest Ophthalmol Vis Sci.

Roehr B (2010). *FDA committee urges tight restrictions on rosiglitazone.* BMJ 341: c3862.

Romeo G, Liu WH, Asnaghi V, Kern TS, Lorenzi M (2002). *Activation of nuclear factor-kappaB induced by diabetes and high glucose regulates a proapoptotic program in retinal pericytes.* Diabetes 51(7): 2241-2248.

Rosen ED, Spiegelman BM (2001). *PPARgamma : a nuclear regulator of metabolism, differentiation, and cell growth.* J Biol Chem 276(41): 37731-37734.

Sakai H, Tani Y, Shirasawa E, Shirao Y, Kawasaki K (1995). *Development of electroretinographic alterations in streptozotocin-induced diabetes in rats.* Ophthalmic Res 27(1): 57-63.

Salam NK, Huang THW, Kota BP, Kim MS, Li YH, Hibbs DE (2008). *Novel PPAR-gamma agonists identified from a natural product library: A virtual screening, induced-fit docking and biological assay study.* Chem Biol Drug Des 71(1): 57-70.

SanGiovanni JP, Chew EY (2005). *The role of omega-3 long-chain polyunsaturated fatty acids in health and disease of the retina.* Prog Retin Eye Res 24(1): 87-138.

Sato T, Iwaki M, Shimogaito N, Wu X, Yamagishi S, Takeuchi M (2006). *TAGE (toxic AGEs) theory in diabetic complications.* Curr Mol Med 6(3): 351-358.

Schmidt AM, Hori O, Brett J, Yan SD, Wautier JL, Stern D (1994). *Cellular receptors for advanced glycation end products. Implications for induction of oxidant stress and cellular dysfunction in the pathogenesis of vascular lesions.* Arterioscler Thromb 14(10): 1521-1528.

Schmidt M, Giessl A, Laufs T, Hankeln T, Wolfrum U, Burmester T (2003). *How does the eye breathe? Evidence for neuroglobin-mediated oxygen supply in the mammalian retina.* J Biol Chem 278(3): 1932-1935.

Schreck R, Albermann K, Baeuerle PA (1992). *Nuclear factor kappa B: an oxidative stress-responsive transcription factor of eukaryotic cells (a review).* Free Radic Res Commun 17(4): 221-237.

Schuller-Levis G, Park E (2006). *Is Taurine a Biomarker?* Adv Clin Chem 41.

Scoditti E, Massaro M, Carluccio MA, Distante A, Storelli C, De Caterina R (2009). *PPARgamma agonists inhibit angiogenesis by suppressing PKCalpha- and CREB-mediated COX-2 expression in the human endothelium.* Cardiovasc Res 86(2): 302-310.

Shen LQ, Child A, Weber GM, Folkman J, Aiello LP (2008). *Rosiglitazone and delayed onset of proliferative diabetic retinopathy.* Arch Ophthalmol 126(6): 793-799.

Siebenlist U, Franzoso G, Brown K (1994). *Structure, regulation and function of NF-kappa B.* Annu Rev Cell Biol 10: 405-455.

Silaeva T, Dokshina GA, Iartsev EI, Iakovleva VV, Arkhangel'skaia TE (1976). *[The effect of taurine on the carbohydrate metabolism of diabetic animals].* Probl Endokrinol (Mosk) 22(3): 99-103.

Silva KC, Rosales MA, Biswas SK, Lopes de Faria JB, Lopes de Faria JM (2009). *Diabetic retinal neurodegeneration is associated with mitochondrial oxidative stress and is improved by an angiotensin receptor blocker in a model combining hypertension and diabetes.* Diabetes 58(6): 1382-1390.

Sivakumar V, Foulds WS, Luu CD, Ling EA, Kaur C (2011). *Retinal ganglion cell death is induced by microglia derived pro-inflammatory cytokines in the hypoxic neonatal retina. J Pathol 224(2): 245-260.*

Sobal G, Menzel EJ, Sinzinger H (2005). *Troglitazone inhibits long-term glycation and oxidation of low-density lipoprotein. J Cardiovasc Pharmacol 46(5): 672-680.*

Song MK, Roufogalis BD, Huang TH (2012a). *Modulation of diabetic retinopathy pathophysiology by natural medicines through PPAR-gamma-related pharmacology. Br J Pharmacol 165(1): 4-19.*

Song MK, Roufogalis BD, Huang TH (2011a). *Modulation of Diabetic Retinopathy Pathophysiology by Natural Medicines through PPAR-gamma-related Pharmacology. Br J Pharmacol 165(1): 4-19.*

Song MK, Roufogalis BD, Huang THW (2012b). *Reversal of the caspase-dependent apoptotic cytotoxicity pathway by taurine from Lycium barbarum (Goji Berry) in human retinal pigment epithelial cells: potential benefit in diabetic retinopathy Evid-Based Compl Alt 2012: 11.*

Song MK, Roufogalis BD, Huang TW (2011b). *Modulation of RAGE and the downstream targets of RAGE signaling cascades by taurine in Lycium barbarum (Goji Berry): protection of human retinal pigment epithelial barrier function and its potential benefit in diabetic retinopathy J Diabetes Metab 2(9): 162.*

Song MK, Roufogalis BD, Huang TW (2012c). *Role of peroxisome proliferator activator receptor γ in diabetic retinopathy pathophysiology. J Diabetes Metab 5(S3).*

Song MK, Salam NK, Roufogalis BD, Huang TH (2011c). *Lycium barbarum (Goji Berry) extracts and its taurine component inhibit PPAR-gamma-dependent gene transcription in human retinal pigment epithelial cells: Possible implications for diabetic retinopathy treatment. Biochem Pharmacol 82(9): 1209-1218.*

Stevens MJ, Hosaka Y, Masterson JA, Jones SM, Thomas TP, Larkin DD (1999). *Downregulation of the human taurine transporter by glucose in cultured retinal pigment epithelial cells. Am J Physiol 277(4 Pt 1): E760-771.*

Stitt AW (2001). *Advanced glycation: an important pathological event in diabetic and age related ocular disease. Br J Ophthalmol 85(6): 746-753.*

Stitt AW (2003). *The role of advanced glycation in the pathogenesis of diabetic retinopathy. Exp Mol Pathol 75(1): 95-108.*

Stitt AW, Li YM, Gardiner TA, Bucala R, Archer DB, Vlassara H (1997). *Advanced glycation end products (AGEs) co-localize with AGE receptors in the retinal vasculature of diabetic and of AGE-infused rats. Am J Pathol 150(2): 523-531.*

Storer PD, Xu JH, Chavis J, Drew PD (2005). *Peroxisome proliferator-activated receptor-gamma agonists inhibit the activation of microglia and astrocytes: Implications for multiple sclerosis. Journal of Neuroimmunology 161(1-2): 113-122.*

Sulistio MS, Zion A, Thukral N, Chilton R (2008). *PPARgamma agonists and coronary atherosclerosis. Curr Atheroscler Rep 10(2): 134-141.*

Sung B, Park S, Yu BP, Chung HY (2006). *Amelioration of age-related inflammation and oxidative stress by PPARgamma activator: suppression of NF-kappaB by 2,4-thiazolidinedione. Exp Gerontol 41(6): 590-599.*

Szabo A, Kenesei E, Korner A, Miltenyi M, Szucs L, Nagy I (1991). *Changes in plasma and urinary amino acid levels during diabetic ketoacidosis in children. Diabetes Res Clin Pract 12(2): 91-97.*

Takatani T, Takahashi K, Uozumi Y, Matsuda T, Ito T, Schaffer SW, et al. (2004). *Taurine prevents the ischemia-induced apoptosis in cultured neonatal rat cardiomyocytes through Akt/caspase-9 pathway. Biochem Biophys Res Commun 316(2): 484-489.*

Tawfik A, Sanders T, Kahook K, Akeel S, Elmarakby A, Al-Shabrawey M (2009). *Suppression of retinal peroxisome proliferator-activated receptor gamma in experimental diabetes and oxygen-induced retinopathy: role of NADPH oxidase. Invest Ophthalmol Vis Sci 50(2): 878-884.*

Timbrell JA, Waterfield CJ, Draper RP (1995). *Use of Urinary Taurine and Creatine as Biomarkers of Organ Dysfunction and Metabolic Perturbations. Comp Haematol Int 5: 112-119.*

Tomi M, Terayama T, Isobe T, Egami F, Morito A, Kurachi M, et al. (2007). *Function and regulation of taurine transport at the inner blood-retinal barrier. Microvascular Research 73(2): 100-106.*

Touyz RM, Schiffrin EL (2006). *Peroxisome proliferator-activated receptors in vascular biology-molecular mechanisms and clinical implications. Vascul Pharmacol 45(1): 19-28.*

Tretiach M, Madigan MC, Wen L, Gillies MC (2005). *Effect of Muller cell co-culture on in vitro permeability of bovine retinal vascular endothelium in normoxic and hypoxic conditions. Neurosci Lett 378(3): 160-165.*

Tu G (1992). *Pharmacopoeia of the People's Republic of China. . edn. Guangdong Science and Technology Press: Guangzhou, China.*

Uchimura K, Nakamuta M, Enjoji M, Irie T, Sugimoto R, Muta T, et al. (2001). *Activation of retinoic X receptor and peroxisome proliferator-activated receptor-gamma inhibits nitric oxide and tumor necrosis factor-alpha production in rat Kupffer cells. Hepatology 33(1): 91-99.*

Uryu S, Harada J, Hisamoto M, Oda T (2002). *Troglitazone inhibits both post-glutamate neurotoxicity and low-potassium-induced apoptosis in cerebellar granule neurons. Brain Research 924(2): 229-236.*

Vilchis C, Salceda R (1996). *Effect of diabetes on levels and uptake of putative amino acid neurotransmitters in rat retina and retinal pigment epithelium. Neurochem Res 21(10): 1167-1171.*

Villarroel M, Ciudin A, Hernandez C, Simo R (2010). *Neurodegeneration: An early event of diabetic retinopathy. World J Diabetes 1(2): 57-64.*

Vincent AM, Perrone L, Sullivan KA, Backus C, Sastry AM, Lastoskie C, et al. (2007). *Receptor for advanced glycation end products activation injures primary sensory neurons via oxidative stress. Endocrinology 148(2): 548-558.*

Wang W, Matsukura M, Fujii I, Ito K, Zhao JE, Shinohara M, et al. (2011). *Inhibition of high glucose-induced VEGF and ICAM-1 expression in human retinal pigment epithelium cells by targeting ILK with small interference RNA. Mol Biol Rep.*

Wang Y, Zhao H, Sheng X, Gambino PE, Costello B, Bojanowski K (2002). *Protective effect of Fructus Lycii polysaccharides against time and hyperthermia-induced damage in cultured seminiferous epithelium. J Ethnopharmacol 82(2-3): 169-175.*

Watson GS, Cholerton BA, Reger MA, Baker LD, Plymate SR, Asthana S, et al. (2005). *Preserved cognition in patients with early Alzheimer disease and amnestic mild cognitive impairment during treatment with rosiglitazone: a preliminary study. Am J Geriatr Psychiatry 13(11): 950-958.*

West AL, Oren GA, Moroi SE (2006). *Evidence for the use of nutritional supplements and herbal medicines in common eye diseases. Am J Ophthalmol 141(1): 157-166.*

Williams R, Airey M, Baxter H, Forrester J, Kennedy-Martin T, Girach A (2004a). *Epidemiology of diabetic retinopathy and macular oedema: a systematic review. Eye 18(10): 963-983.*

Williams R, Airey M, Baxter H, Forrester J, Kennedy-Martin T, Girach A (2004b). *Epidemiology of diabetic retinopathy and macular oedema: a systematic review. Eye (Lond) 18(10): 963-983.*

Winkler BS, Boulton ME, Gottsch JD, Sternberg P (1999). *Oxidative damage and age-related macular degeneration. Mol Vis 5: 32.*

Wong A, Dukic-Stefanovic S, Gasic-Milenkovic J, Schinzel R, Wiesinger H, Riederer P, et al. (2001). *Anti-inflammatory antioxidants attenuate the expression of inducible nitric oxide synthase mediated by advanced glycation endproducts in murine microglia. Eur J Neurosci 14(12): 1961-1967.*

Wu JS, Lin TN, Wu KK (2009). *Rosiglitazone and PPAR-gamma overexpression protect mitochondrial membrane potential and prevent apoptosis by upregulating anti-apoptotic Bcl-2 family proteins. J Cell Physiol 220(1): 58-71.*

Wu QD, Wang JH, Fennessy F, Redmond HP, Bouchier-Hayes D (1999). *Taurine prevents high-glucose-induced human vascular endothelial cell apoptosis. Am J Physiol 277(6 Pt 1): C1229-1238.*

Xie H, Zhang S (1997). *[Determination of taurine in Lycium barbarum L. by high performance liquid chromatography with OPA-urea pre-column derivatization]. Se Pu 15(1): 54-56.*

Xin X, Yang S, Kowalski J, Gerritsen ME (1999). *Peroxisome proliferator-activated receptor gamma ligands are potent inhibitors of angiogenesis in vitro and in vivo. J Biol Chem 274(13): 9116-9121.*

Yam JC, Kwok AK (2007). *Update on the treatment of diabetic retinopathy. Hong Kong Med J 13(1): 46-60.*

Yamagishi S, Nakamura K, Matsui T (2007). *Potential utility of telmisartan, an angiotensin II type 1 receptor blocker with peroxisome proliferator-activated receptor-gamma (PPAR-gamma)-modulating activity for the treatment of cardiometabolic disorders. Curr Mol Med 7(5): 463-469.*

Yanagi Y (2008). *Role of Peoxisome Proliferator Activator Receptor gamma on Blood Retinal Barrier Breakdown. PPAR Res 2008: 679237.*

Yanli H (2005). *The effect on immunisupressive factors VEGF, TGF-beta1 of Lycium barbarum polysaccharide(LBP) in H~2~2-bearing mice. Pharmacology and Clinics of Chinese Materia Medica 21(5): 28.*

Yu MS, Leung SK, Lai SW, Che CM, Zee SY, So KF, et al. (2005). *Neuroprotective effects of anti-aging oriental medicine Lycium barbarum against beta-amyloid peptide neurotoxicity. Exp Gerontol 40(8-9): 716-727.*

Yu X, Chen K, Wei N, Zhang Q, Liu J, Mi M (2007a). *Dietary taurine reduces retinal damage produced by photochemical stress via antioxidant and anti-apoptotic mechanisms in Sprague-Dawley rats. Br J Nutr 98(4): 711-719.*

Yu X, Li C, Li X, Cai L (2007b). *Rosiglitazone prevents advanced glycation end products-induced renal toxicity likely through suppression of plasminogen activator inhibitor-1. Toxicol Sci 96(2): 346-356.*

Yu X, Xu Z, Mi M, Xu H, Zhu J, Wei N, et al. (2008). *Dietary taurine supplementation ameliorates diabetic retinopathy via anti-excitotoxicity of glutamate in streptozotocin-induced Sprague-Dawley rats. Neurochem Res 33(3): 500-507.*

Yuuki T, Kanda T, Kimura Y, Kotajima N, Tamura J, Kobayashi I, et al. (2001). *Inflammatory cytokines in vitreous fluid and serum of patients with diabetic vitreoretinopathy. J Diabetes Complications 15(5): 257-259.*

Zeng HY, Green WR, Tso MO (2008). *Microglial activation in human diabetic retinopathy. Arch Ophthalmol 126(2): 227-232.*

Zeng K, Xu H, Mi M, Chen K, Zhu J, Yi L, et al. (2010). *Effects of taurine on glial cells apoptosis and taurine transporter expression in retina under diabetic conditions. Neurochem Res 35(10): 1566-1574.*

Zeng K, Xu H, Mi M, Zhang Q, Zhang Y, Chen K, et al. (2009). *Dietary taurine supplementation prevents glial alterations in retina of diabetic rats. Neurochem Res 34(2): 244-254.*

Zhang LX, Ino-ue M, Dong K, Yamamoto M (2000). *Retrograde axonal transport impairment of large- and medium-sized retinal ganglion cells in diabetic rat. Current Eye Research 20(2): 131-136.*

Zhao R, Li Q, Xiao B (2005). *Effect of Lycium barbarum polysaccharide on the improvement of insulin resistance in NIDDM rats. Yakugaku Zasshi 125(12): 981-988.*

Zheng L, Howell SJ, Hatala DA, Huang K, Kern TS (2007). *Salicylate-based anti-inflammatory drugs inhibit the early lesion of diabetic retinopathy. Diabetes 56(2): 337-345.*

Expression of Hyaluronan Synthases in Normal and Glaucoma Trabecular Meshwork

Kate E. Keller and Ted S. Acott

1 Introduction

Primary open-angle glaucoma (POAG) is the most common form of a group of optic neuropathies known as the glaucomas. Glaucoma is the second leading cause of blindness in the world and there is an estimated 66 million affected persons (Quigley, 1996). The major risk factors for glaucoma include age, ocular hypertension (elevated intraocular pressure (IOP)), ethnicity, family history and certain medical conditions. IOP is generated by a balance of inflow of aqueous humor fluid and egress of this fluid from the anterior chamber of the eye. When this balance is disrupted, the result is elevated IOP. Persistent elevated IOP leads to optic disc cupping and optic nerve damage, which in turn causes the progressive and irreversible loss of vision (Quigley, 2011). Lowering elevated IOP remains the only effective strategy to halt glaucomatous vision loss. Current therapeutic targets include reducing aqueous humor production by the ciliary body (inflow) or increasing aqueous humor outflow from the anterior chamber (Stamer & Acott, 2012). Aqueous humor exits the eye via the conventional outflow pathway or via the secondary alternative uveal pathway. All current outflow medications increase outflow via the alternative route and no therapy is targeted toward increasing outflow via the conventional pathway, although several conventional route therapies are in clinical trials. Since approximately 80% of aqueous humor exits via the conventional route, this remains an attractive prospect for the development of new therapies (Stamer, 2012).

1.1 Conventional Aqueous Humor Outflow Pathway

Aqueous humor primarily drains from the anterior chamber via the conventional pathway through the trabecular meshwork (TM) (Goel *et al.*, 2010; Stamer & Acott, 2012). TM tissue is composed of a series of fenestrated beams around which the aqueous flows before exiting the anterior chamber via Schlemm's canal (Tamm, 2009). It is a triangular-shaped tissue that sits within the scleral sulcus and extends anteriorly from the cornea to the ciliary body and iris root at the posterior. The TM can be divided into four regions based on anatomical location: the insert region, the outer uveal meshwork, the corneoscleral meshwork, and the juxtacanalicular region, which lies adjacent to Schlemm's canal. The insert region is an area underlying Schwalbe's line and is where TM stem cells reside (Kelley *et al.*, 2009). The beams of the outer uveal and corneoscleral meshworks are composed of extracellular matrix (ECM) and are covered by a continuous monolayer of TM endothelial cells. These cells are responsible for the phagocytic uptake and degradation of debris in the aqueous humor to prevent obstruction of the innermost outflow pathways. The large intertrabecular spaces of the outer meshwork gradually diminish toward Schlemm's canal, which signals the transition into the juxtacanalicular (JCT) region, or cribriform meshwork (Tamm, 2009). This area lies within 20 μm of

Schlemm's canal and is different from the rest of the tissue as it is non-fenestrated and TM cell density is highly reduced compared to the outer beams. The ECM of this region is also different and forms a discontinuous basement membrane. The innermost layer of the JCT abuts Schlemm's canal inner wall cells that form a continuous monolayer around the lumen of the canal (Ethier, 2002; Overby et al., 2009). The eye requires IOP to maintain its form and function. Since aqueous humor inflow rates are relatively constant, physiological IOPs are generated by building an adjustable resistance to aqueous humor outflow. It is generally assumed that the main site of the outflow resistance is in the JCT region (Grant, 1963; Johnson, 2006; Maepea & Bill, 1992; Rosenquist et al., 1989).

1.2 Extracellular Matrix of the Trabecular Meshwork

Elevated IOP arises from impaired aqueous humor outflow through the TM (Acott & Kelley, 2008). The exact molecular identity of the impairment remains somewhat controversial, but ECM is commonly evoked as a source of the normal resistance and of the blockage. ECM of the TM is composed of many molecules including glycosaminoglycan (GAG) chains, proteoglycans, collagens, elastic fiber components, basement membrane proteins and other glycoproteins (Acott & Kelley, 2008). In response to a period of sustained pressure, TM cells in the JCT region sense pressure changes as a stretch/distortion and respond by activating and releasing matrix metalloproteinases (MMPs) to focally degrade the ECM facilitating enhanced aqueous fluid flow through the TM (Bradley et al., 2001; Keller et al., 2009a). Concurrently, new ECM is synthesized to replace that which has been lost in order to maintain the new modified outflow.

The roles of individual ECM components in outflow resistance and IOP regulation is just starting to be realized. Recent studies on various matricellular proteins are particularly intriguing. Matricellular proteins are a family of ECM molecules that are not structural components, but rather they serve as mediators of cell function (Bornstein & Sage, 2002; Rhee et al., 2009). These proteins directly interact with cells, but they can also influence cell signaling pathways and alter surrounding ECM by modulating growth factors, proteases and other ECM proteins. Matricellular protein family members expressed in the TM include SPARC (secreted protein and rich in cysteine), hevin, tenascin C (TNC) and tenascin X (TNX), thrombospondins-1 and -2 (TSP1, TSP2), and osteopontin (OPN). The importance of these matricellular proteins in the TM has been studied using knockout mice. Knockout of SPARC, TSP1 and TSP2 decreased IOP, while knockout of hevin, OPN, TNC and TNX did not significantly affect IOP (Chowdhury et al., 2011; Haddadin et al., 2009; Haddadin et al., 2012; Kang et al., 2011; Keller et al., 2013). The SPARC effect has been studied in more detail and it was found that over-expression of SPARC increases IOP (Oh et al., 2013).

GAG chains have also attracted much attention as a source of the blockage. GAG chains are large sugar chains that usually attach to a protein backbone to generate proteoglycans. The types of GAG chain in the TM are chondroitin sulfate (CS), dermatan sulfate (DS), hyaluronan (HA), keratan sulfate (KS) and heparan sulfate (HS) (Acott et al., 1985; Knepper et al., 1996a). In multiple animal species, enzymatic degradation of GAG chains altered outflow in vitro via the conventional pathway (Barany & Scotchbrook, 1954; Francois et al., 1956; Grant, 1963; Hubbard et al., 1997; Keller et al., 2008; Knepper et al., 1984; Sawaguchi et al., 1992). In human eyes, chemical inhibition of synthesis and decreasing their concentration by RNAi silencing of the enzymes in their biosynthetic pathway decreased outflow rates in perfusion culture (Keller et al., 2008; Keller et al., 2011; Keller et al., 2012b). Moreover, RNAi silencing of versican, a large proteoglycan that is substituted with CS chains and binds HA, increased outflow resistance when applied in *in vitro* perfusion culture of human anterior segments (Keller *et al.*, 2011). Thus, these studies strongly implicate GAGs as a source of outflow resistance.

1.3 Hyaluronan and Hyaluronan Synthases

Hyaluronan (HA) is an acidic GAG chain that is synthesized by TM cells (Camenisch & Mcdonald, 2000; Gong *et al.*, 1994; Keller *et al.*, 2012b; Tammi *et al.*, 2002; Toole, 2004). Unlike other GAG chains, it is not attached to a protein backbone, does not undergo epimerization and it is not sulfated. It is built of repeating disaccharides of glucuronic acid (GlcA) and N-acetyl-glucosamine (GlcNAc). HA chains are usually of high molecular weight, ranging from 10^5 to 10^7 Da, but under certain pathological or physiological conditions, smaller fragments or oligosaccharides can exist. Because of its large size, its ability to interact with water molecules and its random coil structure, HA occupies a large hydrodynamic volume (Camenisch & Mcdonald, 2000). This imbues tissues with lubricating and/or filtering functions. Historically, HA was regarded as an inert space-filling molecule, but more recent studies reveal a molecule with multiple functions that provides microenvironmental cues to regulate cellular behavior (Toole, 2004).

In the TM, HA represents approximately 20-25% of the total amount of GAG chains (Acott *et al.*, 1988; Acott *et al.*, 1985). Using HA-binding protein (HAbp), it was found that HA is located at increased levels in the anterior portion of the TM and in areas of the JCT that are closest to Schlemm's canal (Gong *et al.*, 1994; Keller *et al.*, 2012a; Keller *et al.*, 2012b; Knepper *et al.*, 1996b; Lerner *et al.*, 1997; Lutjen-Drecoll *et al.*, 1990). It has been postulated that HA covering the surfaces of the outflow pathways might prevent adherence of molecules contained in aqueous humor to TM beams and prevent clogging of the outflow pathways (Gabelt & Kaufman, 2005; Lutjen-Drecoll *et al.*, 1990). HA concentrations in the TM are not constant, but are altered during a patient's lifetime. There is a decrease in the amount of HA during aging and a much greater loss in POAG TM (Cavallotti *et al.*, 2004; Knepper *et al.*, 2005; Knepper *et al.*, 1996a; Knepper *et al.*, 1996b). Loss of HA in the aged JCT may render TM cells incapable of launching a normal homeostatic response to adjust outflow and may leave some patients susceptible, directly or indirectly, to elevated IOP. Reconstituted HA *in vitro* was found to be particularly sensitive to increased pressure gradients, although the results remain somewhat controversial (Knepper *et al.*, 2005). Collectively, these observations implicate a major role, directly or indirectly, for HA in outflow resistance and suggest that HA concentration needs to be tightly regulated for the TM to function normally.

HA is synthesized by three HA synthase (HAS) genes called HAS1, HAS2 and HAS3. HASs are integral multipass membrane proteins and they form a pore in the plasma membrane through which the HA chain is extruded directly into the ECM (Itano, 2008; Toole, 2004). This biosynthesis is unlike that of other GAG chains, which are synthesized directly on proteoglycan core proteins in the rough endoplasmic reticulum and Golgi apparatus and secreted much like other glycoproteins. The bacterial homolog, SpHAS, remains the archetype of HA biosynthesis (Itano, 2008; Tammi *et al.*, 2002). Studies on SpHAS elucidated that monosaccharides are likely added to the reducing end of the growing HA chain. Each HAS synthesizes HA chains with different properties. HAS3 synthesizes shorter HA molecules (0.12 – 1 x 10^6 Da), but is more active than HAS1 and HAS2, which produce longer molecules (3.9 x 10^6 Da) (Itano *et al.*, 1999). Once secreted, HA chains are associated with the cell surface via its cell surface receptors (including CD44 and RHAMM) or by prolonged sequestering by its synthase (Ponta *et al.*, 2003; Toole, 2004). Interaction of HA with CD44 mediates cellular responses to their microenvironment and therefore HA-CD44 interactions are tightly regulated. CD44 can exist in active, inducible and inactive states with regard to HA binding and CD44 is also involved in uptake of HA following its degradation into fragments (Knudson *et al.*, 2002; Nagano & Saya, 2004; Ponta *et al.*, 2003; Tammi *et al.*, 2002). If HA is large, or is bound by other proteoglycans, then internalization by CD44 is sterically inhibited (Hua *et al.*, 1993). In the ECM, HA also binds various ligands including versican, brevican and TSG6 (tumor necrosis factor-stimulated gene-6) (Toole, 2004). Our recent manuscript showed that inhibition of HA synthesis reduces levels of certain ECM proteins in TM cells, namely versican and fibronectin (Keller *et al.*, 2012a). Alterations in the levels of numerous ECM genes in response to reduced HA synthesis is directly relevant to glaucoma since HA concentration in glaucomatous TM is greatly reduced compared to normal aged eyes (Knepper *et al.*, 1996b). Thus, the levels of HA synthesized can readily influence ECM interactions and modulate cell-ECM cross-talk.

Increased HAS mRNA expression directly correlates to increases in HA biosynthesis in various cell types (Guo *et al.*, 2007; Tammi *et al.*, 2011). Thus, it is likely that age-related changes of HA concentration may be due to alterations in total HA synthesis by one, two or all three HAS genes. Also, modifying the ratios of expression of each HAS gene likely alters the properties of the HA chain produced. HAS protein distribution in the TM has been studied, but this was prior to the identification of all three HAS isoforms (Rittig *et al.*, 1993). Previously, HAS protein was detected in the uveal and corneoscleral meshworks and luminal side of the inner wall endothelium, but was lacking in the outer corneoscleral and JCT regions of the tissue (Rittig *et al.*, 1993). Analysis of which HAS genes are expressed and their effects on TM cells could provide invaluable information for how HA concentration is regulated in the TM. The purpose of this study is to report alterations in mRNA levels of three HAS genes in normal and glaucoma eyes perfused at physiological and elevated pressure for 24 hours. Confocal microscopy and immunostaining of HAS protein in paraffin-embedded radial sections of human trabecular meshwork was also investigated.

2 Methods

2.1 Anterior Segment Perfusion Culture of Human Eyes

Human eye tissue was obtained from cadavers from Lions Eye Banks, Portland, Oregon. Use of donor eye tissue was approved by Oregon Health & Science University Institutional Review Board and experiments were conducted in accordance with the tenets of the Declaration of Helsinki for the use of human tissue. Diagnosis of glaucoma was listed on a datasheet accompanying the eyes, but no personal identifiers were listed. In some cases, glaucoma medications were listed (Table 1), but no other details regarding disease status was available. If glaucoma was suspect, or listed as "per next of kin", the eyes were excluded. We accepted both normal and glaucomatous eyes that had undergone intraocular lens surgery or had posterior eye diseases, such as age-related macular degeneration, but excluded eyes with anterior segment eye disease.

Human eyes (n=22) were bisected and the iris, ciliary body, lens and aqueous humor were removed by dissection. The anterior segment containing the cornea, trabecular mesh-

Eye ID #	Age (years)	Sex	Disease state	Medications (if known)
2009-0287	88	F	Normal	-
2009-0325	84	M	Normal	-
2008-0182	77	M	Normal	-
2008-0123	78	F	Normal	-
2009-1819	91	M	Normal	-
2010-0317	71	M	Normal	-
2011-1312	69	M	Normal	-
2009-0951	88	M	Normal	-
2007-0157	72	M	Normal	-
2011-0411	90	M	Normal	-
2009-0915	88	M	Normal	-
2009-0925	84	F	Normal	-
2006-1104	67	M	Normal	-
2008-1702	67	M	Normal	-
2010-0300	94	M	Glaucoma	?
2010-0286	95	F	Glaucoma	Xalatan
2009-1813	88	F	Glaucoma	Lumigan, Timolol
2009-2059	80	F	Glaucoma	?
2009-0295	73	M	Glaucoma	?
2009-0371	91	M	Glaucoma	Xalatan
2009-0289	94	M	Glaucoma	Xalatan
2009-0058	80	M	Glaucoma	?

Table 1: Summary of human eyes used in this study.

work and a thin rim of sclera was placed into serum-free organ culture for 5-7 days to allow cellular recovery post-mortem. Several changes of media also aided removal of residual glaucoma medications. The age range of the cadaver eyes was 67 – 95 years, with an average age of 82.2 ± 9.2 years (Table 1). Anterior segments were clamped into a perfusion chamber and perfused with serum-free DMEM at a constant pressure (8 mmHg) until flow rates stabilized at an average flow rate of 1-7 µl/min (Keller *et al.*, 2008; Keller *et al.*, 2011; Keller *et al.*, 2012b). For experiments using increased pressure, the pressure head was doubled in height to provide approximately 16 mmHg for 24 hours (Bradley *et al.*, 1998). One eye of each pair was subject to elevated pressure (2x) while the contralateral control served as a control (1x).

2.2 RNA Isolation and Quantitative RT-PCR

At the end of perfusion, total RNA was isolated. Briefly, the anterior segments were removed from the perfusion apparatus, the TM was dissected from the anterior segment and then it was homogenized with a glass/Teflon tissue homogenizer with 0.5 ml Trizol (Invitrogen). RNA was isolated following the manufacturer's instructions and RNA was quantitated with a Nanodrop 2000 spectrophotometer (Thermo Fisher Scientific, Wilmington, DE). Total RNA was then amplified with the MessageAmp II aRNA amplification kit (Ambion). cDNA was reverse-transcribed from 1 µg of amplified RNA using Superscript III reverse transcriptase (Invitrogen). Quantitative RT-PCR (qRT-PCR) was performed using the HAS primers listed in Table 2 and using methods previously described (Keller *et al.*, 2009b; Keller *et al.*, 2007). Briefly,

2 μl of cDNA was used in a 20 μl reaction with DyNAmo HS Sybr Green qPCR mix (Thermo Fisher Scientific). Products were amplified in a thermal cycler equipped with a Chromo4 detector using 40 cycles (94°C for 30s, 58-60°C [primer dependent] for 30s, and 72°C for 30s). Fluorescence measurements were read following the completion of each cycle and a melting curve was generated immediately following the final amplification cycle. Fluorescence data was analyzed using Opticon Monitor 2 software with a 7-point dilution standard curve. A baseline was subtracted using the average over cycle range method. Relative template concentrations of each unknown sample were determined in duplicate, averaged and plotted as relative fluorescent units (RFUs). Mean results (+/- standard error of the mean) are shown with the number of biological replicates shown in the figure legend. Results were normalized to 18S RNA, which acted as a housekeeping gene. Products were analyzed on agarose gels to verify band sizes and purity (data not shown).

Gene	Forward (5'-3') Reverse (5'-3')	Product size (bp)	Annealing temp (°C)
HAS1	ACTGGGTAGCCTTCAATGTGGA TACCAGGCCTCAAGAAACTGCT	121	58
HAS2	ATCCTCCTGGGTGGTGTGATTT TTCCGCCTGCCACACTTATTGA	164	60
HAS3	TCCTACTTTGGCTGTGTGCAGT TCCAGAGGTGGTGCTTATGGAA	313	58
18S RNA	CGGCTACCACATCCAAGGAA CACCAGACTTGCCCTCCAAT	164	58

Table 2: Primers used in quantitative RT-PCR.

2.3 Immunofluorescence and Confocal Microscopy

For immunostaining, the anterior segments were removed from the perfusion chambers and cut up into 8-10 wedges. Tissue was fixed in 4% paraformaldehyde and then all wedges were embedded into a single paraffin block. Serial radial sections (5 μm) were cut at the histology core facility of the Knight Cancer Center (Oregon Health & Science University). Therefore, each section contained 8-10 regions of tissue from around the entire eye to allow analysis of the whole tissue and to mitigate variability in immunostaining due to potential segmental differences around the eye. Hematoxylin and eosin was used to stain some tissue sections and images were obtained using an Olympus BX51 differential interference contrast (DIC). At least 6 eyes from normal individuals were evaluated.

Immunostaining was performed on radial sections as previously described (Keller *et al.*, 2009b; Keller *et al.*, 2008). Briefly, slides were deparaffinized, hydrated and then blocked using universal CAS blocking buffer (Invitrogen). Sections were incubated overnight with mouse monoclonal anti-HAS1 (1:50; Novus Biologicals, Littleton, CO), goat polyclonal anti-HAS2 (1:50; Santa Cruz Biotechnology, Inc., Santa Cruz, CA) or rabbit polyclonal anti-HAS3 ((1:50; Abcam, Cambridge, MA). For negative controls, the primary antibody was omitted (not shown). The appropriate species secondary antibody conjugated to Alexa Fluor 488 was used. Coverslips were mounted with ProLong gold containing DAPI nuclear stain (Invitrogen). Sections were examined using a Olympus Fluoview 1000 laser scanning confocal microscope (Olympus, San Diego, CA) and 0.5 µm z-slices were acquired. The images shown are compressed z-stacks of 3-5 slices.

3   Results

3.1   HAS Gene Expression in Normal and Glaucomatous TM

HA concentration is reduced in normal aged eyes and is highly reduced in POAG eyes (Knepper *et al.*, 1996b). We hypothesized that this could be a result of altered HAS gene expression. Therefore, we used quantitative RT-PCR to measure the mRNA levels of each HAS gene in normal and glaucomatous TM tissue to investigate whether any differences could be detected. The mRNA levels of each HAS gene were quantitated in normal and glaucomatous human anterior segments perfused at physiological (1x) for 24 hours (Figure 1). The relative abundance of each HAS in TM tissue was HAS2>HAS3>HAS1. This did not differ between normal and diseased eyes. When comparing HAS levels between normal and glaucoma TM, there was a slight decrease in HAS2 mRNA levels in glaucoma TM, but this reduction was not significant. The relative mRNA levels of HAS1 and HAS3 were quite similar between normal and glaucomatous TM.

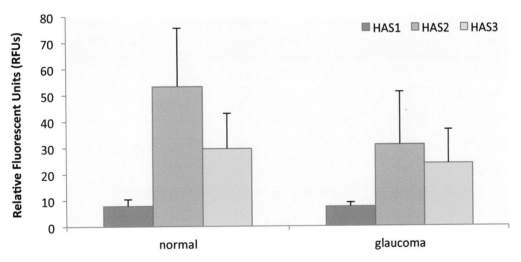

Figure 1: HAS gene expression in normal and glaucomatous eyes. The graph shows mRNA levels of each HAS in normal and glaucoma eyes perfused at physiological 1x pressure and normalized to 18S RNA levels. HAS1, n= 4 (Normal) and 7 (Glaucoma); HAS2, n=6 (Normal) and 6 (Glaucoma); HAS3, n=5 (Normal) and 7 (Glaucoma). Error bars are the standard error of the mean.

3.2   HAS mRNA Regulation in TM Tissue Subject to Elevated Pressure

Next, we investigated HAS mRNA expression in response to elevated IOP. One eye of each pair at physiological (1X) and the contralateral eye at 2X pressure for 24 hours and HAS mRNA expression was quantitated using qRT-PCR. In normal eyes, HAS1 mRNA levels were significantly reduced in normal human anterior segments perfused at 2x pressure (Figure 2). Although HAS2 and HAS3 mRNA were also reduced, the changes were not significant. In glaucoma eyes, the mRNA levels for all 3 HAS genes were highly reduced. This suggests that HAS genes in glaucoma eyes respond differently than in normal eyes in response to elevated pressure.

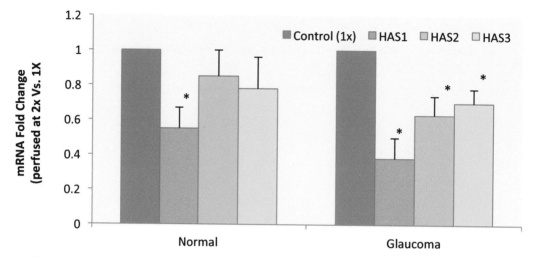

Figure 2: HAS gene expression in normal and glaucoma TM in anterior segments perfused at physiological and elevated pressure (2x) for 24 hours. Graph shows the mRNA fold changes of 2x pressure compared to physiological pressure for each HAS gene. Normal: HAS1, n=6, *p=0.0004; HAS2, n=5, HAS3, n=6. Glaucoma: HAS1, n=5, *p=0.0001; HAS2, n=7, *p=0.006; HAS3, n=8, *p=0.005. Error bars show the standard error of the mean.

3.3 HAS Protein Distribution in Normal TM Tissue

Next, we investigated the distribution patterns of each HAS protein in normal human TM tissue using immunofluorescence and confocal microscopy (Figure 3). Tissue from two different individuals is shown: a 69 year old male (Figure 3A-C, G, H) and an 88 year old male (Figure 3D-F). HAS protein levels by immunofluorescence were consistent with mRNA expression: HAS1 was barely detected, while HAS2 and HAS3 were present at much higher levels. This data is consistent with the relative levels of HAS proteins found in TM cells in cell culture (Keller *et al.*, 2012b). HAS1 was detected at low levels in human TM tissue and the immunostaining that was present was confined to a few punctate dots in the beams of the outer uveal and corneoscleral meshworks (Figure 3A, D). HAS2 protein appeared to be the most abundant HAS and was distributed throughout the TM, both surrounding the beams of the outer uveal and corneoscleral meshworks with somewhat less in the ECM of the JCT region (Figure 3B, E). There was some variability in HAS2 staining in eyes from different individuals, and also in sections from around the circumference of the eye. HAS2 appeared to be more abundant in sections that contained a collector channel (Figure 3E). HAS3 immunostaining seemed to be largely confined more to the corneoscleral meshwork, with less immunostaining of the JCT region. There did not seem to be much variation in HAS3 immunostaining that was dependent on the presence of a collector channel. However, there still appeared to be circumferential variation in different sections from around the eye.

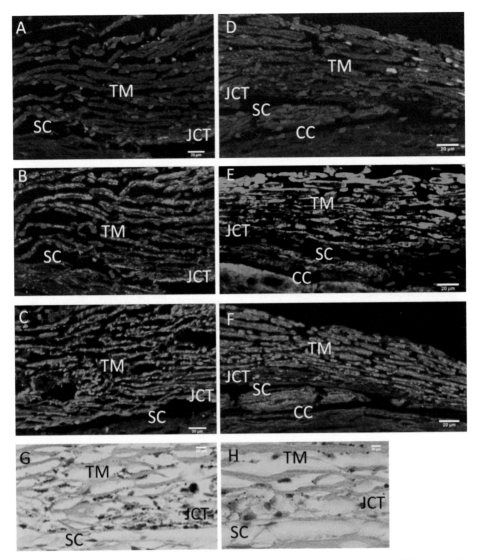

Figure 3: HAS protein immunostaining in radial sections of normal human TM tissue from 2 different individuals (A-C, 69 year old male; D-F, 88 year old male). (A, D) HAS1, (B, E) HAS2 and (C, F) HAS3. (G, H) Hematoxylin and eosin staining of sections from the 69 year old eye shown in (A-C). TM = trabecular meshwork, JCT = juxtacanalicular region, SC = Schlemm's canal, CC = collector channel. DAPI was used to stain nuclei (blue). Scale bars = 20 μm.

4 Discussion

The aim of this study was to investigate HAS gene expression and protein distribution in TM tissue and whether changes in HAS mRNA levels in response to elevated IOP could explain the reduction in HA concentration that is associated with normal aging and in POAG TM tissue. While there may be differences in antibody binding or primer annealing, our results suggest that, at both the mRNA and protein levels, HAS2 is the most abundant HAS expressed in TM tissue, followed by HAS3, with lower HAS1 expression. In other cell types, it is known that each HAS synthesizes unique HA chains: HAS1 and HAS2 synthesize large molecular weight HA chains, while HAS3 synthesizes low molecular weight HA (Adamia *et al.*, 2005; Itano, 2008; Itano *et al.*, 1999). In addition, different activities of each synthase lead to alterations in the amount of each HA chain synthesized. HAS2 and HAS3 produce abundant HA chains, while HAS1 is less active (Itano *et al.*, 1999). Although we did not assess HA size or concentration in this study, the high expression levels of HAS2 is consistent with large amounts of large molecular weight HA being synthesized by TM cells.

HAS mRNA expression directly correlates to HA synthesis in other cell types (Guo *et al.*, 2007; Tammi *et al.*, 2011). Previously, we showed that this was also true for TM cells since there was a decrease in HA concentration and lower HAS protein levels when each HAS gene was individually knocked down using RNAi silencing lentivirus to infect TM cells in culture (Keller *et al.*, 2012a). Thus, HAS gene activity directly relates to HA concentration in TM cell culture. In another study, HA concentration in the JCT of TM tissue of glaucoma eyes was shown to be more depleted than age-matched control eyes (Knepper *et al.*, 1996b). In this study, we found that HAS2 gene expression was decreased in glaucoma eyes compared to normal eyes perfused at physiological pressure, although this decrease was not significant. Based on our cell culture knockdown data, lower HAS mRNA expression may result in lower HAS protein levels in TM tissue, although this was not directly tested here. Nonetheless, this data suggests that most of the depletion of HA in glaucoma eyes is likely due to decreased levels of HAS2, rather than HAS1 or HAS3. This provides one explanation as to why HA concentration is highly reduced in POAG eyes. However, HA concentration can also be reduced by degradation by hyaluronidases. Further studies are required to assess the expression levels, protein distribution and activity of each of the hyaluronidases (HYALs) in order to fully understand the regulation of HA concentration in the TM of normal and POAG eyes.

In response to elevated pressure, we show that expression of all 3 HAS genes was dramatically reduced in POAG eyes, whereas only HAS1 was significantly reduced in normal eyes. This indicates that all three HASs likely contribute to the paucity of HA in glaucoma eyes in response to pressure. Certainly, decreased HAS gene expression dramatically alters outflow facility. This was shown using lentiviruses to silence each HAS individually. These were applied to human anterior segment perfusion culture *in vitro* to test their effects on outflow rates. It was found that individual knockdown of HAS1 and HAS2 significantly decreased outflow rates, which is indicative of increased IOP, but knock down of HAS3 had no effect (Keller *et al.*, 2012a). In POAG eyes, a combined reduction of all 3 HAS genes in response to pressure likely decreases HA concentration in the TM to a greater extent than individual HAS knockdown. This combinatory response, in turn, would profoundly affect outflow resistance. The differential effects on HAS gene expression between normal and glaucoma eyes may help explain why glaucoma eyes develop elevated IOP.

Depletion of HA also may have profound consequences for other ECM molecules. In our prior study, we used 3 different ways to reduce HA concentration in TM cells and tissue: treatment with 4-methylumbelliferone (4-MU), RNAi silencing of each individual HAS gene and using daily hyaluronidase treatment to degrade HA chains (Keller *et al.*, 2012a). In each case, the levels of versican and fibronectin mRNA and protein were concomitantly reduced. Thus, a reduction of HAS gene expression, and therefore HA concentration, in POAG eyes in response to pressure could have secondary effects on the expression levels of other ECM molecules. Moreover, GAG chains also influence the binding interactions of ECM molecules. Our previous studies showed that inhibition of GAG chain sulfation or attachment of GAG chains to their core proteins led to an abnormally high colocalization of tenascin C with fibronectin (Keller *et al.*, 2008). Although these studies do not provide direct evidence for HA because it is not sulfated or attached to a proteoglycan, it does demonstrate the influence that GAG chains have on ECM binding interactions and assembly. Thus, reduced HA concentration could negatively impact ECM form and function in normal aged and POAG eyes

An accumulation of HA in the pericellular matrix creates a hydrated zone that facilitates cell-shape changes (Toole, 2004). Therefore, it is conceivable that a reduction in HA concentration caused by decreased HAS activity may be detrimental to TM cell contractility. Alterations in cell contractility can profoundly influence homeostatic responses to elevated pressure (Tian *et al.*, 2009). Moreover, HA interacts with numerous cell surface receptors. These can bind HA produced by all HAS proteins. However, there is mounting evidence that low molecular weight HA, or HA fragments produced by hyaluronidase degradation of large HA chains, are more efficient at activating cellular signaling pathways via cell surface receptors than high molecular weight HA (Camenisch & Mcdonald, 2000; Lokeshwar & Selzer, 2000). HAS3 is the synthase that produces low MW HA (Itano *et al.*, 1999). Our data shows that HAS3 is significantly reduced in glaucoma eyes in response to pressure. A reduction in low molecular weight HA chains synthesized by HAS3 may have important consequences on the activation or modulation of TM cellular signaling pathways and cell behavior.

Our HAS2 and HAS3 protein distribution was consistent with that of a previous study that showed HAS protein highly expressed in the outer uveal and corneoscleral meshworks with less in the JCT regions of the tissue (Rittig *et al.*, 1993). Glaucomatous tissue was also immunostained with HAS antibodies but no differences in immunostaining patterns was noted compared to normal TM tissue, although these studies were performed on a limited number of samples. Differences in HAS protein immunostaining may indicate individual biological variations, or may reflect regional differences in HAS protein levels around the circumference of the eye. Previously we found that HA binding protein (HAbp), which is a link domain protein that binds to HA, showed somewhat variable staining around the eye (Keller *et al.*, 2008; Keller *et al.*, 2012b). It has been long known that aqueous outflow is not uniform around the circumference of the eye. Several studies utilizing tracer particles e.g. zymosan, latex microspheres, cationic ferritin, fluorescent Qdots, etc indicated that segmental variations in outflow exist (Battista *et al.*, 2008; Buller *et al.*, 1990; De Kater *et al.*, 1989; Ethier & Chan, 2001; Hann *et al.*, 2005; Hann & Fautsch, 2009; Johnson *et al.*, 1990; Keller *et al.*, 2011; Lu *et al.*, 2008; Lu *et al.*, 2011). The TM can therefore been separated into regions of high and low outflow. This geographic outflow segmentation appears to be consistent across species (human, monkeys, bovine, mice) (Zhu *et al.*, 2013). Logically, there must be molecular differences between the components of each region that either affect, or possibly reflect, the geographical outflow pathways. Other studies show variability in the immunostaining patterns of some ECM molecules e.g. fibronectin and HAbp-labeling of HA chains (Floyd *et al.*, 1985; Keller *et al.*, 2008) but at the time the studies were performed, these distributions were not correlated with tracer particles. More recently, we investigated the distribution of versican, a CS-bearing proteoglycan, in the TM of human and porcine eyes (Keller *et al.*, 2011). This study was the first to correlate expression of an ECM molecule with regions of high and low outflow, as delineated using fluorescent tracer particles. We found an inverse relationship between versican levels and outflow: high versican expression was observed in low outflow regions and conversely, low versican expression was found in areas of high outflow (Keller *et al.*, 2011). Another group has suggested that there is an anatomical relationship to segmental outflow since outflow was found to be higher where collector channels were located (Hann & Fautsch, 2009). Together, these studies suggest that morphological and molecular differences contribute to the outflow pathways of the TM. One function of HA is to provide an environment through which aqueous can flow. Our study shows apparently more abundant HAS2 expression in areas with a collector channel inferring that HA concentration may also be higher in areas with collector channels. This immunolocalization data is consistent with increased HA concentration in areas of higher fluid flow. However, further studies will be required to correlate HAS gene expression and HA concentration in regions of high and low segmental outflow using fluorescent tracers.

One limitation of this study was that we only analyzed one time point (24 hours) after pressure treatment. This time point was chosen as it is reflective of the time frame of a homeostatic response to pressure changes. A homeostatic response to pressure typically takes 1-3 days and in this time the TM cells release MMPs to focally degrade existing ECM, while concurrently synthesizing replacement ECM that is slightly different in order to maintain the modified outflow (Keller *et al.*, 2009a; Keller *et al.*, 2007). TM cells also have the ability to discriminate between these sustained pressure increases and more transient pressure changes, for instance if you rub your eyes or bend over to tie your shoe laces. Another limitation of this study was that it was performed in perfusion culture, which is not a live *in vivo* study. However, we chose to use perfusion culture since this is the closest *in vitro* model we have to analyze molecular changes in the TM (Johnson, 2005). Perfusion culture has the advantages that pressure changes can be studied and we can analyze the differences between normal and glaucoma eyes, both of which are not possible with live animal models or in humans.

In summary, our data suggests that HAS2 is the most highly expressed HAS in TM tissue, which is consistent with synthesis of high amounts of large molecular weight HA. Alterations in HAS gene expression may contribute to the paucity of HA in normal aged eyes and in POAG eyes. The combined effects of altered HAS gene expression will deplete HA concentration in the TM, influence aqueous humor outflow resistance and is likely a contributing factor to elevated IOP in glaucoma patients.

Acknowledgements

The authors would like to acknowledge our grant funding sources: NIH grants EY019643 (KEK), EY003279, EY008247, EY010572 (TSA), a grant-in-aid from Fight for Sight, New York, NY (KEK) and by an unrestricted grant to the Casey Eye Institute from Research to Prevent Blindness, New York, NY.

Authors

Kate E. Keller
Oregon Health & Science University, Portland, OR, USA

Ted S. Acott
Oregon Health & Science University, Portland, OR, USA

References

Acott, T. S., & Kelley, M. J. (2008). Extracellular matrix in the trabecular meshwork. Exp Eye Res, 86(4), 543-561.

Acott, T. S., Kingsley, P. D., Samples, J. R., & Van Buskirk, E. M. (1988). Human trabecular meshwork organ culture: morphology and glycosaminoglycan synthesis. Invest Ophthalmol Vis Sci, 29(1), 90-100.

Acott, T. S., Westcott, M., Passo, M. S., & Van Buskirk, E. M. (1985). Trabecular meshwork glycosaminoglycans in human and cynomolgus monkey eye. Invest Ophthalmol Vis Sci, 26(10), 1320-1329.

Adamia, S., Maxwell, C. A., & Pilarski, L. M. (2005). Hyaluronan and hyaluronan synthases: potential therapeutic targets in cancer. Curr Drug Targets Cardiovasc Haematol Disord, 5(1), 3-14.

Barany, E. H., & Scotchbrook, S. (1954). Influence of testicular hyaluronidase on the resistance to flow through the angle of the anterior chamber. Acta Physiol Scand, 30(2-3), 240-248.

Battista, S. A., Lu, Z., Hofmann, S., Freddo, T., Overby, D. R., & Gong, H. (2008). Reduction of the available area for aqueous humor outflow and increase in meshwork herniations into collector channels following acute IOP elevation in bovine eyes. Invest Ophthalmol Vis Sci, 49(12), 5346-5352.

Bornstein, P., & Sage, E. H. (2002). Matricellular proteins: extracellular modulators of cell function. Curr Opin Cell Biol, 14(5), 608-616.

Bradley, J. M., Kelley, M. J., Zhu, X., Anderssohn, A. M., Alexander, J. P., & Acott, T. S. (2001). Effects of mechanical stretching on trabecular matrix metalloproteinases. Invest Ophthalmol Vis Sci, 42(7), 1505-1513.

Bradley, J. M., Vranka, J., Colvis, C. M., Conger, D. M., Alexander, J. P., Fisk, A. S., . . . Acott, T. S. (1998). Effect of matrix metalloproteinases activity on outflow in perfused human organ culture. Invest Ophthalmol Vis Sci, 39(13), 2649-2658.

Buller, C., Johnson, D. H., & Tschumper, R. C. (1990). Human trabecular meshwork phagocytosis. Observations in an organ culture system. Invest Ophthalmol Vis Sci, 31(10), 2156-2163.

Camenisch, T. D., & McDonald, J. A. (2000). Hyaluronan: is bigger better? Am J Respir Cell Mol Biol, 23(4), 431-433.

Cavallotti, C., Feher, J., Pescosolido, N., & Sagnelli, P. (2004). Glycosaminoglycans in human trabecular meshwork: age-related changes. Ophthalmic Res, 36(4), 211-217.

Chowdhury, U. R., Jea, S. Y., Oh, D. J., Rhee, D. J., & Fautsch, M. P. (2011). Expression profile of the matricellular protein osteopontin in primary open-angle glaucoma and the normal human eye. Invest Ophthalmol Vis Sci, 52(9), 6443-6451.

de Kater, A. W., Melamed, S., & Epstein, D. L. (1989). Patterns of aqueous humor outflow in glaucomatous and nonglaucomatous human eyes. A tracer study using cationized ferritin. Arch Ophthalmol, 107(4), 572-576.

Ethier, C. R. (2002). The inner wall of Schlemm's canal. Exp Eye Res, 74(2), 161-172.

Ethier, C. R., & Chan, D. W. (2001). Cationic ferritin changes outflow facility in human eyes whereas anionic ferritin does not. Invest Ophthalmol Vis Sci, 42(8), 1795-1802.

Floyd, B. B., Cleveland, P. H., & Worthen, D. M. (1985). Fibronectin in human trabecular drainage channels. Invest Ophthalmol Vis Sci, 26(6), 797-804.

Francois, J., Rabaey, M., & Neetens, A. (1956). Perfusion studies on the outflow of aqueous humor in human eyes. AMA Arch Ophthalmol, 55(2), 193-204.

Gabelt, B. T., & Kaufman, P. L. (2005). Changes in aqueous humor dynamics with age and glaucoma. Prog Retin Eye Res, 24(5), 612-637.

Goel, M., Picciani, R. G., Lee, R. K., & Bhattacharya, S. K. (2010). Aqueous humor dynamics: a review. Open Ophthalmol J, 4, 52-59.

Gong, H., Underhill, C. B., & Freddo, T. F. (1994). Hyaluronan in the bovine ocular anterior segment, with emphasis on the outflow pathways. Invest Ophthalmol Vis Sci, 35(13), 4328-4332.

Grant, W. M. (1963). Experimental aqueous perfusion in enucleated human eyes. Arch Ophthalmol, 69, 783-801.

Guo, N., Kanter, D., Funderburgh, M. L., Mann, M. M., Du, Y., & Funderburgh, J. L. (2007). A rapid transient increase in hyaluronan synthase-2 mRNA initiates secretion of hyaluronan by corneal keratocytes in response to transforming growth factor beta. J Biol Chem, 282(17), 12475-12483.

Haddadin, R. I., Oh, D. J., Kang, M. H., Filippopoulos, T., Gupta, M., Hart, L., Sage, E.H., & Rhee, D. J. (2009). SPARC-null mice exhibit lower intraocular pressures. Invest Ophthalmol Vis Sci, 50(8), 3771-3777.

Haddadin, R. I., Oh, D. J., Kang, M. H., Villarreal, G., Jr., Kang, J. H., Jin, R., Gong, H., & Rhee, D. J. (2012). Thrombospondin-1 (TSP1)-Null and TSP2-Null Mice Exhibit Lower Intraocular Pressures. Invest Ophthalmol Vis Sci, 53(10), 6708-6717.

Hann, C. R., Bahler, C. K., & Johnson, D. H. (2005). Cationic ferritin and segmental flow through the trabecular meshwork. Invest Ophthalmol Vis Sci, 46(1), 1-7.

Hann, C. R., & Fautsch, M. P. (2009). Preferential fluid flow in the human trabecular meshwork near collector channels. Invest Ophthalmol Vis Sci, 50(4), 1692-1697.

Hua, Q., Knudson, C. B., & Knudson, W. (1993). Internalization of hyaluronan by chondrocytes occurs via receptor-mediated endocytosis. J Cell Sci, 106 (Pt 1), 365-375.

Hubbard, W. C., Johnson, M., Gong, H., Gabelt, B. T., Peterson, J. A., Sawhney, R., Freddo, T., & Kaufman, P. L. (1997). Intraocular pressure and outflow facility are unchanged following acute and chronic intracameral chondroitinase ABC and hyaluronidase in monkeys. Exp Eye Res, 65(2), 177-190.

Itano, N. (2008). Simple primary structure, complex turnover regulation and multiple roles of hyaluronan. J Biochem, 144(2), 131-137.

Itano, N., Sawai, T., Yoshida, M., Lenas, P., Yamada, Y., Imagawa, M., Shinomura, T., Hamaguchi, M., Yoshida, Y., Ohnuki, Y., Miyauchi, S., Spicer, A.P., McDonald, J.A., & Kimata, K. (1999). Three isoforms of mammalian hyaluronan synthases have distinct enzymatic properties. J Biol Chem, 274(35), 25085-25092.

Johnson, D. H. (2005). Trabecular meshwork and uveoscleral outflow models. J Glaucoma, 14(4), 308-310.

Johnson, M. (2006). 'What controls aqueous humour outflow resistance?'. Exp Eye Res, 82(4), 545-557.

Johnson, M., Johnson, D. H., Kamm, R. D., DeKater, A. W., & Epstein, D. L. (1990). The filtration characteristics of the aqueous outflow system. Exp Eye Res, 50(4), 407-418.

Kang, M. H., Oh, D. J., & Rhee, D. J. (2011). Effect of hevin deletion in mice and characterization in trabecular meshwork. Invest Ophthalmol Vis Sci, 52(5), 2187-2193.

Keller, K. E., Aga, M., Bradley, J. M., Kelley, M. J., & Acott, T. S. (2009a). Extracellular matrix turnover and outflow resistance. Exp Eye Res, 88(4), 676-682.

Keller, K. E., Bradley, J. M., & Acott, T. S. (2009b). Differential effects of ADAMTS-1, -4, and -5 in the trabecular meshwork. Invest Ophthalmol Vis Sci, 50(12), 5769-5777.

Keller, K. E., Bradley, J. M., Kelley, M. J., & Acott, T. S. (2008). Effects of modifiers of glycosaminoglycan biosynthesis on outflow facility in perfusion culture. Invest Ophthalmol Vis Sci, 49(6), 2495-2505.

Keller, K. E., Bradley, J. M., Vranka, J. A., & Acott, T. S. (2011). Segmental versican expression in the trabecular meshwork and involvement in outflow facility. Invest Ophthalmol Vis Sci, 52(8), 5049-5057.

Keller, K. E., Kelley, M. J., & Acott, T. S. (2007). Extracellular matrix gene alternative splicing by trabecular meshwork cells in response to mechanical stretching. Invest Ophthalmol Vis Sci, 48(3), 1164-1172.

Keller, K. E., Sun, Y. Y., Vranka, J. A., Hayashi, L., & Acott, T. S. (2012a). Inhibition of hyaluronan synthesis reduces versican and fibronectin levels in trabecular meshwork cells. PLoS One, 7(11), e48523.

Keller, K. E., Sun, Y. Y., Yang, Y. F., Bradley, J. M., & Acott, T. S. (2012b). *Perturbation of hyaluronan synthesis in the trabecular meshwork and the effects on outflow facility. Invest Ophthalmol Vis Sci, 53(8), 4616-4625.*

Keller, K. E., Vranka, J. A., Haddadin, R. I., Kang, M. H., Oh, D. J., Rhee, D. J., . . . Acott, T. S. (2013). *The effects of tenacin C knockdown on trabecular meshwork outflow resistance. Invest Ophthalmol Vis Sci, 54(8), 5613-5623.*

Kelley, M. J., Rose, A. Y., Keller, K. E., Hessle, H., Samples, J. R., & Acott, T. S. (2009). *Stem cells in the trabecular meshwork: present and future promises. Exp Eye Res, 88(4), 747-751.*

Knepper, P. A., Fadel, J. R., Miller, A. M., Goossens, W., Choi, J., Nolan, M. J., & Whitmer, S. (2005). *Reconstitution of trabecular meshwork GAGs: influence of hyaluronic acid and chondroitin sulfate on flow rates. J Glaucoma, 14(3), 230-238.*

Knepper, P. A., Farbman, A. I., & Telser, A. G. (1984). *Exogenous hyaluronidases and degradation of hyaluronic acid in the rabbit eye. Invest Ophthalmol Vis Sci, 25(3), 286-293.*

Knepper, P. A., Goossens, W., Hvizd, M., & Palmberg, P. F. (1996a). *Glycosaminoglycans of the human trabecular meshwork in primary open-angle glaucoma. Invest Ophthalmol Vis Sci, 37(7), 1360-1367.*

Knepper, P. A., Goossens, W., & Palmberg, P. F. (1996b). *Glycosaminoglycan stratification of the juxtacanalicular tissue in normal and primary open-angle glaucoma. Invest Ophthalmol Vis Sci, 37(12), 2414-2425.*

Knudson, W., Chow, G., & Knudson, C. B. (2002). *CD44-mediated uptake and degradation of hyaluronan. Matrix Biol, 21(1), 15-23.*

Lerner, L. E., Polansky, J. R., Howes, E. L., & Stern, R. (1997). *Hyaluronan in the human trabecular meshwork. Invest Ophthalmol Vis Sci, 38(6), 1222-1228.*

Lokeshwar, V. B., & Selzer, M. G. (2000). *Differences in hyaluronic acid-mediated functions and signaling in arterial, microvessel, and vein-derived human endothelial cells. J Biol Chem, 275(36), 27641-27649.*

Lu, Z., Overby, D. R., Scott, P. A., Freddo, T. F., & Gong, H. (2008). *The mechanism of increasing outflow facility by rho-kinase inhibition with Y-27632 in bovine eyes. Exp Eye Res, 86(2), 271-281.*

Lu, Z., Zhang, Y., Freddo, T. F., & Gong, H. (2011). *Similar hydrodynamic and morphological changes in the aqueous humor outflow pathway after washout and Y27632 treatment in monkey eyes. Exp Eye Res, 93(4), 397-404.*

Lutjen-Drecoll, E., Schenholm, M., Tamm, E., & Tengblad, A. (1990). *Visualization of hyaluronic acid in the anterior segment of rabbit and monkey eyes. Exp Eye Res, 51(1), 55-63.*

Maepea, O., & Bill, A. (1992). *Pressures in the juxtacanalicular tissue and Schlemm's canal in monkeys. Exp Eye Res, 54(6), 879-883.*

Nagano, O., & Saya, H. (2004). *Mechanism and biological significance of CD44 cleavage. Cancer Sci, 95(12), 930-935.*

Oh, D. J., Kang, M. H., Ooi, Y. H., Choi, K. R., Sage, E. H., & Rhee, D. J. (2013). *Overexpression of SPARC in human trabecular meshwork increases intraocular pressure and alters extracellular matrix. Invest Ophthalmol Vis Sci, 54(5), 3309-3319.*

Overby, D. R., Stamer, W. D., & Johnson, M. (2009). *The changing paradigm of outflow resistance generation: towards synergistic models of the JCT and inner wall endothelium. Exp Eye Res, 88(4), 656-670.*

Ponta, H., Sherman, L., & Herrlich, P. A. (2003). *CD44: from adhesion molecules to signalling regulators. Nat Rev Mol Cell Biol, 4(1), 33-45.*

Quigley, H. A. (1996). *Number of people with glaucoma worldwide. Br J Ophthalmol, 80(5), 389-393.*

Quigley, H. A. (2011). *Glaucoma. Lancet, 377(9774), 1367-1377.*

Rhee, D. J., Haddadin, R. I., Kang, M. H., & Oh, D. J. (2009). *Matricellular proteins in the trabecular meshwork. Exp Eye Res, 88(4), 694-703.*

Rittig, M., Flugel, C., Prehm, P., & Lutjen-Drecoll, E. (1993). *Hyaluronan synthase immunoreactivity in the anterior segment of the primate eye. Graefes Arch Clin Exp Ophthalmol, 231(6), 313-317.*

Rosenquist, R., Epstein, D., Melamed, S., Johnson, M., & Grant, W. M. (1989). *Outflow resistance of enucleated human eyes at two different perfusion pressures and different extents of trabeculotomy. Curr Eye Res, 8(12), 1233-1240.*

Sawaguchi, S., Yue, B. Y., Yeh, P., & Tso, M. O. (1992). *Effects of intracameral injection of chondroitinase ABC in vivo. Arch Ophthalmol, 110(1), 110-117.*

Stamer, W. D. (2012). *The cell and molecular biology of glaucoma: mechanisms in the conventional outflow pathway. Invest Ophthalmol Vis Sci, 53(5), 2470-2472.*

Stamer, W. D., & Acott, T. S. (2012). *Current understanding of conventional outflow dysfunction in glaucoma. Curr Opin Ophthalmol, 23(2), 135-143.*

Tamm, E. R. (2009). *The trabecular meshwork outflow pathways: structural and functional aspects. Exp Eye Res, 88(4), 648-655.*

Tammi, M. I., Day, A. J., & Turley, E. A. (2002). *Hyaluronan and homeostasis: a balancing act. J Biol Chem, 277(7), 4581-4584.*

Tammi, R. H., Passi, A. G., Rilla, K., Karousou, E., Vigetti, D., Makkonen, K., & Tammi, M. I. (2011). *Transcriptional and post-translational regulation of hyaluronan synthesis. FEBS J, 278(9), 1419-1428.*

Tian, B., Gabelt, B. T., Geiger, B., & Kaufman, P. L. (2009). *The role of the actomyosin system in regulating trabecular fluid outflow. Exp Eye Res, 88(4), 713-717.*

Toole, B. P. (2004). *Hyaluronan: from extracellular glue to pericellular cue. Nat Rev Cancer, 4(7), 528-539.*

Zhu, J. Y., Ye, W., Wang, T., & Gong, H. Y. (2013). *Reversible changes in aqueous outflow facility, hydrodynamics, and morphology following acute intraocular pressure variation in bovine eyes. Chin Med J (Engl), 126(8), 1451-1457.*

Quality of Life in Nigerian Glaucoma Patients

Chigozie Anuli Mbadugha and Adeola Olukorede Onakoya

1 Introduction

Glaucoma is an optic neuropathy associated with retinal ganglion cell loss, characteristic optic nerve head changes and corresponding visual field defects with intra-ocular pressure as a modifiable risk factor. It is the leading cause of irreversible blindness globally (Quigley & Broman, 2006) and it is estimated that by the year 2020, 79.6 million people will have glaucoma and 11.2 million will be bilaterally blind from glaucoma. Several studies have reported that in people of African descent, glaucoma has a higher prevalence (Tielsch et al., 1990; Racette et al., 2003) and earlier onset (Wilson et al., 1985). Glaucoma in blacks also appears to be more severe (Racette et al., 2003) and more refractory to medical therapy (Murdoch, 1996) with a higher risk of visual impairment or blindness (Munoz et al., 2000). About two million people are thought to develop glaucoma annually and more than 50% of people who have glaucoma in the developed world (Tielsch et al., 1991; Mitchell et al., 1997) are undiagnosed while in developing countries, more than 90% are outside care (Ramakrishnan et al., 2003).

Kyari et al. (2009) and the Nigerian National Blindness and Visual Impairment Study Group reported that glaucoma was the second leading cause of blindness after cataract and was responsible for 16.7% of blindness in the study population. The prevalence of blindness for Nigeria was reported to be 4.2% and ranged from 2.8% - 6.1% in the six geo-political zones of the country. The cause-specific prevalence of blindness due to Glaucoma was 0.7%. Primary open angle glaucoma (POAG) is the commonest type of glaucoma seen in Nigeria (Omoti, 2005; Enock et al., 2010) and is characteristically symptomless in its early stages. It is therefore not uncommon for glaucoma patients to be bilaterally blind at presentation to hospitals in the Southern part of Nigeria (Omoti et al., 2002; Nwosu, 1996).

1.1 Effect of Blindness

Blindness has far-reaching effects on people's ability to function independently in virtually every sphere of their lives. It affects the physical, mental and social well-being of people. Poor vision can affect the ability of patients to carry out activities of daily living and personal care and can cause poor orientation and mobility. All these ultimately lead to loss of self-confidence and independence. Good vision is required for many jobs and patients with advanced glaucoma, who have severe visual loss, may need to be rehabilitated to acquire skills for other jobs or crafts which are less visually demanding than their present employment.

Traditionally, glaucoma patients have been monitored over time using physician based outcomes (Massof & Rubin, 2001) such as intra-ocular pressures, visual field assessments and more recently, objective tests of optic nerve head or retinal nerve fibre layer structure such as confocal scanning laser ophthalmoscopy and retinal nerve fibre layer analysis. These have been used to assess efficacy of treatment (Sawada et al., 2011), evaluate disease severity and progression (Hyman *et al.*, 2005) and indirectly represent patients' ability to function. Though essential, it has been advocated that physician based outcomes are no longer adequate for a holistic evaluation of patients (Cassell, 1982; Wilson *et al.*, 1998; Hartman & Rhee, 2006) as they do not reflect the impact of glaucoma on the functional status and quality of life (QOL) of the patient.

1.2   Quality of Life

The World Health Organization (WHO Anonymous, 1993) defines Quality of life (QOL) as "an individual's perception of their position in life in the context of the culture and value systems in which they live and in relation to their goals, expectations, standards and concerns." It is the subjective perception of wellbeing and wholeness. QOL is a broad, complex and multidimensional concept which includes an assessment of the ability of the patient to meet their needs and how they react to the restrictions they experience. It is therefore subjective, individualised and difficult to measure but its assessment is crucial to a holistic understanding of patients. QOL is affected by the environmental, socio-economic and health conditions in which an individual finds himself. The components or dimensions of QOL include psychological health, physical health, social relationships and environment. Several QOL theories exist and include the classical theory and the item response theory.

Health related QOL is the functional effect of a medical condition and its consequent therapy upon a patient. It is an important indicator which when measured can be used to quantify the degree to which a disease and its treatment affect the patients' life. Its measurement alongside traditional clinical measures captures a more comprehensive picture of the burden of disease experienced by patients.

Ophthalmologists use the term "vision-related QOL" to distinguish the fact that their area of primary interest is the effect of visual loss or impairment and the treatment of eye disease on patients' ability to function optimally. Vision related QOL has been defined as 'a person's satisfaction with their visual ability and how their vision impacts on their daily life' (Asaoka *et al.*, 2011). Vision-related QOL in glaucoma patients has been studied extensively by different authors (Labiris *et al.*, 2010; Goldberg *et al.*, 2009; Magacho *et al.*, 2004; Nelson *et al.*, 2003; Lester & Zingirian, 2002; Wilson *et al.*, 1998; Sherwood *et al.*, 1998; Gutierrez *et al.*, 1997; Jampel, 2001).

QOL domains may differ depending on the questionnaire being used or the research question being studied but essentially, most questionnaires try to include aspects of life which may affect the quality of one's life. This list can be excessively cumbersome; therefore an attempt is often made to include important domains while maintaining brevity. That way, one ensures that the questionnaire remains relevant and suitable for use even in a busy clinical setting. The QOL research unit of the University of Toronto[1] defined QOL simply as the degree to which a person enjoys the important possibilities of his or her life. They identified three major domains of QOL as: (1) The Being Domain; (2) The Belonging Domain; (3) The Becoming Domain. Table 1 describes the domains, components of the sub-domains and the possible effect of poor vision on each of these components.

Patrick & Erickson (1988) on the other hand, outlined opportunity, health perceptions, functional status, impairments, death and duration of life as important concepts to be studied.

---

[1] Global Development Research Centre [online]. 2007 [cited 23/11/2008]: http://www.gdrc.org/ucm/qol-define.html

QOL Domains	Sub-domains & Components	Effect of poor vision on QOL
Being Domain	**Physical Being:** mobility, personal hygiene, Nutrition, grooming.	Decreased mobility & independence; poor hygiene & growth, Tardy appearance
	Psychological Being: feelings, self esteem	Low self-esteem, depression, anger & irritability.
	Spiritual Being: spiritual beliefs, personal value	Despair, lack of faith, hopelessness.
Belonging Domain	**Physical Belonging:** interactions at work & home	Decreased interaction, loss of job & livelihood.
	Social Belonging: acceptance by friends & family	Neglect, decreased social circle
	Community Belonging: access to community resources	Decreased mobility, increased dependence on others to access resources.
Becoming Domain	**Practical Becoming:** employment, activities of daily living	Loss of job & livelihood.
	Leisure Becoming: relaxation, socialization	Lack of relaxation, withdrawal from social circles.
	Growth Becoming: skill & knowledge acquisition & maintenance	Lack of zeal & zest for life; stagnancy & feeling of lack of progress or achievement.

Table 1: Interaction between vision & quality of life.

The abbreviated form of the QOL assessment questionnaire designed by the World Health Organisation, the WHOQOL-Bref Questionnaire (Skevington *et al.*, 2004) has the following domains: physical health, psychological health, environment and social relationships.

The social relationships domain of the WHOQOL-Bref questionnaire explores patients' personal relationships, sexual activity and social support. This is important because even though overtly one may not see the essence of asking ophthalmology patients questions relating to sexual health, it is pertinent to note that topical beta-blockers which are commonly used in glaucoma patients can affect libido and sexual health. Patients, who experience this side effect, may not volunteer this information to their ophthalmologist because they may feel it is not their terrain and may not have made the connection between the use of the eye drop and their complaint. If they present to a urologist or a gynaecologist, they may not inform the attending physician of the eye drops they use. Most ophthalmology patients in Nigeria do not see eye drops as drugs. The answer to the question 'Are you on any routine medications prescribed by a doctor?' in the past drug history component of the medial history is usually in the negative unless one is specific enough to ask about eye drop usage. So these patients may present as a diagnostic dilemma to their attending physician and be subjected to a barrage of unnecessary investigations.

Several multidimensional factors influence QOL. The socio-demographic characteristics of individuals (age, gender, and educational status), life experiences and culture may affect an individual's QOL. Individualised characteristics such as patient's temperament, personality

(Warrian *et al.*, 2009) and life expectations also influence QOL. Wrosch & Scheier (2003) reported that dispositional optimism in a person's personality facilitates subjective wellbeing and good health which is mediated by a person's coping behaviour. This explains why some patients who have an easy going cheerful disposition being managed for advanced or end-stage remain hopeful with less decrease in their QOL than expected given the stage or severity of the disease. Conversely, some patients with early or mild glaucoma and minimal visual field loss who have an anxious or panicky disposition tend to be more psychologically affected by a diagnosis of glaucoma. These fears should neither be dismissed nor ignored but should be elucidated so that adequate psychological support could be given to patients who need it.

A patient's perception, belief system and experiences may also affect his/her QOL. A patient with a first degree relative who became blind from glaucoma is more likely to be afraid of going blind from glaucoma. This fear of blindness can have several effects on the patient's outlook. It may create a healthy caution that makes the patient extremely compliant and adherent to drug usage and follow-up visits which is beneficial or it could make the patient despondent and uninterested in whatever therapy is being offered to them with consequent poor drug compliance and irregular attendance at scheduled clinic visits. Conversely, patients with early or mild glaucoma who do not have a first degree relative with poor vision as a result of glaucoma are more likely to have difficulty accepting their diagnosis and understanding the need for strict compliance and adherence to treatment regimen and hospital visits.

The potential effect of spiritual, religious and personal beliefs on QOL is evidenced by the recent development of a short term measure to assess spiritual, religious and personal beliefs (SPRB) within QOL (Skevington *et al.*, 2013). Nigerian patients are often very religious and are usually quick to 'reject' a diagnosis of glaucoma and deny the need for other family members to screen for glaucoma. They strongly believe that their family members are not at risk and are unlikely to convey the need for periodic glaucoma eye screening to their relatives.

The culture or way of life of a group of people influences their belief system or outlook about life. The culture also influences QOL by the role definition and responsibilities it ascribes to members of the community. Patients often define personal success or failure based on their ability to fulfil these roles and responsibilities and their emotional response to the restrictions they experience impact on their QOL. Culture also dictates the extent of family or communal support available to members of the community. Nigerians communities have been known to have a strong extended family support system which can be useful in times of crises but with modernisation and urban migration, this support system is gradually weakening (Fajemilehun & Odebiyi 2011; Adebowale *et al.*, 2012). Nigerians do not have a strong reading culture and therefore may not accurately respond to QOL questions regarding difficulties encountered when reading newspapers, magazines or novels. However being quite religious, they are more likely to complain about difficulties experienced when reading spiritual books and devotionals. The cinema culture in Nigeria had been moribund for years and the ready availability of digital cable stations and Nigerian films recorded on digital versatile discs reduced people's desire to visit the cinema for entertainment at an extra cost. It is only in the last five to ten years that there has been a reawakening of the cinema culture with the establishment of modern cinema halls which are largely patronised by youths, the elite and the rich. Questions regarding difficulty experienced when going to the cinema may therefore not be very appropriate for the older generation and the low or middle income earners. Such QOL questions could be made more culturally relevant in Nigeria by replacing them with questions on whether they have difficulty attending age-group, family, and religious group meetings.

Gureje *et al.* (2008) identified loss of independence, inability to participate in family and community activities and loss of contact with family members and friends as important social factors affecting QOL in elderly Nigerians.

The presence of adequate housing, safe environment, guaranteed income and freedom has also been identified as factors that can influence QOL (Patrick & Bergner 1990). Most houses in Nigeria are built by self-effort for either personal use or tenancy and there is presently a deficit of affordable low-cost houses for low and middle-income earners. The unemployment rate in Nigeria is currently at its peak and for most people, income is far from guaranteed. These social factors could negatively affect QOL of glaucoma patients in Nigeria.

1.2.1   Effect of Glaucoma on QOL

Glaucoma may affect patients' QOL for several reasons (Lester & Zingirian, 2002). There is the psychological effect of being diagnosed with a potentially blinding disease and several studies have identified anxiety and depression in glaucoma patients (Mabuchi *et al.* 2008, Dawodu *et al.* 2004; Skalicky & Goldberg 2008; Akindipe *et al.*, 2011). Odberg *et al.* (2001) reported that 80% of patients experienced negative emotions at diagnosis: 64% were anxious; 33% were afraid of going blind and 23% experienced depression. Anxiety was commoner amongst the younger patients in this study. Janz *et al.* (2007) studied fear of blindness in glaucoma patients over time and reported that the most significant correlate over time was the perceived impact of the disease on an individual's ability to perform visual tasks. They noted a reduction from 34% of patients who were afraid of going blind at the onset to 11–12% after 5 years. They attributed this reduction to reassurance, more knowledge about the low risk of blindness with treatment and adaptation to the diagnosis. Hamelin *et al.* (2002) reported that 11% of glaucoma cases in a study had severe anxiety which necessitated the use of prescription drugs and Heijl (2001) has advised physicians to keep in view the psychological needs of glaucoma patients.

The visual loss associated with progression of glaucoma such as visual field loss, impaired colour vision and stereopsis, reduced contrast sensitivity and ultimately decrease in visual acuity in advanced stages of the disease affects orientation, mobility, driving, independence and activities of daily living. Glaucoma patients may experience difficulty recognising faces, reading, watching television, noticing objects in their peripheral vision and adapting to different levels of lighting. Glaucoma patients are at a higher risk of falls and accidents (Gutierrez *et al.*, 1997; Ivers *et al.*, 1998; Haymes *et al.*, 2007). Drivers diagnosed with glaucoma are three to four times more likely to be involved in a car crash compared to those without the disease (Haymes *et al.*, 2008). Reduced walking speed (Altarangel *et al.*, 2006; Friedman *et al.*, 2007), slower reading speed (Ramulu *et al.*, 2013), postural instability and impaired balance (Shabana *et al.*, 2005; Black *et al.*, 2008; Friedman *et al.*, 2007) restrict patients' ability to perform activities of daily living and reduce their satisfaction with their lifestyle (Turano *et al.*, 2002).

Living with a chronic disease like glaucoma that requires periodic life-long observation and monitoring irrespective of the treatment modality employed has economic implications for patients (Bramley *et al.*, 2008). The follow-up visits are time consuming and some patients with poor vision need to be accompanied to the clinic resulting in an increase in indirect costs through the loss of working hours or earnings for the patient and the companion as well. The periodic investigations and treatment (laser, medical & surgical) are often expensive and in countries like Nigeria where an adequate welfare system is not yet in place, the economic burden of glaucoma is immense. Studies on the economic burden or cost of living with glaucoma have been carried out in different locations globally such as in Nigeria (Adio & Onia 2012); in

Ireland (Knox *et al.* 2003) and in Egypt (Eldaly *et al.,* 2007). Adio & Onia (2012) reported that some middle income earners spent 50% of their monthly income on glaucoma treatment while low income earners, could spend their entire monthly income on glaucoma treatment. Cost has been identified as a significant barrier to adherence to therapy in glaucoma patients (Friedman *et al.,* 2008; Sleath *et al.,* 2006). It is therefore not surprising that compliance and adherence rates are lower amongst Nigerian glaucoma patients (Omoti & Waziri-Erameh, 2003; Ashaye & Adeoye, 2008) than in advanced countries. Non-compliance rates for Nigerian glaucoma patients are as high as 60% (Omoti & Waziri-Erameh 2003) while that in other countries they range from 8%-44% (Tsai *et al.,* 2003; Jampel *et al.,* 2003; Deokule *et al.,* 2003).

The daily use of anti-glaucoma eye drops is sometimes inconvenient and a regular reminder of the fact that one is being managed for a potentially blinding eye disease. The convenient once daily dosing regimen of prostaglandin analogues and the development of newer combination drugs have simplified the dosing schedule for most glaucoma patients but for those on multiple medical therapies, complex dosing schedules may interfere with other activities. These drugs have side effects, may be difficult to instil for the elderly and have been associated with the ocular surface disease experienced by glaucoma patients (Leung *et al.,* 2008; Badouin 2008). Patients who have had surgery and have a cystic filtering bleb may complain of discomfort and a gritty sensation and are at risk of ocular infection in the operated eye.

1.2.2   Benefits of QOL Assessment

Measurement of QOL in glaucoma patients is crucial for several reasons. Primary open angle glaucoma (POAG) which is commoner than angle closure glaucoma in most populations outside the Asian continent is essentially symptomless, can lead to irreversible blindness if untreated and requires life-long follow up irrespective of the treatment modality employed. There is no cure for glaucoma and vision lost from glaucoma cannot be restored with the level of knowledge available at present although research is on-going.

The goal of treatment in glaucoma is therefore to improve clinical outcome by preventing further progression of the disease and ultimately preserve or improve the patients' QOL. It is impossible to preserve or improve something that has not been measured. Vandenbroeck *et al.* (2011) advocate that the patient's perspective is important and should be more fully integrated into clinical practice and research evaluations. This is even more important in a disease like glaucoma where some treatment effects may only be detectable by patients. QOL assessments have been included in several glaucoma clinical trials (Janz *et al.,* 2001; Wren *et al.,* 2009; Hyman *et al.,* 2005; Gedde *et al.,* 2005) such as the Collaborative Initial Glaucoma Treatment Study (CIGTS), the Early Manifest Glaucoma Trial (EMGT) and the primary tube versus trabeculectomy study. QOL assessment has the following advantages:

a)   It improves the holistic management of patients by assessing the impact of the disease on a patient's daily life (burden of disease) and how they are coping with it.

b)   It improves the physician's understanding of patient's challenges with performance of everyday tasks requiring good vision.

c)   It helps identify individual priority areas so that patient management can be customised and it can provide a basis for advocacy for provision of services.

d)   It generates information about how glaucoma affects QOL and how these effects are modified by treatment. This information is useful for patient counselling which helps patients make informed treatment choices in the course of their management (Mills 1998).

e)   QOL assessment process may help assess the economic impact of current and new therapies.

f)   It may help in describing the natural history of the disease (Greenfield & Nelson, 1992).

g)   May assist in assessing the quality of care given to patients.

h)   It may assist in the evaluation of treatment modalities and their efficacy by providing insight into the effect of treatment modalities on QOL.

i)   May be useful for interpreting clinical outcomes.

j)   May guide decision making on priorities, resource allocation and policy implementation.

k)   Enhances patient-provider relationship and the rapport between physicians and patients and this can improve treatment adherence (Nassiri *et al.*, 2013)

l)   Sequential QOL assessments may assist physicians monitor the effect of disease and treatment on QOL.

m)   It can assist clinicians suspect other problems if there is a discrepancy between QOL scores and severity of disease.

n)   It can be used to quantitatively assess patient's satisfaction or to detect increasing visual burden.

QOL assessments are subjective evaluations and therefore are liable to the inherent weaknesses of self-reported assessments. They are highly variable and unpredictable and it is not unusual to find two patients with the same degree of visual loss but markedly different QOL scores. There is no ideal QOL instrument and most QOL tools actually assess functional ability as an indirect measure of QOL.QOL is influenced to a great extent but to variable degrees by socio-demographic variables and psychological concepts which are difficult to assess and measure quantitatively.

1.3   Measurement of QOL

QOL is multidimensional and highly subjective and for this reason, its measurement is difficult. QOL questionnaires are also called tools, measures or instruments. They measure multiple characteristics referred to as scales, domains or constructs and are comprised of questions known as items. QOL assessment tools are quantitative measures which allow comparable, reproducible, responsive and valid functional health status determination to be made. Measurement of QOL is done using either preference based or function based instruments. Preference based instruments assess the value placed by patients on their QOL while function based tools use items to grade the degree of difficulty patients experience while performing vision-related tasks but do not explore the relative priority placed on the performance of these tasks by patients (Aspinall *et al.*, 2007).

1.3.1   Preference based QOL Tools

Preference based measures allow patients to hypothetically give up valuable items (money, time, risk of death) to obtain a cure for a disease. It is derived from economic theory and gives an insight into the burden of the disease as it affects QOL (Leeyaphan *et al.*, 2011). Using preference based measures, patients are asked to choose between alternative life situations. The choices they make are then used to derive the relative importance or value (Aspinall *et al.*, 2007) they place on various tasks. The importance or value placed on these tasks by patients is often determined by their life circumstances, occupational needs and the severity of disease (Gupta *et al.*, 2011). Information on relative priority is crucial for resource allocation and for planning rehabilitation strategies for patients (Massof 1998).

Utility values are preference-based measures that quantify the QOL associated with a health state or disease condition (Brown *et al.*, 1999, Kupfer *et al.*, 2006). They provide an objective measurement of QOL of patients by quantifying their preferences. A utility value of 1.0 is associated with perfect health while a utility value of 0.0 is associated with death (Kymes 2008). The closer the utility value is to 1.0, the better the QOL of the patient. Utility values closer to 0.0 imply a poor QOL. Utility valuation permits patients' objective assessment of the desirability of a disease state according to their perception of their own lives (Brown GC *et al.*, 2000). Utility values are a component of cost-effective or health economic analysis (Aspinall *et al.*, 2007, Drummond *et al.*, 1997). They allow a comparison of widely disparate medical specialties (Brown GC *et al.*, 2001) and are thought to be comprehensive QOL measures since they take into account factors such as anxiety, support systems, socio-economic status and psychological overlay (Redelmeier & Detsky, 1995; Brown MM *et al.*, 1999).

1.3.2   Function based Measures

Functional assessment involves evaluating a patient's ability to perform tasks in domains being investigated and is often used as a surrogate for QOL measurement. It assesses the level of difficulty experienced by patients in carrying out specified activities which require vision. This assessment may be objective or subjective. Objective function based measures involve observing patients carrying out specific tasks and scoring the patient's performance. Tasks which can be observed include balance, range of motion, reading or walking speed, visuo-motor coordination and the time taken to complete an activity. Table 2 summarises the methods and instruments available for the measurement of QOL.

1.3.3   Properties of an Ideal QOL Instrument

An ideal QOL instrument should be sensitive, valid, responsive and reliable. It should have good internal consistency, give a low respondent/ administrative burden and have an easily interpretable scoring system. A sensitive instrument is able to detect differences between varying patient groups such as cases and controls.

The validity of an instrument can be defined as how well it measures what it was intended to measure. Criterion validity can be determined by comparing an instrument to an established gold standard (Tosh *et al.*, 2012). Construct validity can be assessed by evaluating if an instrument is able to distinguish between groups of patients with a defining criteria for categorising them such as patients with varying degrees of severity of disease. Convergent validity can be defined as the extent to which an instrument correlates with another instrument which measures the same concept. It can be assessed by observing the correlation between the individual subscales or domains of the instrument being validated and the overall score from an alternative instrument. Concurrent validity is present if there is an association between the scores obtained from an instrument and clinical measures of visual function like worsening QOL with reduction in visual acuity orprogression of visual field loss in glaucoma.

Instruments for Measuring QOL	Examples
Preference based Tools	Time trade off
	Standard Gamble
	Linear Rating
	Choice based Conjoint Analysis
	Willingness to pay
Questionnaires measuring priorities indirectly	EuroQOL quality of life scale EQ5D
	Glaucoma Utilities Index
	SF-6D
Function Based measures	
Objective function based	AFREV questionnaire
Subjective function based	
Generic instruments	36 item Short Form Questionnaire (SF 36)
	20 item Short Form Questionnaire (MOS 20)
	Sickness Impact Profile (SIP)
	WHO-QOL Bref
Vision-related QOL instruments	51 item, 25 item and 19 item National Eye Institute Visual Function Questionnaires: NEIVFQ51, NEIVFQ25, NEIVFQ19.
	14-item visual functioning index (VF14)
	Visual Activities Questionnaire (VAQ)
	Activities of Daily Vision Scale (ADVS)
Disease specific instruments	15 item Glaucoma QOL questionnaire (GQL-15)
	Glaucoma Symptom scale (GSS)
	Viswanathan et al.'s Questionnaire
	Glaucoma Health Perceptions Index (GHPI)
Therapy specific	COMTOL
	TSS-IOP
	GLAUSAT
	Outcome expectation scale
	Glaucoma Self-efficacy scale

Table 2: Methods of measuring QOL.

Other less stringent facets of validity are face validity and content validity. An instrument has face validity if on perusal the scales it is designed to measure look correct and there is content validity if it appears to cover the relevant items.

Responsiveness refers to the ability of an instrument to detect changes in visual status over time. An instrument should detect a change in QOL with progression of a disease or with improvement in visual function after an intervention such as cataract extraction or provision of low vision aids. The reliability of an instrument is defined as its ability to reproduce results when measurements are repeated on an unchanged population (Brazzier & Deverill, 1999). It can be assessed by observing the consistency of the scores on re-administering the instrument after a period of time (test-retest-reliability) or across conditions of re-administration such as mode of instrument administration or interviewer administering the instrument (inter-observer reliability).

The measurement of QOL in glaucoma patients in developing countries like Nigeria is important as it can help improve the quality of eye care given to patients by identifying priority areas for intervention in each individual patient. Given the lean resources available it may provide justification for health care expenditure in the identified areas. Glaucoma is of public health importance in Nigeria being the second leading cause of blindness (Kyari *et al.*, 2009) and a significant cause of bilateral blindness in patients presenting to the eye clinic. Oluleye *et al.* (2006) reported that 29% of bilaterally blind patients attending a general hospital in South-west Nigeria were blind from glaucoma.

2   The Study on QOL of Nigerian Glaucoma Patients

The QOL of glaucoma patients in Nigeria was evaluated because a paucity of data on QOL in this group of patients was noted in spite of an increasing recognition of the need to consider the glaucoma patient's life from his or her perspective in order to obtain a holistic picture of the burden or impact of the disease on the patient's life (Odberg *et al.*, 2001; Lee 1996). This is particularly important in a developing country like Nigeria with a low human development index and which is ranked 153rd out of 187 countries using the United Nations Human Development Index[2]. The average life expectancy for the Nigerian male is very low (48.95 years) and is only slightly higher for the Nigeria female (55.35 years)[3]. This low life expectancy as well as the unacceptably high infant, under-five and maternal mortality rates suggests that health care in Nigeria is faced with several challenges. Nigeria also has no formal structure for social benefits in place presently and the National Health Insurance Scheme (NHIS) is still evolving and is grossly undersubscribed. Medical expenses are therefore often settled by out of the pocket payment by majority of the citizens (Gureje *et al.*, 2008). This is worrisome as nearly 70% of Nigerians are estimated by the World Bank[4] to be living below the poverty line with a high rate of labour force unemployment[5]. Nigerian glaucoma patients have to contend with these socio-economic challenges while struggling to cope with the impact of the disease on their QOL and the potential risk of going blind from glaucoma.

The study was carried out in the glaucoma clinic of the ophthalmic unit of the University of Lagos Teaching Hospital, Lagos, Nigeria. Lagos was the capital of Nigeria until 1991 when the capital was moved to Abuja but remains the commercial nerve centre of the country and is a densely populated urban metropolitan state with an estimated population of 21 million. It is often referred to as the Centre of Excellence and is regarded as a reference point for other states in terms of infrastructure, health policies and job opportunities.

The aim of the study was to evaluate the QOL of Nigerian patients with varying stages of severity of POAG and compare it to the QOL of age and sex matched controls with corrected refractive errors only. Function based methods were chosen for the assessment of QOL in this study because it was felt the Time Trade Off (TTO) and Simple Gamble preference based methods would not be culturally acceptable in Nigeria as death and lifespan are not topics that are discussed freely. An open discussion of death has been reported to be a taboo for Asians (McLaughlin & Braun 1998; Wu *et al.*, 2002). Carr & Robinson (2003) and Wee *et al.* (2008) advocate that the acceptability, feasibility and appropriateness of any tool should al-

---

[2]United Nations Human Development Index [Online]. Cited [24/10/2013]. Available from URL: http://www.hdrstats.undp.org/en/countries/profiles/NGA.html
[3]Index Mundi Nigeria's Demographic profile 2013 [Online] cited [24/10/2013]. Available from URL: http://www.inndexmundi.com/nigeria
[4] World Bank Country Data [Online] cited [24/10/2013]. Available from URL: www.data.worldbank.org/country/nigeria
[5] Economy watch [Online] cited [14/10/2013]. Available from URL: http://www.economywatch.com

ways be considered when selecting a tool for a study. Wee *et al.* (2008) found that religious beliefs influenced some participants' health preferences and that based on their religious beliefs, giving up life years was not an option for them. Some participants even declined to participate after hearing that the survey involved a discussion on death.

A disease specific instrument: 15-item Glaucoma Quality of Life questionnaire (GQL-15) and a non-disease specific instrument: the 25-item National Eye Institute Visual Function Questionnaire (NEIVFQ25) were used for this evaluation. The NEIVFQ25 was chosen because it measures the impact on patients' performance of everyday activities, independence, social relationships and emotional wellbeing (Elliot *et al.*, 2007). It also addresses impairment, participation restriction and activities limitations which are recommended by the World Health Organisation's International Classification of Functioning and Disability & Health (WHO-ICF) as components that are important for assessing health-related components of a disease (McGougall *et al.*, 2010). The GQL-15 was selected because it is a glaucoma-specific questionnaire and has the advantage of being short enough to be included in busy clinical practices with relative ease.

The study hoped to show that QOL assessment is an important complementary aspect of eye care which needs to be incorporated into the clinical management of patients to enable them enjoy meaningful quality lives. This need is greater in a disease that is chronic, progressive and potentially blinding like glaucoma and in patients that the ophthalmologist is likely to manage for the rest of their lives. It hoped to elucidate socio-demographic factors which influence QOL and compare the ability of two vision specific questionnaires to measure QOL in this study population.

3   Methods

The study on QOL in Nigerian glaucoma patients was carried out using a cross-sectional analytical study design. It was a hospital based study. From consecutive patients attending the eye clinic of a tertiary institution in Lagos, Nigeria two groups of 132 participants each with a confirmed diagnosis of Primary Open Angle Glaucoma (POAG) and corrected refractive errors were recruited as cases and controls respectively. The cases and controls were matched by 5-year age categories and by sex. Table 3 lists the inclusion and exclusion criteria for cases and controls in this study.

POAG was defined as the presence of glaucomatous optic nerve head changes, open anterior chamber angles, and visual field loss with or without an elevated IOP in one or both eyes (Mbadugha *et al.*, 2012). The glaucoma patients (cases) were further divided into three groups of 44 participants each based on a modification of the Hodapp-Parrish-Anderson classification (Hodapp *et al.*, 1993) of severity of visual field loss. The value of the mean deviation was noted and patients with mean deviations (MD) less than or equal to -6 decibels (dB) were classified as having mild glaucoma while those with MD greater than -6 dB but less than -12 dB were classified as having moderate glaucoma. Those with MD greater than -12 dB were grouped as patients with severe glaucoma. For patients with asymmetric disease, the more severe eye was used to classify the patient. Enrolment into the different subgroups of glaucoma patients was consecutive and stopped as soon as the pre-determined sample size for the subgroups (44 participants) was reached. The extra time needed to complete the recruitment of participants into other subgroups after completing the recruitment into one did not exceed an extra clinic session.

CASES

INCLUSION CRITERIA

Patients with POAG who were at least 40 years old at the time of diagnosis of POAG in one or both eyes, who were on medical therapy or who had had trabeculectomy at least 3 months before the commencement oft he study.

Patients who met inclusion criteria with mean deviation (MD) cut off values ranging from -0.1dB to -6dB were classified as mild glaucoma cases, >-6dB to less than -12dB as moderate glaucoma cases, >12dB as severe glaucoma cases. Patients with poor vision who could not perform a central visual field test were also classified as having severe glaucoma.

EXCLUSION CRITERIA

History of any intraocular surgery other than glaucoma filtration surgery.

History of a trabeculectomy within the 3 months preceding the study period;

Presence of other eye diseases such as retinopathies, maculopathies, optic neuropathies or visually significant lens opacities defined as greater than stage 2 of the Lens Opacities classification III [LOCS III] (Chylack et al., 1993).

Closed anterior chamber (AC) angles (defined as less than or equal to grade II Shaffer's grading of the anterior chamber angles).

Presence of any other conditions which could be responsible for visual field defects similar to that seen in glaucoma.

History of chronic systemic illnesses such as hypertension, diabetes mellitus, heart disease, mental illness or immunosuppression.

Presence of cognitive, hearing or mobility disability.

CONTROLS

INCLUSION CRITERIA

Age and sex-matched patients with spherical refractive errors less than 5Dioptres Sphere (DS) from emmetropia and/or cylindrical errors less than 2Dioptres Cylinder (DCyl) of astigmatism corrected to at least 6/9, normal optic discs and visual fields.

EXCLUSION CRITERIA

High refractive errors (greater than 5DS from emmetropia and/or cylindrical errors greater than 2DCyl of astigmatism

Best corrected visual acuity less than 6/9

Presence of suspicious optic discs, abnormal visual fields or ocular hypertension (defined as IOP greater than 21mmHg in either eye),

Presence of visually significant lens opacities,

History of glaucoma or unexplained blindness in a first-degree relative

History of chronic systemic illnesses such as hypertension, diabetes mellitus, heart disease, mental illness or immunosuppression.

Presence of cognitive, hearing or mobility disability.

Table 3: Inclusion and Exclusion Criteria for cases & controls.

The October 2008 revision of the declaration of Helsinki was adhered to and ethical approval was obtained from the institutional ethical committee. All participants provided written informed consent and were informed of the general aim of the study and requirements. They were also told that should they decide to withdraw from the study at any time, their decision would not affect any aspect of the care they were receiving from the institution.

A thorough medical and ophthalmic history was obtained and a comprehensive ocular examination was carried out on all participants which included assessment of distance and near visual acuity using a Snellen's chart at 6 metres and a reading booklet at 33cm; colour vision assessment with the City University online colour vision test; stereopsis assessment using a TNO test and contrast sensitivity assessment using a Pelli-Robson chart. Gonioscopy using a 2 mirror gonioscopy lens (Ocular Instruments, Belluvue, CA, USA), tonometry (using a hand-held Perkins applanation tonometer) and dilated funduscopy (after instillation of 3 drops of Gutts Tropicamide over a half hour period) were also carried out. Stereoscopic optic nerve head assessment was done using a Haag Streit slit-lamp and a Volks +78 diopter sphere (DS) lens.

Standard achromatic perimetry using a full threshold central 30-2 strategy (Optifield Sinemed lnc, Benicia, CA) was performed on a separate day. The same central visual field machine operated by a single perimetrist was used throughout the duration of the study. Visual field results were adjudged reliable if the false positive or negative errors were less than 30% and if the fixation losses were less than 20%. Patients whose visual acuity was too poor for them to visualise the fixation targets were classified as having severe glaucoma and were noted. Using a modification of the formula by Nelson-Quigg et $al.$ (2000) a mean deviation value representative of both eyes (MD OU) was calculated as follows:

$$MD\ OU = (MD\ RE^2 + MD\ LE^2)^{1/2}.$$

Quality of life assessment was done after ascertaining that the participants met the eligibility criteria for either cases or controls. Two trained interviewers administered the NEIVFQ25 and the GQL-15 questionnaires. Two utility questions rating vision and general health on a linear scale were selected from the NEIVFQ25 appendix and were also administered in addition to the 25 items in the body of the NEIVFQ25 questionnaire. The same interviewer administered the NEIVFQ25 first and then the GQL-15in a single sitting. Participants were unaware that two different QOL tools were being administered.

The NEIVFQ25 assesses twelve domains. Five are nonvisual domains while seven are visual domains. The visual domains are: general vision (GV), near vision (NV), colour vision (CV), ocular pain (OP), distance vision (DV), peripheral vision (PV) and driving (DRIV). The non-visual domains are mental health (MH), social function (SF), role difficulty (RD), general health (GH) and dependency (DEP). The NEIVFQ25 is an abridged version of the NEIVFQ51 questionnaire which has 51 items. It is a broad instrument developed by the Research and Development (RAND) Corporation to assess QOL in patients with various visual disorders. The NEIVFQ has been shown to be a reliable QOL assessment tool to which newer QOL tools can be compared.

The NEIVFQ25 was scored using the scoring method designed by RAND which involved assigning scores to individual items. The minimum score was zero and the maximum score for each item was 100. A higher score signified a better QOL. The score for individual items was used to calculate the average score for each domain. The average of the domain scores with the exclusion of the general health domain score was defined as the summary NEIVFQ25 score.

The GQL-15 is a 4 domain; 15-item questionnaire designed specifically for glaucoma patients and was designed with the effect of binocular visual field loss on visual function in mind (Nelson et $al.$, 2003). The domains comprise of near vision, peripheral vision, outdoor mobility and glare and dark adaptation. It has been shown to be reliable and has good internal consistency (Goldberg et $al.$, 2009). One of its limitations is that it is not as broad as the

NEIVFQ25 which has domains which assess other concepts which can influence QOL such as general health, social function, dependency, role difficulty and mental health.

Higher GQL-15 scores indicate poorer QOL. The GQL-15 item level responses were coded on a scale of 0 to 5: 5 represented severe difficulty due to visual reasons, 1 indicated no difficulty with performing the activity, and 0 signified abstinence from activity for nonvisual reasons. Summation of the item response scores of the GQL-15 provided the summary scores. To calculate the subscale scores for the four domains of the GQL-15, the item level responses were scored on a numerical interval scale ranging from 0, indicating no difficulty, to 100, indicating severe difficulty. The subscale score for each domain was calculated using an average of the scores generated for the component item-level responses. Higher subscale scores were indicative of increasing difficulty with vision-related activities and poorer QOL. A measure of the degree of difficulty in performing visual tasks outlined in the GQL-15 was depicted by corresponding visual performance (Nelson *et al.*, 2003). This score was obtained by first subtracting the subscale scores from the total possible score × 100 (1500). The product was thereafter converted to a percentage.

The NEIVFQ25 and the GQL-15 questionnaires were translated into Yoruba, Igbo, and Hausa, which are the three most prominent indigenous Nigerian languages for respondents who were not literate in English. Care was taken to reduce any bias that could occur because of translation. Competent bilingual translators used forward and back-translation methods to ensure accuracy.

Data was entered into Microsoft Excel for Windows XP Professional and later uploaded and analysed using the Statistical Package for the Social Sciences version 15 (SPSS, Chicago III). The mean, median, standard deviation and range of QOL scores for the two questionnaires were calculated and compared for the subgroups of participants. The internal consistency of the NEIVFQ25 and the GQL-15 questionnaires was assessed using Cronbach's alpha. Correlations were assessed using Spearman's rank correlation coefficients. A modest or weak correlation was defined as rho values less than or equal to 0.31; values ranging from 0.32 – 0.55 were defined as moderate correlation, and rho values greater than 0.55 showed strong correlation. Chi-square tests and Mann Whitney U tests were used to compare categorical and ordinal variables respectively. One-way analysis of variance was done using the F test to evaluate the significance of group differences. *P*-values equal to or less than 0.05 were considered statistically significant.

4   Results

Majority of the respondents (97%) were fluent in English and responded to the English version of the NEIVFQ25 & the GQL-15 questionnaires. Only eight participants (3%) responded to the translated versions of the NEIVFQ25 and GQL-15 questionnaires. Data analysis was carried out with all participants included initially and then with the exclusion of the 8 participants who responded to the translated versions of the NEIVFQ25 and GQL-15 questionnaires which are yet to be validated. When the results were reviewed, there was no significant difference in the results. The results and data presented here are those of all the participants irrespective of which version of the questionnaires they responded to.

There were 81 female (61.4%) and 51 male participants (38.6%) in each group with ages ranging from 40-79 years. Table 4 shows the socio-demographic characteristics of the controls and cases with mild, moderate or severe glaucoma and shows p-values for the variation within the subgroups. The mean age for severe glaucoma cases (62.67years) was higher than that for the mild (52.81years) and moderate (59.11years) glaucoma cases. No statistically significant difference was noted for ethnicity, religion and educational status in this study population.

Table 4 also shows that there was a statistically significant difference between the living situation and marital status of the subgroup of participants. More controls were still living with their spouses (22.7%) compared to patients with mild glaucoma (13.6%), moderate glaucoma (4.5%) and severe glaucoma (6.9%). There were also more patients with moderate (13.6%) and severe glaucoma (9.1%) living alone compared to controls (6.1%). None of the patients with mild glaucoma in this study population was living alone. There was no statistically significant difference in these groups of participants in relation to living with family members. More patients with severe (20.5%) and moderate (25%) glaucoma were widowed compared to 15.9% of controls and 4.5% of patients with mild glaucoma but no significant difference was noted in the subgroups for separation or divorce. There were more patients with mild glaucoma (45.5%) in paid employment than moderate (18.2%) or severe glaucoma cases (18.2%) and more retirees among the cases with moderate (34.1%) and severe glaucoma (54.5%) than among mild glaucoma cases (11.4%).

4.1   Summary QOL Scores

Lower GQL-15 summary scores signify a better QOL. The mean GQL-15 QOL score was lower for controls: 15.75 (SD ± 1.85) and higher: 24.07 (SD ± 12.4) for cases signifying better QOL in controls. The corresponding visual performance (CVP) which is a measure of the level of difficulty experienced by respondents when performing the tasks described in the GQL-15, signifies less difficulty when the values are higher and vice versa. The CVP for cases was 84.54% (SD ± 21.65) and 98.75% (SD ± 3.02) for controls suggesting that controls reported less difficulty with tasks than cases. Higher NEIVFQ25 scores signify better QOL. The mean NEIVFQ25 QOL score was higher in controls: 96.7 (SD ± 2.34) than in cases, 85.2 (SD ± 16.07) also depicting better QOL in controls than cases. These differences were all statistically significant (p < 0.001).

There was a statistically significant trend of decreasing QOL with increasing severity of disease (p < 0.001). The NEIVFQ25 scores were highest in mild glaucoma cases (92 ± 6.83) followed by mean scores for moderate glaucoma cases (89.26 ± 10.44) and then than that for the severe glaucoma cases subgroup (74.34 ± 21.13). With the GQL-15, summary QOL scores followed the same order being lowest for the mild glaucoma cases (18.98 ± 6.14) and highest for severe glaucoma cases (32.65 ± 14.95). The mean GQL-15 summary score for moderate glaucoma cases was 20.58 (SD ± 9.7). The corresponding visual performance (CVP) scores reduced with increasing severity of disease (depicting increasing visual disability). Mild cases had a CVP of 93.06 (SD ± 11.08), moderate cases scored 90.72 (SD ± 16.42) while severe glaucoma cases scored 69.85 (SD ± 26.51).

4.2   NEIVFQ25 & GQL-15 Subscale Scores

Higher GQL-15 subscale scores signify worse QOL. The mean GQL-15 subscale scores were higher for cases than controls in all the domains of the GQL-15 questionnaire. The glaucoma cases ranked the domains as follows: Glare & dark adaptation (20.04 ± 24.54); Central and near vision (13.96 ± 23.33); Peripheral vision (12.85 ± 21.52) and Outdoor mobility (10.21 ± 23.98). The mean GQL-15 scores for controls were: Glare & dark adaptation (1.63 ± 4.09); Peripheral

	CONTROLS n=132	mild n=44	moderate n=44	severe n=44	p value
Mean Age (years)	58.61	52.81	59.11	62.67	p=0.41
Education [No patients (%)]					
Nil	3 (2.3)	2 (4.5)	6 (13.6)	2 (4.5)	p=0.31
Completed primary	25 (19)	9 (20.5)	7 (15.9)	12 (27.3)	p=0.78
Completed secondary	35 (26.5)	6 (13.6)	12 (27.3)	8 (18.2)	p=0.29
Completed tertiary	42 (31.8)	20(45.5)	13 (29.5)	18 (40.9)	p=0.44
Postgraduate	27 (20.5)	7 (15.9)	6 (13.6)	4 (9.1)	p=0.37
Religion [No patients (%)]					
Christian	106 (80.3)	35 (79.5)	35(79.5)	39 (88.6)	p=0.67
Muslim	26 (18.3)	9 (20.5)	8 (18.2)	5 (11.4)	p=0.69
Others 0	0	1 (2.3)	0	NA	
Living Situation [No patients (%)]					
Alone	8 (6.1)	0	6 (13.6)	4 (9.1)	p=0.001
Spouse	30(22.7)	6 (13.6)	2(4.5)	3(6.9)	p=0.003
Family	94(71.2)	38 (86.4)	36 (81.8)	37 (84.1)	p=0.14
Ethnicity [No patients (%)]					
Hausa	0	0	0	0	NA
Igbo	36 (27.3)	10 (22.7)	8(18.2)	16 (36.4)	p=0.39
Yoruba	82 (62.1)	28 (63.6)	28 (63.6)	22 (50)	p=0.66
Others	14 (10.6)	6 (13.6)	8 (18.2)	6 (13.6)	p=0.82
Marital Status [No patients (%)]					
Single	4 (3.0)	1 (2.3)	1 (2.3)	0	p=0.204
Married	104 (81.67)	36 (81.8)	30 (68.2)	34 (77.3)	p=0.67
Separated/Divorced	3 (2.3)	5 (11.4)	2 (4.5)	1 (2.3)	p=0.458
Widow(er)	21 (15.9)	2 (4.5)	11 (25)	9 (20.5)	p=0.013
Employment [No patients (%)]					
Unemployed	8 (6.1)	2 (4.5)	4 (9.1)	1 (2.3)	p=0.63
Employed	61 (46.2)	20 (45.5)	8 (18.2)	8 (18.2)	p<0.001
Self-employed	33 (25)	17 (38.6)	17(38.6)	11 (25)	p=0.303
Retired	30 (22.7)	5(11.4)	15 (34.1)	24 (54.5)	p<0.001

The percentages are column percentages and are in parenthesis.
P values are for chi-square tests for categorical variables and fisher's exact test where indicated.
One-way analysis of variance was used for continuous variables.

Table 4: Socio-demographic characteristics of Mild, Moderate & Severe Glaucoma cases & Controls.

vision (0.87 ± 2.96) and Outdoor mobility (0.73 ± 4.07) and Central and near vision (0.21 ± 1.6).

Higher NEIVFQ25 subscale scores signify better QOL. The mean NEIVFQ25 subscale scores were lower for cases than for the controls. The lowest NEIVFQ25 subscale scores for cases were in the driving domain (65.74 ± 36.79) followed by the general vision domain (67.35 ± 17.79) and then the general health domain (67.45 ± 18.61). The mental health domain was the fourth most affected domain for cases with a mean subscale score of 82.23 (SD ± 22.44). The mean score for the mental health domain was lower that of peripheral vision (87.92 ± 21.25), distance (87.31 ± 20.70) and near activities (85.94 ± 21.96) domains. The most affected subscales for the control group were General health (76.5 ± 15.87), General Vision (81.5 ± 11.97), Mental health (91.1 ± 4.73) and ocular pain (92.0 ± 11.2). There was a clear trend of decreasing NEIVFQ25 subscale scores with increasing severity of disease for all the subscales of the NEIVFQ25 except for the general health (GH) and ocular pain (OP) subscales (see Table 5).

NEIVFQ25 SUBSCALES	CONTROLS n=132	MILD GLAU-COMA n=44	MODERATE GLAUCOMA n=44	SEVERE GLAUCOMA n=44	P values
General Health	76.50 (± 15.87)	71.24 (± 16.76)	64.75 (± 18.20)	66.38 (± 20.50)	P<0.001
General Vision	81.50 (± 11.97)	75.88 (± 10.85)	68.94 (± 16.47)	57.25 (± 19.86)	P<0.001
Ocular Pain	92.00 (± 11.20)	86.19 (± 13.82)	86.25 (± 16.46)	82.81 (± 18.06)	P=0.239
Near Activities	99.38 (± 2.89)	94.48 (± 12.06)	86.79 (± 15.85)	73.55 (± 25.16)	P<0.001
Distance Activities	99.10 (± 3.39)	94.09 (± 17.09)	92.82 (± 12.34)	75.01 (± 25.16)	P<0.001
Social Functioning	100 (± 0.00)	98.50 (± 6.09)	95.31 (± 13.78)	86.56 (± 21.63)	P<0.001
Mental Health	91.10 (± 4.73)	87.46 (± 17.76)	87.81 (± 13.94)	71.41 (± 29.1)	P<0.001
Role Difficulty	99.48 (± 2.99)	94.19 (± 12.95)	92.11 (± 17.15)	71.23 (± 32.18)	P<0.001
Dependency	99.58 (± 2.12)	94.90 (± 15.81)	94.58 (± 12.30)	78.54 (± 29.53)	P<0.001
Driving	94.55 (± 6.75)	82.62 (± 22.75)	75.93 (± 31.04)	38.52 (± 39.25)	P<0.001
Colour Vision	100.0 (± 0.00)	100.0 (± 0.00)	96.87 (± 8.37)	88.12 (± 24.01)	P<0.001
Peripheral Vision	100.0 (±0.00)	95.63 (± 12.52)	92.50 (± 15.19)	75.63 (± 27.44)	P<0.001

Table 5: NEIVFQ25 subscale scores across subgroups of disease severity.

The trend was statistically significant with p values of F test of one-way analysis of variance <0.001. For the GH subscale, patients with mild glaucoma had the highest score (71.24 ± 16.76) followed by patients with severe glaucoma (66.38 ± 20.51) and then moderate glaucoma cases (64.75 ± 18.20). These differences were statistically significant (p < 0.001) even though the scores did not follow the trend of decreasing scores with increasing severity of disease as in the other subscales (excluding the OP & MH subscales). The OP subscale was the only NEIVFQ25 subscale in which the difference in the average subscale scores for the subgroups of cases: mild (86.19 ± 13.82), moderate (86.25 ± 16.46) and severe (82.81 ± 18.06) was not statistically significant (p = 0.556) and in this subscale moderate glaucoma cases had slightly higher QOL scores than mild glaucoma cases. Moderate glaucoma cases also had slightly higher scores than mild glaucoma cases in the Mental Health subscale.

GQL-15 subscale scores increased with increasing severity of disease signifying worsening QOL. All the cases irrespective of the degree of severity of their visual field defect had the greatest difficulty with tasks associated with glare and dark adaptation. Figure 1 is a bar chart comparing the CVP and the GQL-15 subscale scores in cases with increasing severity of disease. The error bars are for standard errors of mean and the p values show comparison of scores across disease severity subgroups. A comparison of the mean NEIVFQ25 subscale scores of cases with mild, moderate and severe glaucoma showed that patients with mild and moderate glaucoma reported the greatest difficulty with the general health, general vision and the driving subscales. Table 6 depicts the NEIVFQ25 & GQL-15 subscales that controls and patients with mild, moderate or severe glaucoma reported having the most difficulty with.

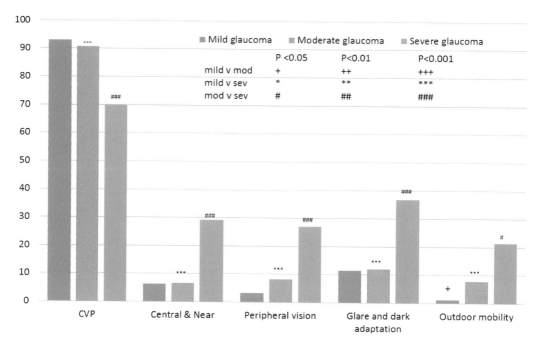

CVP- Corresponding visual performance with GQL-15; GQL-15 Subscales
CNV- Central and near vision; PV- Peripheral vision;
GDA- Glare and Dark Adaptation; OM- Outdoor mobility

Figure 1: Bar chart of mean GQL-15 subscale scores & CVP for mild, moderate & severe glaucoma cases.

4.5   QOL scores for Mild Glaucoma Cases &Controls

A comparison of the summary QOL scores for mild glaucoma cases and age and sex-matched controls showed a statistically significant difference between the two groups of participants for the NEIVFQ25 summary scores (p<0.001); the GQL-15summary scores (p = 0.002) and CVP (p = 0.002). There was also a statistically significant difference between the NEIVFQ25 and GQL-15 subscale scores as shown in Table 7 for all the GQL-15 domains except outdoor mobility and all the NEIVFQ25 domains except colour vision and social functioning.

Subscales	Mild Glaucoma	Moderate Glaucoma	Severe Glaucoma	Controls
NEIVFQ25 subscales	General Health	General Health	Driving	General Health
	General Vision	General Vision	General Vision	General Vision
	Driving	Driving	General Health	Mental Health
	Ocular pain	Ocular pain	Role difficulty	Ocular pain
	Mental health	Near Activities	Mental Health	Driving
GQL-15 subscales	Glare Dark Adaptation	Glare Dark Adaptation	Glare Dark Adaptation	Glare Dark Adaptation
	Central Near Vision	Peripheral Vision	Central Near Vision	Peripheral Vision
	Peripheral Vision	Outdoor Mobility	Peripheral Vision	Outdoor Mobility
	Outdoor Mobility	Central Near Vision	Outdoor Mobility	Central Near Vision

Table 6: Most affected NEIVFQ25 & GQL-15 subscales across subgroups of disease severity.

Scores	Mild Cases n= 44	Age & Sex Matched Control n=44	P Value QOL (t-test)
GQL-15			
Summary scores	18.97 (± 6.14)	15.83 (± 2.09)	p<0.001
Subscales Scores			
Central & Near Vision	6.25 (±11.32)	0.31 (±1.98)	p<0.001
Peripheral Vision	3.34 (±10.65)	1.36 (±4.26)	p<0.001
Glare & Dark Adaptation	11.46 (±15.12)	1.67 (±5.56)	p<0.001
Outdoor Mobility	1.25 (±7.91)	1.25 (±5.52)	p=1
NEIVFQ25			
Summary Scores	92.00 (± 6.83)	96.98 (±2.43)	p<0.001
Subscale Scores			
General Health	71.24 (±16.76)	76.50 (±15.87)	p<0.001
General Vision	75.88 (±10.85)	81.50 (±11.97)	p<0.001
Ocular Pain	86.19 (±13.82)	92.00 (±11.20)	p<0.001
Near Activities	94.48 (±12.06)	99.38 (±2.89)	p<0.001
Distance Act.	94.09 (±17.09)	99.10 (±3.34)	p<0.001
Vision Specific			
Social functioning	98.50 (±6.09)	100.0 (±0.00)	p=0.07
Mental Health	87.46 (±17.76)	91.10 (±4.73)	p<0.001
Role Difficulty	94.19 (±12.95)	99.48 (±2.99)	p<0.001
Dependency	94.90 (±15.81)	99.58(±2.12)	p<0.001
Driving	82.62 (±22.75)	94.55 (±6.75)	p<0.001
Colour Vision	100.00 (±0.00)	100.0 (±0.00)	p=1
Peripheral Vision	95.63 (±21.25)	100.0 (±0.00)	p<0.001

All results are mean values with the Standard deviation in parenthesis

Table 7: A Comparison of NEIVFQ25 & GQL-15 summary & subscale scores for mild glaucoma cases and age & sex-matched controls.

4.6   Correlation of QOL Scores with Visual Function

4.6.1   Correlation with Laterality &Visual Field Indices

Correlations were evaluated using Spearman's rank coefficients. Rho values less than or equal to 0.31 were modest or weak correlations; between 0.32 and 0.55 were moderate while values greater than 0.55 were regarded as strong correlations. Most of the glaucoma cases had bilateral disease (90.9%), and binocular visual field defects were demonstrated in 93.94% of the patients. There was no significant correlation between the NEIVFQ25 QOL scores and laterality (Spearman's rho: –0.123; p = 0.18). For the GQL-15, the Spearman's rho was 0.100 (p = 0.28).

The visual field indices evaluated were mean deviation worse eye (MDWE); mean deviation for both eyes after summation (MD OU) and pattern standard deviation (PSD). There was a moderate correlation of the QOL scores for both questionnaires with MDWE (NEIVFQ25 Spearman's rho = 0.32; GQL-15 rho = –0.32). NEIVFQ25 and GQL-15 summary scores had slightly higher correlations with the binocular summation of mean deviation MD OU (NEIVFQ25 Spearman's rho = –0.36; GQL-15 rho = 0.37) than MDWE. The correlation with PSD was weak for the NEIVFQ25 with rho values ranging from: –0.09 to –0.25. For the GQL-15, the association was also weak with Spearman's rho values ranging from 0.09 to 0.19.

For both questionnaires, the worse the mean deviation (MD) the worse the QOL (lower scores for the NEIVFQ25 and higher scores for the GQL-15). This is depicted in Figures 2 and 3 which are scatter plots of the MD worse eye (MDWE) and the GQL-15 QOL scores and the MD worse eye and the NEIVFQ25 QOL scores respectively. The blue lines represent the line of equality or best fit with the adjacent red lines depicting 95% confidence intervals.

The above scatter plot shows that there is a negative correlation between the MD worse eye (MDWE) and the GQL-15 score. As the MD worse eye increases (better visual field), the GQL-15 scores decrease (better QOL). The slope in this case is a negative slope. Plotting the MD Worse eye against the CVP will give a positive slope with a similar interpretation. The scatter plot in Figure 3 shows that there is a positive correlation between the MD worse eye and the NEIVFQ25 score. As the MD worse eye increases (better visual field), the NEIVFQ25 scores also increases (better QOL). The slope in this case is a positive slope.

4.6.2   Correlation with Contrast Sensitivity Scores

The correlation between the mean contrast sensitivity score (CSS) and the summary NEIVFQ25 score (Spearman's rho: 0.42, p < 0.001) was the highest amongst the visual function measures assessed in this study. The GQL-15 summary scores also had moderate correlations with mean CSS (Spearman's rho: -0.37, p < 0.001).

Figures 4 and 5 are graphic illustrations of the correlation between the mean contrast sensitivity scores CSS and the NEIVFQ25 scores and the GQL-15 scores. As the CSS increases, the QOL as measured by both instruments improves. As can be seen from Figure 4, the NEIVFQ25 v Mean CSS scatter plot has a positive slope because higher values of CSS signify better contrast sensitivity and higher values of NEIVFQ25 signify better quality of life. The GQL-15 v Mean CSS scatter plot (Figure 5) shows a negative slope signifying that as the Mean CSS increases (better contrast sensitivity), the GQL-15 score decreases (better QOL).

4.6.3   Correlation with Visual Acuity

After adjusting for age, NEIVFQ25 correlated more significantly with mean logMAR VA worse eye (Spearman's rho = 0.41, p < 0.001) than mean logMAR VA better eye. (rho = 0.37, p

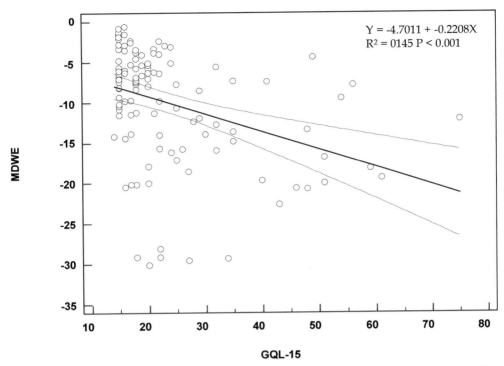

Figure 2: Scatter plot showing the correlation between the GQL-15 scores and the MD Worse Eye.

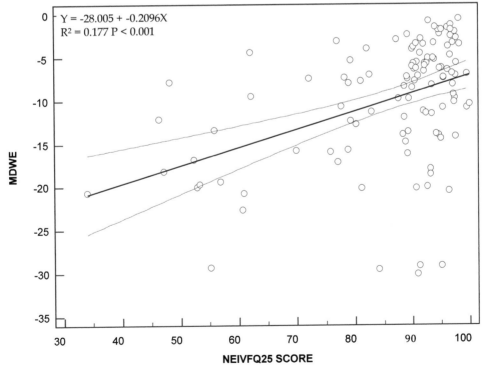

Figure 3: Scatter Plot showing the correlation between the MD Worse eye (MDWE) and the NEIVFQ25 scores.

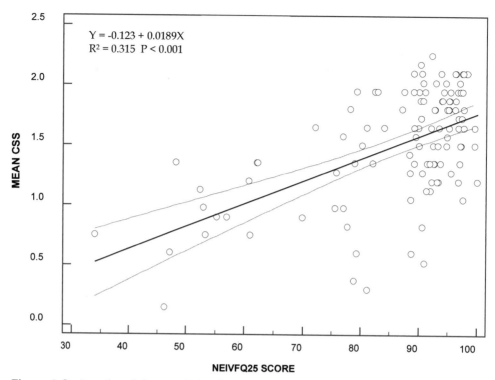

Figure 4: Scatter plot of the correlation between the Mean CSS and the NEIVFQ25 scores. CSS-contrast sensitivity score.

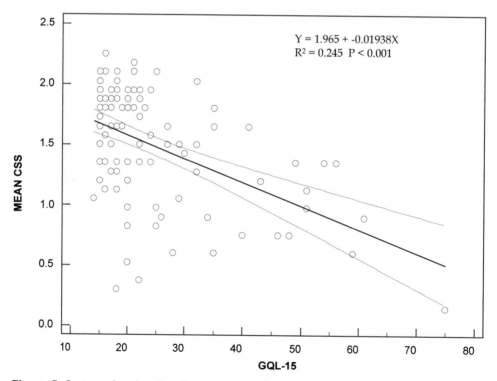

Figure 5: Scatter plot showing the correlation between the Mean CSS and the GQL-15 scores. CSS- Contrast Sensitivity score.

< 0.001). The reverse was the case with the GQL-15 which had a stronger correlation with mean logMAR VA better eye (rho: –0.45, p < 0.001) than mean logMAR VA worse eye (rho: –0.32, p < 0.001).

4.6.4   Correlation with Structural Index: Cup-Disc-Ratio

The NEIVFQ25 summary score showed a strong negative correlation with the Cup-Disc-Ratio (CDR) of the right eye (rho: –0.660; p < 0.001) and the CDR left eye (rho: –0.663; p < 0.001). Increasing CDR (increased severity of disease) was associated with reduction in NEIVFQ25 scores (worse QOL). The GQL-15 summary score also had a strong but positive correlation with the CDR right eye (rho: 0.621; p < 0.001) and the CDR left eye (rho: 0.642; p < 0.001). Increasing CDR (increased severity of disease) was associated with increasing GQL-15 scores (worse QOL).

4.7   Influence of Socio-demographic Variables on QOL Scores

The only three socio-demographic variables that significantly influenced QOL scores in this study were Age, Sex and Education. Younger participants had better QOL scores than older participants using both questionnaires. This effect affected all the GQL-15 subscale scores and eight of the twelve subscales of the NEIVFQ25. The NEIVFQ25 subscales that were not influenced by age were mental health, role difficulty, colour vision and ocular pain. Females generally had better QOL scores than males in this study. Participants who had better education had better NEIVFQ25 and GQL-15 QOL scores than less educated participants.

Figures 6 and 7 are regression analysis plots illustrating the relationship between age and QOL scores using the GQL-15 and the NEIVFQ25. Older patients tended to report more QOL-related difficulties. This finding was similar for both the GQL-15 and the NEIVFQ25. In Figure 6, only one outlier is visible above the GQL-15 score 45 for respondents within the age range of 40 – 50 years, compared to 11 outliers above score 45 for respondents aged 50 and above. There are also only 5 outliers above GQL-15 score 25 for respondents aged 40-50 years compared to 30 outliers for those aged 50 and above. Figure 7 shows only 2 outliers below NEIVFQ25 score 80 within the 40 – 50 years age range compared to 28 outliers within the 50 – 80 age range.

4.8   Comparison of the NEIVFQ25 & GQL15 Questionnaires

It took about 12 minutes to administer the lengthier NEIVFQ25 questionnaire and 5 minutes, on average to administer the GQL-15. Both questionnaires had high internal consistency with Cronbach's alpha of 0.93 for the NEIVFQ25 and 0.94 for the GQL-15. The reliability of the questionnaires was assessed during the pilot phase of the study. Test-retest reliability was 0.89 for the NEIVFQ25 and 0.92 for the GQL-15. Inter-observer reliability measured by Kappa statistics was quite high ranging from 0.82 to 0.87 for both questionnaires. The responsiveness of the two questionnaires was not assessed.

Both questionnaires appeared sensitive and differentiated clearly between cases and controls. There was a clear trend of worsening QOL summary & subscale scores (lower scores for the NEIVFQ25 and higher scores for the GQL-15) with increasing severity of disease (see table 5). The only NEIVFQ25 subscale in which there was no statistically significant difference in the QOL scores across patients with mild, moderate and severe glaucoma was the ocular pain subscale (p = 0.556).

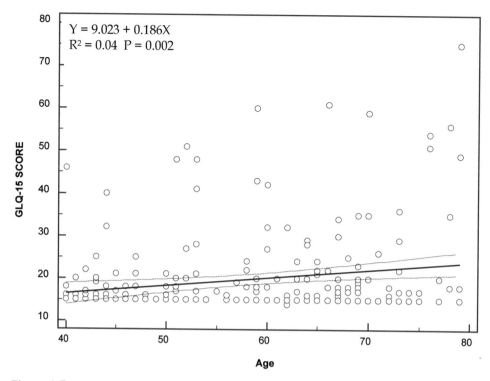

Figure 6: Regression analysis plot showing the relationship between GQL-15 and Age.

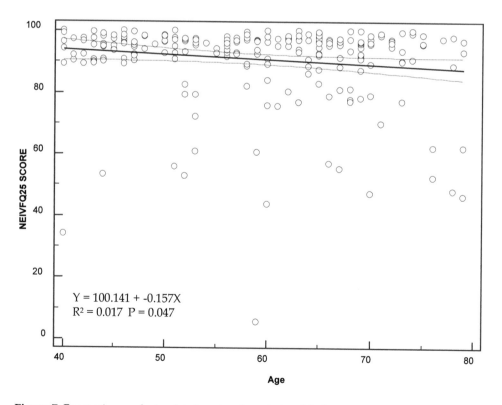

Figure 7: Regression analysis plot showing the relationship between NEIVFQ25 and Age.

4.8.1 Correlations

The GQL-15 and the NEIVFQ25 summary scores showed strong correlation across a wide range of subgroups in the study: cases, mild cases, moderate cases, severe cases and total study population with Spearman's rho ranging from 0.748 to 0.836. The scores however showed a moderate correlation (rho: –0.378) when the summary QOL scores of controls were evaluated. The correlation between the subscales of the NEIVFQ25 and the domains of the GQL-15 were all statistically significant at the 0.01 level (2 tailed) and ranged from weak correlations between the Central near vision domain of the GQL-15 (rho: –0.185) and the General Health subscale of the NEIVFQ25 to strong correlations between the GQL-15 central near vision domain and the near activities subscale of the NEIVFQ25 (rho: -0.731). Table 8 shows the Spearman's rank correlation coefficients between the NEIVFQ25 and the GQL-15 summary and subscale scores.

	GQL-15 summary score	Outdoor Mobility	Peripheral vision	Glare & Dark Adaptation	Central & Near Vision
NEIVFQ25 summary score	-0.753	-0.451	-0.688	-0.707	-0.615
General Health	-0.245	-0.198	-0.280	-0.235	-0.185
General Vision	-0.492	-0.395	-0.545	-0.447	-0.433
Ocularpain	-0.348	-0.199	-0.264	-0.325	-0.305
Near activities	-0.633	-0.489	-0.621	-0.591	-0.731
Distance activities	-0.685	-0.510	-0.709	-0.656	-0.655
Social functioning	-0.548	-0.614	-0.584	-0.541	-0.688
Mental Health	-0.603	-0.434	-0.542	-0.565	-0.535
Role difficulty	-0.577	-0.614	-0.558	-0.580	-0.618
Dependency	-0.531	-0.596	-0.565	-0.508	-0.570
Driving	-0.633	-0.452	-0.488	-0.644	-0.526
Colour Vision	-0.418	-0.585	-0.461	-0.416	-0.515
PeripheralVision	-0.565	-0.620	-0.639	-0.520	-0.588

Table 8: Correlation between NEIVFQ25 and GQL-15 summary & subscale scores.

The NEIVFQ25 and the GQL-15 showed good group validity in that they were able to discriminate between subgroups of cases with varying levels of disease severity categorised using MD values of standard automated perimetry. The summary scores differentiated between patients with mild & severe glaucoma (p < 0.001), moderate & severe glaucoma (p<0.001) but did not show a statistically significant difference between patients with mild & moderate glaucoma (p = 0.92 for the NEIVFQ25 & p = 0.25 for the GQL-15). Table 9 shows the p values of the comparison between the disease severity subgroups for summary and subscale scores of the NEIVFQ25 and the GQL-15 questionnaires. A comparison of the NEIVFQ25 scores for mild and moderate glaucoma cases for the General Vision and the Near Activities subscale was statistically significant (Table 9). The Outdoor mobility domain scores for mild and moderate glaucoma cases also differed significantly as can be seen from Tables 5 and 9.

4.8.2 Concurrent Validity

The NEIVFQ25 and the GQL-15 showed good concurrent validity by demonstrating moderate correlations with several measures of visual function as has been discussed above. They both correlated moderately with Mean CSS, MD OU, MD WE, logMAR VA better eye and worse eye. They exhibited a weak correlation with PSD. Both questionnaires showed a strong correlation with Cup-Disc Ratios in both eyes.

	Mild v Moderate Glaucoma	Moderate v Severe Glaucoma	Mild v Severe Glaucoma
NEIVFQ25 summary score	P=0.92	P<0.001	P<0.001
General Health	P=0.101	p=0.708	P=0.249
General Vision	P=0.029	P<0.005	P<0.001
Ocularpain	P=0.986	P=0.376	P=0.350
Near activities	P=0.017	P=0.013	P<0.001
Distance activities	P=0.704	P<0.001	P<0.001
Social functioning	P=0.184	P=0.034	P=0.001
Mental Health	P=0.922	P=0.002	P=0.004
Role difficulty	P=0.542	P<0.001	P<0.001
Dependency	P=0.920	P=0.002	P=0.003
Driving	P=0.275	P<0.001	P<0.001
Colour Vision	P=0.472	P=0.033	P<0.001
PeripheralVision	P=0.288	P<0.001	P<0.001
GQL-15summary score	P=0.25	P<0.001	P<0.001
Outdoor Mobility	P=0.046	P=0.026	P<0.001
Peripheral vision	P=0.091	P<0.001	P<0.001
Glare & DarkAdaptation	P=0.891	P<0.001	P<0.001
Central & Near Vision	P=0.917	P<0.001	P<0.001

Table 9: Comparison of level of significant difference in NEIVFQ25 and GQL-15 summary and subscale scores across subgroups.

5   Discussion

To our knowledge this is the first Nigerian study on QOL in glaucoma patients. Assessing QOL in this population of POAG patients in Nigeria provided an insight into the burden of the disease on POAG patients living in Lagos Nigeria. The results are a reflection of the QOL of other Nigerian POAG patients living in urban areas or capital cities but may not be generalizable to the rural population in Nigeria. This is because living in rural parts of Nigeria has been associated with a poorer QOL (Tran HM et al., 2011). This may be due to the lack of infrastructural development and social amenities in some rural areas in Nigeria.

Reduced NEIVFQ25 QOL scores and increased GQL-15 scores in cases compared to controls demonstrated clearly that glaucoma affects the QOL of POAG patients in Nigeria. A population-based study done in Nigeria (Tran HM et al., 2011) reported that patients blind from glaucoma had worse visual function and QOL scores than patients blind from cataract. There was no explanation given for this but glaucoma patients may have worse QOL if they are aware that blindness due to glaucoma is irreversible. This was also reported in the ProyectoVer Eye Project (Broman et al., 2002) in which subjects with glaucoma had worse vision-related QOL scores compared to subjects with cataract and diabetic retinopathy. A trend of worsening QOL scores with increasing severity of disease was noted in this study and suggests that QOL worsens with progression of disease. This has previously been reported.

(Sherwood *et al.*, 1998; Janz *et al.*, 2001; Nelson *et al.*, 2003; Gutierrez *et al.*, 1997; Parrish 1996; Skalicky & Goldberg 2008; Goldberg *et al.*, 2009).

GQL-15 scores obtained in this study were lower (signifying better QOL) in all sub groups of participants than that obtained in Goldberg *et al.* (2009) and Skalicky & Goldberg (2008). However, in Nelson *et al.* (2003), the severe glaucoma cases had lower QOL scores (24.9) than the cases with severe glaucoma in this study (32.65) suggesting better QOL in that study population. The patients with mild and moderate glaucoma in this study had lower GQL-15 scores than those in Nelson *et al.* (2003) suggesting better QOL in the Nigerian patients with mild and moderate glaucoma. The different eligibility criteria, categorisation methods and cultural influences in these studies may account for this finding. Nelson *et al.* (2003) excluded patients with severe glaucoma who had poor vision while visual acuity was not one of the criteria used in recruiting patients in this study. The GQL-15 was also not designed with the Nigerian population in mind and may not have considered QOL indices relevant to this group of patients and so may not have provided an accurate assessment of their QOL.

On the other hand, Nigerians are known to be resilient, optimistic people with a very positive outlook despite obvious daunting challenges. They may therefore have had better QOL scores than their Australian counterparts in the study by Goldberg *et al.* (2009) because of better coping strategies and a more positive outlook. It is also possible that the Nigerian patients with mild and moderate glaucoma who had better QOL scores than the participants in the Nelson *et al.* (2003) study, coped better in the early stages of the disease than the later stages.

5.1   Subscale Scores

The trend of decreasing NEIVFQ25 subscale scores (worse QOL) with increasing severity of disease was observed in nine subscales of the NEIVFQ25 (see Table 5). This trend was not observed in the General Health (GH), Ocular Pain (OP) and the Mental Health (MH) subscales. In the GH subscale, the scores were highest for mild glaucoma cases (71.24 ± 16.76), followed by severe glaucoma cases (66.38 ± 20.51) and then moderate glaucoma cases (64.7 ± 18.20). The reason for this is unclear. However, if patients with moderate glaucoma had more age-related health complaints or were of a more anxious or pessimistic disposition, they would have lower QOL scores in this subscale. The latter reason is however not supported by the fact that moderate glaucoma cases had the highest scores in the MH subscale (87.81 ± 17.76) followed closely by mild glaucoma cases (87.46 ± 13.94) and then severe glaucoma cases (71.41 ± 29.1). Similarly, in the OP subscale, the moderate glaucoma cases had the highest scores (see Table 5) followed by the mild glaucoma cases and then the severe glaucoma cases. This is unusual because even though pain is not a feature of POAG, if one assumes the ocular discomfort reported as pain is a feature of ocular surface disease resulting from the use of anti-glaucoma topical medications, mild glaucoma cases would be expected to have the highest subscale scores. This is because they are less likely to be on multiple medications compared to patients with moderate or severe glaucoma.

Driving was the NEIVFQ25 subscale that was most affected among glaucoma cases in this study. This was also the finding in the Los Angeles Latino Eye Study (McKean-Cowdin *et al.*, 2008). This difficulty observed did not cut across the subgroups of disease severity. Patients with mild and moderate glaucoma ranked the driving subscale 3rd after the general health and general vision subscales. Tables 5 and 6 show that patients with severe glaucoma ranked the driving subscale 1st with QOL scores (38.52 ± 39.25) that were much lower than the scores for patients with mild (82.61 ± 22.75) and moderate glaucoma (79.93 ± 31.04).

In the present study, 4.55% of patients with mild glaucoma and 9.52% of moderate glaucoma patients had stopped driving for visual reasons. In the subgroup of patients with severe glaucoma, 25% of patients had stopped driving because of poor vision and over half (53.85%) of those who still drove, had stopped driving at night while 15.38% had stopped driving during rush hours or in heavy traffic for visual reasons. This finding is in agreement with a study by Ramulu et al. (2009) which reported that glaucoma is associated with frequent driving cessation and limitation. Mental health and role difficulty were both in the top five NEIVFQ25 subscales patients reported difficulty with and is a pointer to the potential psychological difficulty patients with glaucoma may have. Green et al. (2002) and De Leo et al. (1999) pointed out that even if the ophthalmologist is not able to restore vision to a patient, visual disability can cause depression which can be alleviated by the use of drugs, psychotherapy or both.

It is interesting to note that peripheral vision which is the first area of the visual field affected in glaucoma was not one of the first five NEIVFQ25subscales that patients reported difficulty with in this study. This was also the case in several other studies (Mangione et al., 2001; Labiris et al., 2010; Wu et al., 2008). It was only in Suzukamo et al. (2005) that the NEIVFQ25 peripheral vision subscale was ranked as the 3rd most affected subscale by glaucoma patients. This buttresses the importance of QOL assessments. It could have been taken for granted that visual disability due to field restriction as assessed by items in the peripheral vision subscale of the NEIVFQ25, would top the ranking of affected subscales by glaucoma patients. The least affected NEIVFQ25 subscales for glaucoma patients in this study were colour vision, social functioning and dependency. This is similar to the findings in other studies (Parrish et al., 1997; Hyman et al., 2005; Labiris et al., 2008; Wu et al., 2008). Interestingly, peripheral vision subscale was the third least affected subscale in the study by Labiris et al. (2010). It is not surprising that dependency was one of the least affected subscales in this study because Nigerian culture encourages depending on one's extended family members for help in difficult situations. Family members on the other hand are expected to provide assistance to relations in need therefore the patients are unlikely to prioritise their dependence on family as a problem.

Glare and dark adaptation related visual difficulty was identified as a crucial area which needs to be addressed as part of the clinical management of glaucoma. All the subgroups of cases: mild, moderate and severe, reported the greatest difficulty with tasks related to glare and dark adaptation which worsened with increasing severity of disease. These results have been published previously (Mbadugha et al., 2012; Onakoya et al., 2012). Other studies have reported similar findings. (Nelson et al., 2003; Goldberg et al., 2009; Viswanathan et al., 1999; Skalicky & Goldberg 2008; Burr et al.,2007; Zhou et al., 2013). Mangione et al. (1998) reported that 82% of glaucoma subjects had difficulty seeing in the dark compared to 32% of controls. There may be need to explore modifying lighting conditions for work or recreation using suitable filters or environmental modification for patients who have difficulty with glare and dark adaptation.

5.2   QOL in Patients with Mild Glaucoma

The results of this study challenge the earlier belief that POAG being symptomless in the early stages does not affect QOL until there is some degree of visual impairment. Patients with mild glaucoma exhibited worse NEIVFQ25 & GQL15 QOL scores compared to age and sex-matched controls in this study (see Table 7) and suggests that QOL is reduced significantly early in the course of the disease. This has previously been reported (Nelson *et al.*, 2003: Odberg *et al.*, 2001). In the Los Angeles Latino Eye Study (LALES), QOL was lower in participants with glaucoma compared to those without and McKean-Cowdin *et al.* (2008) that 75% (n=160) of cases who did not know they had glaucoma had reduced QOL even before the diagnosis was revealed to them and so that this was clearly a disease effect. Janz *et al.* (2001) in the Collaborative Initial Glaucoma Treatment Study (CIGTS) reported a drop in the QOL of patients immediately after diagnosis and initiation of treatment and this supports the previous studies which report that QOL is decreased early in the course of the disease. This suggests therefore that administration of QOL questionnaires to glaucoma suspects may assist in detecting glaucoma earlier.

Table 7 shows that in ten NEIVFQ25 subscales there was a statistically significant difference between mild glaucoma cases and age and sex matched controls. The two NEIVFQ25 subscales in which the difference in the scores between the two groups of patients was not statistically significant were Social Functioning (SF) and Colour Vision (CV). It is not surprising that no difference was noted in the SF subscale as the level of visual disability experienced by mild glaucoma patients is unlikely to be severe enough to affect their social interactions. The early preferential affectation of blue-yellow retinal ganglion cells is the basis for the development of Short Wavelength Automated Perimetry. It is therefore a little surprising that no significant difference was noted in the colour vision subscale of the NEIVFQ25 in these two groups of patients. However colour vision abnormalities may be so subtle in the early stages of the disease that they may go unnoticed by the patient with mild glaucoma.

For the GQL-15, there was no difference between Outdoor Mobility domain scores of mild glaucoma cases and age & sex-matched controls. This may be because the level of visual impairment in the mild glaucoma cases had not started to affect their ability to function outdoors. Also, if most of the patients with mild glaucoma are introverts who are not very outgoing by nature, they are unlikely to notice any challenges when they are outdoors.

The clear demonstration of reduction in QOL in mild glaucoma patients in Nigeria suggests that administration of QOL questionnaires to glaucoma suspects may assist in identifying patients with mild glaucoma before they are diagnosed clinically. This is especially helpful in a developing country like Nigeria where availability and cost may be a barrier to undergoing tests that assess retinal nerve fibre layer and optic nerve head structure. The administration of vision-related QOL questionnaires during routine annual medical check-ups in the developed world may also assist in the earlier detection of glaucoma by increasing the index of suspicion of health workers reviewing such questionnaires.

5.3   Correlation of QOL Scores with Laterality, Visual Function Tests& Cup-Disc-Ratio

Our study did not find a significant correlation between laterality and QOL scores. This may have resulted from the fact that over 90% of the patients in this study had binocular glaucoma. In the LALES study (McKean-Cowdin *et al.*, 2007) even mild (2-6dB) unilateral visual field loss was associated with worse QOL scores. Chan *et al.* (2013) reported that unilaterality was associated with worse vision-specific functioning while bilaterality was not. Goldberg *et al.* (2009) reported that individuals with bilateral visual field loss from glaucoma have worse QOL scores than patients with unilateral disease.

The present study showed a moderate correlation between NEIVFQ25 & GQL-15 scores and mean deviation. For both questionnaires, progression of disease (depicted by worsening visual field defects) was associated with a reduction in QOL (lower NEIVFQ25 and higher GQL-15 scores). The clinical implication of this finding is that halting disease progression through aggressive management can prevent further deterioration of QOL of patients. The finding of a significant correlation between worse visual field defects and reduced QOL has been reported previously (Chan *et al.*, 2013; Lester & Zingiran, 2002; Parrish *et al.*, 1997; Nelson *et al.*, 2003; Goldberg *et al.*, 2009).

The correlation was slightly higher when the MDOU values were used instead of MDWE. This suggests that the quality of binocular vision may be more predictive of QOL than the quality of vision in the worse eye depicted by MDWE. Kulkarni *et al.* (2012) however, report a significant correlation between QOL scores and visual function measures in the better eye and suggest that the amount of binocular visual field loss and the status of the better eye are more accurate predictors of QOL and functional ability. Some studies show significant correlations with visual function measures in both the better eye and the worse eye (Wren *et al.*, 2009; van Gestel *et al.*, 2010).

There was also a moderate correlation between GQL-15 summary scores and mean logMAR VA more for the better eye than the worse eye. The reverse was the case with the NEIVFQ25. Goldberg *et al.* (2009) also found moderate correlation between GQL-15 summary and domain scores with visual acuity. The NEIVFQ25 and GQL-15 QOL scores had slightly higher Spearman's rho values (NEIVFQ25 Spearman's rho = 0.42; GQL-15 rho = -0.37) when correlated with CSS than MDWE (NEIVFQ25 Spearman's rho = 0.32; GQL-15 rho = -0.32). This suggests that loss of contrast sensitivity is a major contributor to the visual disability and reduced QOL experienced by glaucoma patients. Routine evaluation of contrast sensitivity & QOL in glaucoma clinics can help identify patients who need intervention to reduce the effect of loss of contrast sensitivity on their activities of daily living. This was however different from the finding of Nelson *et al.* (2003) in which the correlation of GQL-15 scores with MD (rho = -0.6) was much higher than for contrast sensitivity (rho = -0.45).

The finding of strong correlations between QOL scores and cup-disc ratios in this study is highly significant for a developing country like Nigeria where visual function assessment tests may not be widely available or accessible. A thorough and astute assessment of the optic nerve head periodically in remote or rural areas may be used to detect disease progression and knowing that worsening cup-disc ratios strongly correlate with QOL scores as demonstrated in this study, treatment should be more aggressive.

5.4   Influence of Socio-demographic Variables

5.4.1   Age

In this study, younger Nigerian glaucoma patients had better QOL scores than older patients. Several reasons could account for this. Younger patients had early or mild glaucoma and therefore better QOL as shown by the fact that the mean age for patients with mild glaucoma (53.80 ± 9.23 years) was much less than that for moderate (59.18 ± 11.5 years) or severe glaucoma (62.75 ± 8.75 years) cases. Younger patients may also have had a higher educational status than older patients in this study and therefore a better understanding of the disease, less fear and better QOL. Tran HM *et al.* (2011) and Magacho *et al.* (2004) also reported that younger patients in their study had better QOL. However, Odberg *et al.* (2001) reported that anxiety was commoner in younger glaucoma patients and suggested that there could have been a tendency for older patients to report less difficulty and presume the difficulties they were experiencing were part of the aging process. Janz *et al.* (2001) and Goldberg *et al.* (2009) also reported that the younger glaucoma patients in their studies reported greater vision-related problems than older patients with glaucoma. Younger patients may have worse QOL and greater anxiety over the diagnosis of glaucoma if they may feel that their lives are just beginning and may be worried about the loss of opportunities, unharnessed potentials and unachieved dreams that may be their lot if they lose their sight. Lester & Zingiran (2002) did not find any difference in QOL across ages. These conflicting reports show that while age does appear to influence QOL there is a likely interplay of multiple factors affecting the QOL of these patients. Patient psychology and personality type are not dependent on age and can influence QOL. Upbeat adaptable people usually report better QOL than pessimistic people. Life's experiences, culture, role definition and coping ability can also affect QOL.

5.4.2 Gender

Females in this study had better QOL scores than the male glaucoma patients. The reason for this is unclear but several factors may have contributed to this. A higher proportion of females than males had mild glaucoma and the study location Lagos is an urban metropolitan city with possibly the highest proportion of educated and economically emancipated women in Nigeria. There was no difference in the educational (p = 0.13) or employment (p = 0.45) status of the males and females in this study and though the women were slightly younger than the men, this difference was not statistically significant (p = 0.06). Details of this data were not shown. A population-based study in Nigeria (Tran HM et al., 2010) reported that the women in their study had worse QOL compared to the men. The authors did not proffer a reason for this finding but reported that living in the Northern geopolitical zones and rural areas in the country was associated with worse QOL. Our study participants were predominantly urban dwellers in Southern Nigeria and this may have contributed to the different findings in the two studies. The findings in Tran HM et al. (2011) are similar to that reported from a study in rural Tanzania. Women reported poorer QOL and greater burden of age-related physical disability than men which the authors attributed to gender biases in relation to economic power.

Akinyemi & Aransiola (2010) reported that QOL measures were likely to favour elderly Nigerian females more than males because the Nigerian society is a largely male dominated and patriarchal system which ascribes greater social responsibility & challenges to the Nigerian male. In the Nigerian culture, the male is considered responsible only if he is able to provide for the basic needs of his household. The woman is permitted to be a financial liability or to depend on her husband to provide for her and even if she works and is financially empowered, her role is that of a helper or secondary provider. Even though both parents work in most Nigerian homes in the urban areas, the cultural role definition for men still stands and while wives assist their husbands, the financial burden of catering for the family often rests more on the male than the female. This may account for the worse QOL in the male glaucoma patients in this study who have the additional financial burden of the costs of living with glaucoma. In addition, Fajemilehin & Odebiyi (2011) reported that elderly females in Nigeria enjoyed more social support than males, continued to work longer than males and had a closer relationship with their children and grandchildren because they often had to provide child care support for their married children.

Woods et al. (2005) reported that women rely more on feelings of discomfort during physical activity in reporting health-related Quality of Life (HRQoL) as compared to males. POAG is characteristically not associated with pain and this may partly explain why females reported fewer symptoms than males in this study. Labiris et al. (2010) reported that female glaucoma patients had worse QOL (lower NEIVFQ scores) than male patients but noted that males had higher QOL scores only in the Ocular Pain (OP) and Social Functioning (SF) sub-scales. Odberg *et al.* (2001) reported that the women were more dissatisfied than the men. Generally, females felt their vision was lower, had more adverse side effects and problems with the instillation of eye drops and felt their needs of care met to a lesser degree. Janz *et al.* (2007) reported that females in their study had increased fear of blindness over time, and that fear of blindness was significantly greater in women than in men at 60 months.

5.4.3   Educational Status

More educated patients had better QOL scores in this study and this is an important finding because Table 4 did not show any significant difference in the proportion of participants with various levels of education across subgroups of disease severity. This suggests that the better QOL in more educated participants is more likely to have been as a result of better awareness and understanding of the disease than earlier presentation. Omoti *et al.* (2002) had previously reported that more educated patients presented earlier with less visual field defects than less educated patients. Odberg *et al.* (2001) found that less educated patients were more afraid of going blind from Glaucoma. Janz *et al.* (2007) reported that higher levels of education were associated significantly with less fear at all the four time points they evaluated.

5.4.4   Living Situation

The living situation for the subgroups varied significantly for those living alone or with their spouse. None of the patients with mild glaucoma lived alone. This may have been due to the fact that they were younger (see Table 4) and more likely to have younger family members residing with them who have not left home for educational or job pursuits or marriage. Cases with moderate or severe glaucoma were less likely to be living with their spouses (p = 0.003) as shown in Table 4. While this may suggest that glaucoma may have put some strain on their marriages, there was no statistically significant difference in the proportion of each of the sub-groups that was separated or divorced (p = 0.458). However more patients with moderate and severe glaucoma were widows and widowers (p = 0.001). These two groups had higher mean ages compared to patients with mild glaucoma or controls (see Table 4). The fact that the proportion of patients in each subgroup that live with family members did not vary significantly (p = 0.14) suggests that the family support system in Nigeria is still viable as families are often compelled by cultural role definitions to cater for visually impaired members of the family.

5.4.5   Employment

Table 4 also shows that a higher proportion of patients with mild glaucoma (45.5%) and controls (46.2%) were in paid employment compared to patients with moderate (18.2%)) and severe glaucoma (18.2%). This could be a pointer to the difficulty and challenges Nigerian glaucoma patients have in remaining in paid job positions. More patients with moderate (34.1%) and severe glaucoma (54.5%) had retired compared to other subgroups (p < 0.001). This could be due to the fact that the mean ages of the moderate and severe glaucoma cases were higher or could suggest that the burden of living with glaucoma may have forced these groups of patients into early retirement.

While the present study did not find any influence of religion or marital status on QOL, Tran HM *et al.* (2011) reported that married respondents had better QOL scores than unmarried ones and respondents who belonged to some religious groups appeared to have better QOL scores than others. No reason was proffered by the authors for this finding.

5.5 Comparison of the NEIVFQ25 and GQL-15 questionnaires

The NEIVFQ25 is a broader but lengthier instrument which assesses other aspects of life that influence QOL. The GQL-15 on the other hand is more specific for glaucoma, shorter and is more likely to be used in a busy clinical setting. Both questionnaires demonstrated good reliability and validity indices in this study. Further details of the comparison have been previously published (Mbadugha *et al.*, 2012).

5.6 Limitations & Strengths of the study

The study was a cross-sectional one and so changes in QOL over time and reproducibility of the QOL tools could not be assessed. Information on the effects of treatment and natural course of the disease on QOL could not be observed using this study design. A multicentre study may have added some variation to the participants but the sample size was robust enough to allow some heterogeneity. Random sampling technique was not used as participants were recruited consecutively as they presented to the clinic. Self- reported QOL assessments as was carried out in this study are typically subjective with the inherent potential for recall bias but correlating these subjective responses to measures of visual function may have reduced this effect. The absence of a replication dataset is a limitation to this study but an attempt has been made to explain the methodology in enough detail to permit replication by other researchers.

The robust sample size and use of an equal number of cases and controls strengthened the study design. The strict eligibility criteria used reduced the effect of possible confounders on the results from this study. The eligibility criteria did not limit participation to only patients fluent in English or patients with good vision and therefore allowed patients with varying levels of literacy and visual disability to participate. Using interviewers allowed respondents to ask for clarification about questions they did not understand thereby reducing the amount of missing data. The QOL interviewers were masked as to the status of the participants (cases/controls) at the time of the interviews. The ophthalmic examination was carried out by one investigator to reduce inter-observer errors.

5.7 Recommendations

There should be a clear protocol on how to use the information obtained from QOL assessments. Trained counsellors could be employed to run counselling units or sessions for glaucoma patients. This will help reduce the burden on the clinician and give patients freedom of expression without undue time-constraints. Professional psychological support and low vision care should be provided for patients who need it.

Inclusion of contrast sensitivity, glare & dark adaptation assessment in routine clinical management of glaucoma patients is advocated since they have been identified as potential areas of vision-related difficulty in performing everyday tasks. This suggestion is buttressed by the fact that Nassiri *et al.* (2013) suggested that items that evaluate contrast sensitivity, glare and dark adaptation should be added to the NEIVFQ to increase its responsiveness to changes in vision-related QOL in glaucoma patents. Regular periodic QOL assessment is helpful to identify individual areas of need which can be addressed.

The authors suggest that vision-related QOL questionnaires should be made readily available to primary, secondary and tertiary level eye care centres in Nigeria. When glaucoma is suspected and facilities for further investigation are not readily available or accessible, paramedical staff and ophthalmic assistants can administer these questionnaires and if the NEIVFQ25 summary score is equal to or less than 89 and the GQL-15 is equal to or greater than 22, urgent referral to a secondary or tertiary level eye care centre should be made. The suggested cut-off value for the summary QOL scores are mean QOL scores for patients with mild glaucoma minus one standard deviation. The suggested cut-off for summary NEIVFQ25 score (89) is close to the mean NEIVFQ25 summary score for patients with moderate glaucoma (89.26 ± 10.44). The suggested GQL-15 cut-off score (22) is slightly higher than the mean GQL-15 score obtained for patients with moderate glaucoma (20.58 ± 9.7). It is believed that QOL assessment may help identify glaucoma suspects who have pre-perimetric glaucoma and who may need urgent referral for more comprehensive assessment and more aggressive glaucoma management strategies.

6   Conclusion

POAG reduced QOL even in the early stages of the disease in this group of Nigerian POAG patients. Early detection and aggressive treatment of early or mild glaucoma should be optimized to prevent progression of the disease and decrease in QOL. QOL assessment can broaden the perspective of physicians and enable them identify individual patient needs and provide customised care based on the expressed areas of concern in the patient's life. A better understanding of how glaucoma affects QOL & disability is helpful for decision–making and comprehensive glaucoma patient care.

Authors

Chigozie Anuli Mbadugha
Department of Ophthalmology, General Hospital Isolo, Lagos, Nigeria

Adeola Olukorede Onakoya
Department of Ophthalmology, Lagos University Teaching Hospital, Idi-Araba, Lagos, Nigeria

References

Adebowale SA, Atte O, Ayeni O. (2012). *Elderly wellbeing in a rural community in North Central Nigeria, Sub Saharan Africa. Public Health Research; 2(4): 92-101.*

AdioAO, Onia AA (2012). *Economic burden of glaucoma in Rivers State Nigeria.Clinical Ophthalmology; 6: 2023-2031.*

Akindipe TO, Aina OF, Onakoya AO (2011).*Risk of Depression And Subjective Quality of Life Among Attendees Of A West African Glaucoma Clinic. International Journal of Medicine and Medical Sciences; 1 (2): 31-34.*

AkinyemiA, Aransiola J. (2010) *Gender perspectives in self-assessment of Quality of Life of the elderly in South-Western Nigeria. Are there variations in QOL among ageing men and women? Journal of Comparative Research in Anthropology & Sociology; (1): 107-120.*

Altarangel U, Spaeth GL, Steinmann WC (2006). *Assessment of function related to vision (AFREV). Ophthalmic Epidemiol; 13 (1): 67–80.*

Asaoka R, Crabb DP, Yamashita T, Russell RA, Wang YX, Garway-Heath DF (2011) Patients have two eyes! :binocular versus better eye visual field indices. Invest Ophthalmol Vis Sci; 52: 7007–7011.

Ashaye AO, Adeoye AO(2008)Characteristics of patients who dropout from a glaucoma clinic. J Glaucoma; 17(3):227-232.

Aspinall PA, Hill AR, Dhillon B, Armbrecht AM, Nelson P, Lumsden C, Farini-Hudson E, Brice R, Vickers A, Buchholz P (2007). Quality of life & relative importance: a comparison of time-trade off and conjoint analysis methods in patients with age-related macular degeneration.Br J Ophthalmol; 91: 766-772.

Aspinall PA, Johnson ZK, Azuara-Blanco A, Montarzino A, Brice R, Vickers A. (2008). Evaluation of Quality of Life & priorities of patients with glaucoma. Invest. Ophthalmol Vis Sci 49; 1907-15.

Baudouin C. (2008) Detrimental effect of preservatives in eyedrops: implications for the treatment of glaucoma. Acta Ophthalmologica; 86:718-726.

Black AA, Wood JM, Lovie-Kitchin JE, Newman BM ((2008). Visual Impairment and postural sway among older adults with glaucoma. Optom Vis Sci; 85:489-497.

Bramley T, Peeples P, Walt JG, Juhasz M, Hansen JE.(2008).Impact of vision loss on costs and outcome in Medicare beneficiaries with glaucoma. Arch Ophthalmol; 126: 849-856.

Brazier J, Deverill M (1999). A checklist for judging preference-based measures of health-related quality of life: learning from psychometrics. Health Econ. 8:41-51.

Broman AT et al. (2002). The impact of visual impairment and eye disease on vision-related QOL in a Mexican-American population: ProyectoVer Eye Project. Inv Ophthalmol Vis Sci; 43(11): 3393-3398.

Brown MM, Brown GC, Sharma S, Garrett S. (1999). Evidence based medicine, utilities and quality of life. Curr Opin Ophthalmol; 10: 221-226.

Brown GC, Sharma S, Brown MM, Kistler J. (2000).Utility values & ARMD. Arch Ophthalmol; 118(1):47-51.

Brown GC, Brown MM, Sharma S, Beauchamp G, Hollands H. (2001) The reproducibility of Ophthalmic Utility Values. Tr Am Ophth Soc; 99: 199-204.

Burr JM, Kilonzo M, Vale L, Ryan M (2007). Developing a preference-based glaucoma utility index using a discrete choice experiment. Optom Vis Sci; 84: 797–808.

Carr AJHI, Robinson PG (2003). Qualityof Life. London. BMJ Books.

Cassel EJ (1982). The nature of suffering and the goals of medicine. N Engl J Med; 306: 639-645.

Chan EW, Chiang PPC, Wong TY, Saw SM, Loon SC, Aung T, Lamoureux E (2013). Impact of Glaucoma Severity & Laterality on Vision-Specific Functioning. The Singapore Malay Eye Study. Invest Ophthalmol Vis Sci; 54 (2): 1169-1175.

Chylack LT Jr, Wolfe JK, Singer DM, Leske MC, Bullimore MA, Bailey IL, Friend J, McCarty D, Wu SY (1993). The Lens Opacities Classification System III.The Longitudinal Study of Cataract Study Group. Arch Ophthalmol.; 111:831–836.

Dawodu OA, Otakpor AN, Ukpomwan CU (2004).Common psychiatric disorders in glaucoma patients as seen at the University of Benin Teaching Hospital, Benin City, Nigeria. Journal of Medicine and Biomedical Research; 3 (1): 42-47.

De Leo D, Hickey PA, Meneghel G, Cantor CH (1999). Blindness, fear of sight loss and suicide.Psychosomatics; 40:339-344.

Deokule S, Sadiq S, Shah S (2004). Chronic Open angle Glaucoma: patient awareness of the nature of the disease, topical medication, compliance and the prevalence of systemic symptoms. Ophthamic Physiol Opt 24: 9-15.

Drummond MF, O'Brien BJ, Stoddart GL, Torrance GW (1997).Cost Utility Analysis. In: Drummond MF, O'Brien BJ, Stoddart GL, Torrance GW, eds. Methods for the Economic Evaluation of Health Care Programmes (2nd ed.) Oxford: Oxford University Press, pp 139-204.

Eldaly M, Hunter M, Khafagy M (2007). The socio-economic impact among Egyptian glaucoma patients. Br J Ophthalmol; 91:1274-1275.

Elliot DB, Pesudovs K, Mallinson T (2007).Vision-Related Quality of life. Optom Vis Sci; 84: 656-658.

Enock ME, Omoti AE, Momoh RO (2010) Glaucoma in a suburban tertiary care hospital in Nigeria. J Ophthalmioc Vis Res; 5: 87-91.

Fajemilehin BR, Odebiyi AI. (2011). Predictors of elderly person's quality of life & health practices in Nigeria.International Journal of Sociology & Anthropology. 3 (7): 245-252.

Friedman DS, Freeman E, Munoz B,Jampel HD, West SK (2007).Glaucoma and Mobility performance: the Salisbury Eye Evaluation Project.Ophthalmology.114: 2232-2237.

Friedman DS, Hahn SR, Gelb L et al. (2008) Doctor-patient communication and health-related beliefs: Results from The Glaucoma Adherence and Persistency Study (GAPS). Ophthalmology.115: 1320-1327.

Gedde SJ, Schiffman JC, Feuer WJ, Parrish RK, 2nd, Heuer DK, Brandt JD(2005); Tube Versus Trabeculectomy Study Group. The tube versus trabeculectomy study: design and baseline characteristics ofstudy patients. Am J Ophthalmol; 140:275-287.

Goldberg I, Clement CI, Chiang TH, Walt JG, Ravelo A, Graham S, Healey PR (2009).Assessing quality of life in patients with glaucoma using the GQL-15 questionnaire. J Glaucoma; 18 (1):6–12.

Green J, Siddah H, Murdoh I (2002). Learning to live with glaucoma: a qualitative study of diagnosis & the impact of sight loss. Soc SciMed; 55:257-267.

Greenfield S, Nelson EC (1992). Recent developments and future issues in the use of health status assessment measures in clinical settings. Med Care; 30:MS23-MS41.

Gupta V, Dutta P, Ov M, Kapoor KS, Sihota R. Kumar G (2011). Effect of glaucoma on the QOL of young patients. Invest Ophthal & Vis Science; 25 (11): 8434-8437.

Gureje O, Kola L, Afolabi E, Olley BO (2008). Determinants of quality of life of elderly Nigerians; results from the Ibadan Study of Ageing. Afr J Med Med Sci 37(3): 239-247.

Gutierrez P, Wilson MR, Johnson C, Gordon M, Cioffi GA, Ritch R, Sherwood M, Meng K, Mangione CM (1997). Influence of glaucomatous visual field loss on health-related quality of life. Arch Ophthalmol; 115:777-784.

Hamelin N, Blatrix C, Brion FMathieu C, Goemaere I, Nordmann JP (2002). How do patients react when glaucoma is diagnosed?J Fr Ophthalmol; 25 (8) :795-798.

Hartmann CW, Rhee DJ (2006). The patient's journey: glaucoma. BMJ; 333(7571): 738–739.

Haymes SA, Leblanc RP, Nicolela MT, Chiasson LA, Chauhan BC (2007). Risk of falls and motor vehicle collisions in glaucoma. Invest Ophthalmol Vis Sci; 48: 1149-1155.

Haymes SA, Leblanc RP, Nicolela MT, Chiasson LA, Chauhan BC (2008). Glaucoma and on-road driving performance. Invest Ophthalmol Vis Sci; 49(7):3035-3041.

Heijl A (2001). Delivering a diagnosis of glaucoma: are we considering the patient oronly his eyes? Acta Ophthalmol Scand; 79: 107.

Hyman LG, Komaroff E, Heijl A, Bengtsson B,Leske MC. (2005) for Early Manifest Glaucoma Trial Group. Treatment and vision-related quality of life in the early manifest Glaucoma Trial. Ophthalmology; 112: 1505-1513.

Hodapp E, Parrish RK II, Anderson DR (1993). Clinical Decisions in Glaucoma. St Louis: Mosby: 53–61.

Ivers RQ, Cumming RG, Mitchell P, Attebo K (1998). Visual impairment and falls in older adults: the Blue Mountains Eye Study. J Am Geriatr Soc.; 46:58-64.

Jampel HD (2001). Glaucoma Patients' Assessment of Their Visual Function and Quality of Life. Tr Am Ophth Soc; 99:301-317.

Jampel HD, Schwartz GF, Robin AL et al. (2003) Patient preferences for eye-drop characteristics: a willingness to pay analysis. Arch Ophthalmol 121:540-546.

Janz NK, Wren PA, Lichter PR, Musch DC, Gillespie BW, Guire KE (2001). Quality of life in newly diagnosed glaucoma patients: the Collaborative Initial Glaucoma Treatment Study. Ophthalmology; 108 (5):887–897.

Janz NK, Wren PA, Guire KE, Musch DC, Gillespie BW, Lichter PR for the Collaborative Initial Glaucoma Treatment Study (2007). Fear of Blindness in the Collaborative Initial Glaucoma Treatment Study: patterns and correlates over time. Ophthalmology; (114) 12: 2213-2220.

Knox FA, Barry M, O'Brien C (2006). The rising cost of glaucoma drugs in Ireland 1996-2003. Br J Ophthalmol; 90: 162-165.

Kulkarni KM, Mayer JR, Lorenzana LL, Myers JS, Spaeth GL (2012). Visual field staging systems in glaucoma and the activities of daily living. Am J Ophthalmol; 154: 445-51.

Kupfer H, Jofre-Bonet M, Gilbert C (2006). Economic evaluation for Ophthalmologists. Ophthamic Epidemiol; 13: 393-401.

Kyari F, Gudlavalleb MVS, Sivsubramaniam S, Gilbert CE, Abdull MM, Eritekume G, Foster A (2009); The Nigeria National Blindness and visual impairment study group. Prevalence of Blindness and visual impairment in Nigeria; the National Blindness and visual impairment survey. Invest Ophthalmol Vis Sci; 50: 2033-2039.

Labiris G, Katsanos A, Fanariotis M, Tsirouki T, Pefkianaki M, Chatzoulis D, Tsironi E(2008). Psychometric properties of the Greek version of the NEI-VFQ 25. BMC Ophthalmol; 8:4.

LabirisG, KatsanosA, Fanariotis M, Zacharaki F, ChatzoulisD, KozobolisVP (2010). Vision-specific quality of life in Greek glaucoma patients. J Glaucoma; 19: 39-43.

Lee BL (1996). Outcomes and end points in Glaucoma. J Glaucoma; 5: 295-297.

Lester M & Zingirian M (2002).Quality of life in patients with early, moderate and advanced glaucoma.Eye; 16: 44-49.

Leung EW, Medeiros FA, Weinreb RN. (2008). Prevalence of ocular surface disease in glaucoma patients. J Glaucoma; 17(5):350-355.

Mabuchi F, Yoshimura K, Kashiwagi K, Shioe K, Yamagata Z, Kanba S, Lijima H, Ysukahara S (2008). High Prevalence of anxiety and depression in patients with primary open angle glaucoma. J Glaucoma; 552-557.

Magacho L,Lima FE, Nery ACS, Sagawa A, Magacho B, Avila MP.(2004). Quality of life in Glaucoma patients: regression analysis and correlation with possible modifiers. Ophthalmic Epidemiol; 11: 263-270.

Mangione CM, Lee PP, Pitts J, Gutierrez P, Berry S, Hays RR (1998). The NEIVFQ Field Test Investigators.Psychometric properties of the National Eye Institute Visual Function Questionnaire (NEIVFQ).Arch Ophthal.; 116 (11):1446–1504.

Mangione CM, Lee PP, Pitts J, Gutierrez P, Berry S, Hays RR (2001). The NEIVFQ Field Test Investigators.Development of the 25-item National Eye Institute Visual Function Questionnaire (NEIVFQ).Arch Ophthal.;119(7):1050–1058.

Massof RW (1998) A systems model for low vision rehabilitation II. Measurement of vision disabilities. Opt Vis Sci; 75: 349-373.

Massof WR, RubinGS.(2001) Visual Function Assessment Questionnaires. Survey of Ophthalmology; 45 (6): 531-547.

Mbadugha CA, Onakoya AO, Aribaba OT, Akinsola FB. (2012). A comparison of the NEIVFQ25 and GQL-15 questionnaires in Nigerian glaucoma patients. Clinical Ophthalmology: 6:1411-1419.

McDougall J, Wright V, Rosenbaum P (2010). The ICF model of functioning and disability: incorporating quality of life and human development. Dev Neurorehabil; 13:204-211.

McKean-Cowdin R, WangY, Wu J, Asen SP,Varma R (2008); and the Los Angeles Latino Eye Study Group. Impact of visual field loss on health-related QOL in glaucoma. The Los Angeles Latino Eye Study. Ophthalmol; 115(6):941–948.

McLaughlin LA, Braun KL (1998). Asian and Pacific islander cultural values: consideration for health care decision making. Health Soc. Work; 23: 116-126.

Mills RP (1998). Correlation of QOL with clinical symptoms and signs at the time of glaucoma diagnosis. Tr Am Ophth Soc.

Mitchell P, Smith W, Chey T, Healey PR (1997). Open angle glaucoma and diabetes: the Blue Mountains eye study, Australia. Ophthalmology; 104: 712-718.

Munoz B, West SK, Rubin GS, Schein OD, Quigley HA, Bressler SB, Bandeen-Roche K (2000). Causes of blindness and visual impairment in a population of older Americans: the Salisbury Eye Evaluation Study. Arch Ophthalmol; 118 (6): 819-825.

Murdoch I (1996). Epidemiology and POAG. Journal of Community Eye Health; 9: 19-22.

Mwanyangala MA, Mayombana C, Urassa H, Charles J, Mahutang C, Abdullah S, Nathan R (2010). Global Health Action; 2. DOI: 10.3402/gha.v310.2142.

Nassiri N, MehravaranS, Nouri-Mahdavi K, Coleman AL (2013). National Eye Institute Visual function Questionnaire: usefulness in Glaucoma. Optom & Vis Sci 90 (8): 745-753.

Nelson P, Aspinall P, Papasoulitis O, Worton B, O'Brien C (2003). Quality of life in glaucoma and its relationship with visual function.J Glaucoma; 12(2):139–150.

Nelson-Quigg J, Cello K, Johnson CA (2000). Predicting binocular visual field sensitivity from monocular visual fieldresults. Invest Ophthalmol Vis Sci; 41: 2212-2221.

Nwosu SNN (1996). Visual fields in glaucoma patients in Nigeria. Nigerian Journal of Ophthalmology.1996; 4:23-26.

Odberg T, Jakobsen JE, Hultgren SJ, HalseideR (2001). The impact of glaucoma on the quality of life of patients in Norway I: results from a self-administered questionnaire. Acta Ophthamol Scand; 79: 116-120.

Oluleye TS, Ajaiyeoba AI, Akinwale MO, Olusanya BA (2006). *Causes of blindness in South-Western Nigeria: a general hospital clinic study*. Eur J Ophthalmol; 16:604-607.

Omoti AE, Waziri-Erameh MJM, Osahon AJ (2002). *The relationship between socio-demographic factors and severity of visual field loss in glaucoma patients at initial presentation in Benin City Nigeria*. Sahel Medical Journal; 5 (4):195-198.

Omoti AE, Waziri-Erameh MJM(2003). *Compliance with medical therapy in patients with primary open angle glaucoma*. Journal of Medicine & Biomedical research; 2 (1):46-53.

Omoti AE (2005). *A review of the choice of treatment in Primary Open Angle Glaucoma*. Niger J Clin Pract.; 8: 29-34.

Onakoya AO, Mbadugha CA, Aribaba OT, Ibidapo OO (2012). *Quality of life of Primary Open Angle Glaucoma Patients in Lagos, Nigeria: Clinical and Socio-demographic correlates*. J Glaucoma; 21 (5): 287-295.

Patrick DL, Erickson P (1988). *Assessing health related quality of life for clinical decision making*. In: Walker SR, Lancaster RM eds. Quality of life, Assessment & Application. London MTP Press pgs 9-49.

PatrickDL, Bergner M (1990). *Measurement of health status in the 1990s*. Ann Rev PublicHealth;11: 165-183.

Parrish RK, 2ⁿᵈ (1996). *Visual Impairment, visual functioning and quality of life assessments in patients with glaucoma*. Trans Am Ophthalmol Soc. 94: 919-1028.

Parrish RK 2nd, Gedde SJ, Scott IU, Feuer WJ, Schiffman JC, Mangione CM, Montenegro-Piniella A (1997). *Visual function and quality of life among patients with glaucoma*. Arch Ophthalmol; 115 (11): 1447-1455.

Quigley HA, Broman AT (2006). *The number of people with glaucoma worldwide in 2010 and 2020*. Br J Ophthalmology; 90: 262-267.

Racette L, Wilson MR, Zangwill LM, Weinreb RN, Pamela A (2003). *Primary Open Angle in Blacks: a review*. Surv Ophthalmol; 48: 295-313.

Ramakrishnan R, Nirmalan PK, Krishnadas R, Thulasiraj RD, Tielsch JM, Katz M, Friedman DS, Robin AC (2003). *Glaucoma in a rural population of Southern India: the Aravind Comprehensive eye survey*. Ophthalmology; 110:1484-1490.

Ramulu PY, Swenor BK, Jeffreys JL, Friedman DS, Rubin GS (2013). *Difficulty with out-loud and silent reading in glaucoma*. Invest Ophthalmol Vis Sci.; 54 (1): 666-672.

Ramulu PY, West SK, Munoz B, Jampel HD, Friedman DS (2009) *Driving cessation and driving limitation in glaucoma: the Salisbury Eye Evaluation Project*.Ophthalmology; 116: 1846-1853.

Redelmeier DA, Detsky AS (1995). *A clinician's guide to utility measurement*. In Bergus GR, Cantor SB, eds. Primary Care Clinics in Office Practice. Philadelphia. WB Saunders; 22: 271-280.

Sawada H, Fukuchi T, Abe H (2011). *Evaluation of the relationship between quality of vision and visual function in Japanese glaucoma patients*. Clin Ophthalmol; 5:259–267.

Shabana N, Comilleau-Peres V, Droulez J(2005). *Postural Stability in Primary Open Angle Glaucoma*. Clin Experiment Ophthalmol; 33:264-273.

Sherwood MB, Garcia-Sieharizza A, Melteer MI, Hebert A, Burns AF, McGorray S(1998)*Glaucoma's impact on QOL and its relation to clinical indicators: a pilot study*. Ophthalmology; 105: 361-366.

Skalicky S, Goldberg I (2008). *Depression and Quality of life in patients with glaucoma: a cross-sectional analysis using the geriatric depression scale15, assessment of function related to vision and the glaucoma quality oflife-15*.J Glaucoma; 17 (7): 546-551.

Sleath B, Robin AL, Covert D, Byrd JE, Tudor G, Svarstad B (2006). *Patient reported behaviour and problems in using glaucoma medications*. Ophthalmology 113 (3): 431-436.

Suzukamo Y, Oshika T, Yuzawa M, Tokuda Y, Tomidokoro A, Oki K, Mangione CM, Green J, Fukuhara S (2005). *Psychometric properties of the 25-item National Eye Institute Visual Function Questionnaire (NEI VFQ-25), Japanese version*. Health Qual Life Outcomes; 3:65.

Skevington SM, Lotfy M, O'Connell KA; WHOQOL Group (2004). *The World Health Organization's WHOQOL-BREF quality of life assessment: psychometric properties and results of the international field trial. A report from the WHOQOL group*. Qual Life Res.; 13 (2):299-310.

Skevington SM, Gunsen KS, O'Connell KA (2013). *Introducing the WHOQOL-SRPB BREF: developing a short form instrument for assessing spiritual, religious and personalbeliefs within QOL*. Quality of Life Research; 22 (5): 1073-1083.

Stewart AL, Sherbourne C, Hays RD. (1992). *Measuring Functioning and Well-Being: The Medical Outcomes Study Approach*. Durham, NC: Duke University Press.: 345–371.

Tielsch JM, Sommer A, Witt K Katz J, Royall M. (1990). *Blindness and Visual impairment in an American Urban population: the Baltimore Eye Survey*. Arch Ophthalmol; 108: 286-290.

Tielsch JM, Sommer A, Katz J, Royall RM, Quigley HA, Javitt J (1991). *Racial variations in the prevalence of Primary Open Angle Glaucoma: the Baltimore Eye Study*. JAMA.; 266: 396-476.

Torrance GW, Thomas WH, Sachett DL (1972). *A utility maximization model for the evaluation of health care programs*. Health Serv Res; 7: 118-133.

Tosh J, Brazzier J, Evans P, Longworth L (2012). *A review of generic preference-based measures of health related Quality of life in visual disorders*. Value Health; 15 (1): 118-127.

Tran HM, Mahdi AM, Sivasubramaniam S, Gudlavalleti MVS, Gilbert CE, Shah SP, Ezelum CC, Abubakar T, Bankole OO on behalf of the Nigerian National Blindness & Visual Impairment Study Group. (2011) *Quality of Life & visual function in Nigeria: findings from the National Survey of Blindness & Visual Impairment*. Br J Ophthalmol; 95: 1646-1651.

Tsai JC, McClure CA, Ramos SE et al.(2003). *Compliance barriers in glaucoma: a systemic classification*. J Glaucoma 12: 393-398.

Turano KA, Massof RW, Quigley H (2002). *A self-assessment instrument designed for measuring independent mobility in Retinitis Pigmentosa patients: generalizability to glaucoma patients*. Invest Ophthalmol & Vis Sci.; 43: 874-2881.

Warrian KJ, Spaeth GL, Lankaranian D, Lopes JF, Steinmann WC (2009). *The effect of personality on measures of QOL related to vision in glaucoma patients*. Br J Ophthalmol; 93 (3): 310-315.

Wee H, Li S, Xie F, Zhang X, Luo N, Feeny D, Cheung Y, Machin D, Fong K, Thumboo J (2008). *Validity, feasibility and acceptability of Time Trade off and Standard Gamble assessments in Health Valuation Studies: A study in a multi-ethnic Asian population in Singapore*.Value in Health; (2): S3-S10.

WHO Anonymous (1993). *Study Protocol for the World Health Organization project to develop a Quality of Life Assessment Instrument (WHOQOL)*. Qual Life Res; 2: 153-159.

Wilson R, Richardson TM, Hertzmark MA, Grant WM (1985). *Race as a risk factor for progressive glaucomatous damage*. Ann Ophthalmol; 653-659.

Woods R, Gardner Re, Ferachi KA, King C, Ermolao A, Cherry KE, Cress ME, Jazwinski SM (2005). *Physical function & Quality of life in older adults: sex differences*. Southern Medical Journal; 98 (5), 504-512.

Wren PA, Musch DC, Janz NK, Niziol LM, Guire KE, Gillespie BW (2009). CIGTS Study Group. *Contrasting the use of 2 vision-specific quality of life questionnaires in subjects with open-angle glaucoma*. J Glaucoma; 18: 403-11.

Wrosch C, Scheier ME (2003). *Personality and Quality of life: the importance of optimism and goal adjustment*. Qual Life Res; 12 (Suppl 1): 59-72.

Wu AM, Tang CS, Kwok TC(2002). *Death, anxiety among Chinese elderly people in Hong Kong*.J Aging Health; 14: 42-56.

Wu SY, Hennis A, Nemesure B, Leske MC; Barbados Eye Studies Group (2008). *Impact of glaucoma, lens opacities, and cataract surgery onvisual functioning and related quality of life: the Barbados Eye Studies*. Invest Ophthalmol Vis Sci; 49: 1333-1338.

Vandenbroeck S, De Geest S, Zeyen T, Stalmans I, Dobbels F (2011). *Patient-reported outcomes (PRO's) in glaucoma: a systematic review*. Eye; 25, 555–577.

vanGestel A, Webers CA, Beckers HJ, van Dongen MC, Severens JL, Hendrikse F, Schouten JS (2010). *The relationship between visual field loss in glaucoma and health-related quality-of-life*. Eye (Lond);24: 1759-69.

Viswanathan AC, McNaught AI, Poinoosawmy D, Fontana L, Crabb DP, Fitzke FW, Hitchings RA(1999). *Severity and stability of glaucoma: patient perception compared with objective measurement*. Arch Ophthalmol; 117(4): 450–454.

Zhou C, Qian S, Wu P, Qiu C. (2013) *Quality of Life of glaucomapatients in China: socio-demographic, clinical and psychological correlates- across sectional study*. Quality of Life Research; DOI 10.1007/s11136-013-0518-2.

Neuro-ophthalmologic Assessment: A Comprehensive Approach to Visual Pathway Disorders

Ana Valverde and Sara Machado

1 Functional Anatomy Of The Visual System

As the eye is part of the brain and many neurological disorders can affect vision, neurological assessment involves a complete examination of the visual function.

The diagnostic approach is identical to other branches of neurology. An accurate history with an appropriate examination will allow the identification of the anatomical localization and timing of onset that will guide the techniques selected to make a correct diagnosis. Lesions in each area of the visual pathway cause distinct patterns of visual loss. Anatomical and physiological knowledge of visual pathways are essential to achieve this goal.

1.1 Anatomy of the Visual System

The anatomo-physiology of the visual system begins at the retina that extends anteroposteriorly from the *ora serrata* to the posterior pole of the eyeball. Two independent systems of photo-receptors, the rods and the cones, are the first neuronal elements that react to visible light and produce electrical activity. The rods, more numerous and distributed throughout the retina except the macula, are specialized in low light levels because of their pigment, rhodopsin. The cones, more concentrated in the macular region, especially in its center (the fovea), react to higher light levels and are important for visual discrimination (Cooper & Metcalfe, 2009).

Because of the optical properties of the eye, the nasal retina receives visual information from the temporal visual field, while the temporal retina receives visual information from the nasal visual field (Figure 1). Similarly, the superior retina receives information from the inferior visual field, and vice versa. The electrical activity produced by the receptors is conveyed by bipolar and amacrine cells to ganglion cells. There are two types of ganglion cells, M and P cells. M cells are concerned with the location of the object, depth perception and contrast sensitivity. P cells, with their macula predominance, are responsible for object characteristics and color contrast sensitivity. The position of the axons of ganglion cells in the optic nerve depends on their origin in the retina. The macular fibers move to a central position, with the superior retinal fibers above and the inferior fibers below. Temporal and nasal fibers retain these positions into the optic nerve (Cooper & Metcalf, 2009).

At the chiasm, axons originating in nasal retina ganglion cells of each eye cross to the contralateral optic tract. Fibers from the inferior part of nasal retina are ventral in the chiasm and loop into the proximal portion of contralateral optic tract (Wilbrand's knee). The existence of this "knee" has been discussed as it was described in enucleated eyes, but clinical cases continue to suggest its existence. Fibers from the superior nasal retina are dorsal in the chiasm

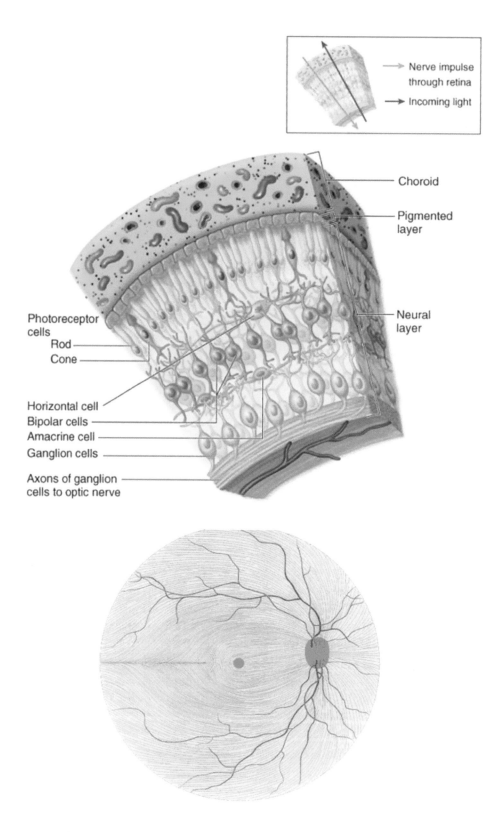

Figure 1: Retinal ganglion cell axons transmitting on the optic nerve head.

and become medial in the optic tract. Uncrossed fibers, originating from the temporal retina, maintain their dorsal or ventral position in the chiasm.

The optic tracts extend from the dorsolateral corners of the chiasm to the lateral geniculate nuclei (LGN). These thalamic structures provide a relay station before the visual cortex.

These nuclei are medial to the temporal lobe and are over the perimesencephalic cisterns. The post-chiasmatic shift in position of optic fibers persists in the geniculate bodies, optic radiations and visual cortex. The optic radiations go from here around the temporal horn of the lateral ventricles (Meyer's loop). Three bundles are described, which correspond to the macula, superior and inferior retina, and finish in different parts of the calcarine fissure.

In the medial region of occipital lobe, cortical area 17 of Brodmann represents the primary visual cortex. Because of a distinctive streak of white matter on the cross section of the cortex (the line of Gennari), it is known as "the striate cortex". Each occipital lobe receives information from the two halves of the retina on the same side as the lobe. The superior and inferior retina are represented over and below the calcarine fissure respectively. The macula and the fovea project to the posterior pole of the occipital lobe, while the peripheral retina is represented anteriorly at the parieto-occipital fissures.

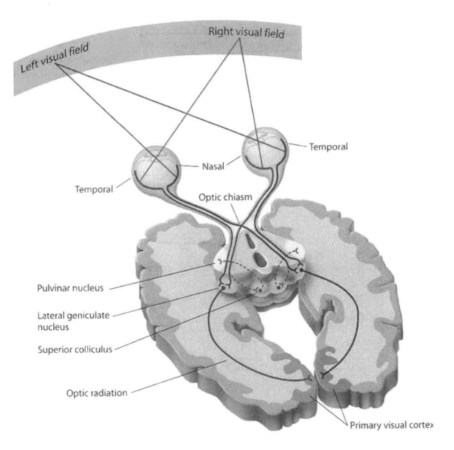

Figure 2: Visual pathways.

The defining qualities of objects, which together form a coherent whole, are processed beyond V1 in the extrastriate areas. To simplify the complex higher visual function network, the idea of two "streams" of vision flowing out from V1 was proposed in the 1980s. The ventral (temporal) stream, referred to as the "what" stream, is concerned with visual objects and face recognition, as well as reading. The dorsal (parietal) stream, or "where" stream, encompasses visual motion and detects multiple items in a scene (Cooper, 2012).

2   Neuro-Ophthalmological Examination

The aim of neuro-ophthalmological examination is to make a neurological diagnosis. Visual acuity and color vision, pupil responses, visual fields and ophthalmoscopy are basic clinical tests useful for this purpose.

2.1   Visual Acuity

Visual acuity is one of the measures of optic nerve function. It must be tested separately with each eye and with the best possible optical correction. If the patient uses corrective lenses, they should be worn. Vision through a pinhole may improve a defect when it is due to refractive error, because it permits only central rays to enter to the eye, minimizing their disruption. (Cornblath, 2009). In neurologic processes or in case of opacities of the media, vision will not improve with a pinhole (Campbell, 2005).

Vision should be measured both at a standard (usually 6 meters or 20 feet) and at near (0.33m or 1 foot) distance. The result, by conventional notation, is expressed by a fraction where the numerator is the distance from the chart and the denominator the distance at which the smallest character is seen by a person with a normal acuity (Thurtell & Tomsak, 2012). Distance vision can be measured with charts such as the Snellen chart in hospital rooms or neurology clinics where there is enough space to test. There are pocket cards for near vision tests. Two types of cards (Figure 3) are available: one has numbers and the other has written text. In neurological practice, the text card measures not only visual acuity but also reading ability. Disparity results with both types of cards suggest a disturbance of language function (Thurtell & Tomsak, 2012).

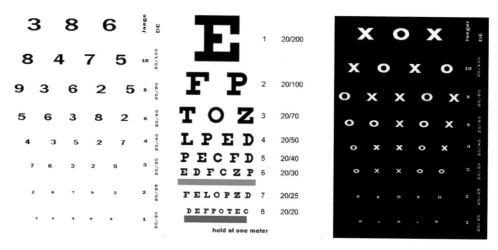

Figure 3: Near vision cards.

2.2 Contrast Vision Testing

Tests for contrast vision check the ability to distinguish adjacent areas of different luminance (light and dark). Special charts such as Pelli-Robson or other new, computerized versions are needed (Thayaparan *et al.*, 2007). It can be evaluated by the perception of lines or optotypes of different sizes with varying degrees of contrast. Eye or retrobulbar pathway problems may show impaired contrast vision (Thurtell & Rucker, 2009).

2.3 Color Vision Testing

Color or pseudoisochromatic plates (Ishihara or similar) assess color vision (Figure 4). In neurologic diseases, red perception is usually lost first (Campbell, 2005). A gross color vision defect is identifiable at the bedside by assessing for red desaturation. A reduced brightness in one eye may suggest nerve dysfunction. Red is normally brighter in the center of the visual field than in periphery. Inversion of this pattern suggests impairment of central vision (Campbell, 2005).

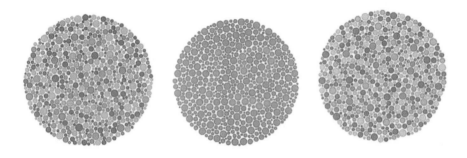

Figure 4: Ishihara plates.

2.4 Pupil Examination

Examination of the pupils involves assessing pupil size, shape, equality and pupillary reflexes. Pupillary size depends on the balance between sympathetic and parasympathetic innervation and the level of illumination. A pupil gauge or a millimeter ruler should be used, and it should be assessed with dim light with the patient fixing on an immobile distant target. A normal pupil is between 2 and 6 mm in diameter. Pupils less than 2 mm are called myotic and more than 6 mm, mydriatic (Campbell, 2005).

A normal pupil is round, with a regular outline. Gross shape abnormalities can be seen in ocular diseases. Slight changes may be significant for neurologic diagnoses.

Pupil size is generally equal for both eyes. A difference of 2 mm is considered significant, while physiologic anisocoria is noted in cases with less than 1 mm of difference between the two sides. In non-physiologic anisocoria cases, pupil size should be measured in darkness and bright light, to allow differentiation between sympathetic and parasympathetic dysfunction.

The pupillary reflexes that must be examined are the light and the near responses. For light reaction, the brightest light available will be the best. The accommodation reflex or near response is elicited by gazing into the distance and then shifting gaze to a close object (e.g. own finger at a distance of 15 to 30 cm). The response consists of thickening of the lens, convergence of the eyes and myosis (Campbell, 2005). In light-near dissociation, the direct light reaction is less than the near reaction. It may happen with small pupils (1 to 2 mm) due to periaqueductal or midbrain lesion (Argyll-Robertson pupil), or with larger pupils because of parasympathetic denervation of the pupil (e.g. Adie tonic pupil or midbrain lesion) (Thurtell & Rucker, 2009).

When testing for light reflex, the amplitude of initial constriction and subsequent escape must be judged by comparing both eyes. Pupil light reflex is considered as an indicator of optic nerve pathology. The abnormal pupillary dilatation or weak response with direct light stimulation, called Marcus-Gunn pupil or "relative afferent pupillary defect" (RAPD), may be amplified by moving the light back and forth between the two eyes. This swinging light test is sensitive in mild optic neuropathy cases. The RAPD term is used to emphasize the difference between the state of the afferent system and light reflex activity from one to the other. This defect may occur in case of bilateral optic nerve involvement, only if significant asymmetry is present. Media opacities will not cause afferent pupil defect, or there will be a slight defect in severe maculopathy or retinopathy cases compared with optic neuropathy (Campbell , 2005).

Other pupillary reflexes such as ciliospinal reflex may be tested. This consists of dilatation of the pupil with painful stimulation of the ipsilateral neck skin. Local cutaneous stimulus activates the sympathetic pathway through connections with the ciliospinal center at C8-T2. An intact reflex confirms brainstem integrity in comatose patients (Campbell , 2005).

Pupil disorders can be divided into pathologic mydriasis or myosis, which can be unilateral or bilateral.

There are two main conditions which can result in a unilateral mydriatic pupil: a third cranial nerve palsy or a parasympathetic denervation (Holmes-Adie tonic pupil). In third nerve palsy, the large pupil does not react to light nor to accommodation. The pupil is more affected than other functions in third nerve palsy, but other signs are usually present. Compressive causes such aneurisms affect the pupil early because of the peripheral position of the parasympathetic fibers on the nerve as it exits the brainstem. This "pupil rule" is not absolute: there are aneurisms that spare the pupil (up to 10% of cases) and diabetic palsies with pupil involvement (up to 25%) (Campbell , 2005).

In Holmes-Adie tonic pupil, there may be a slow reaction to light after prolonged illumination. Once constricted, the tonic pupil returns to normal size very slowly, causing a transient reversal of anisocoria. The accommodation reaction, although slow, is present. It is common in young women, with a suddenly mydriatic pupil, without other symptoms. The pathology is a parasympathetic denervation in the ciliary ganglion or short ciliary nerves, which leads to a supersensitivity. Pupils may constrict with pilocarpine or methacholine solutions that would not cause constriction in a normal eye.

The term "tectal pupils" is used in mydriatic pupils with light near dissociation in upper midbrain lesions. There are several causes for bilateral mydriatic pupils: age, pharmacologic (systemic drugs with anticholinergic effects). A unilateral myotic pupil can be the result of Horner syndrome or neurosyphilis. Horner's syndrome has as its characteristic signs: ptosis, myosis and anhidrosis. Sympathetic denervation to the accessory lid retractors, cause ptosis that may simulate a partial third nerve palsy. Because of lower lid retractor loss of action, the palpebral fissure narrows resulting in an apparent enophthalmos. The myotic pupil scarcely dilates in the dark. This pupillary asymmetry is greater in the dark, contrasting with third nerve palsy and Adie's pupil in which asymmetry is greater in the light.

Pharmacologic tests are useful to determine if a myotic pupil is caused by Horner's syndrome. Cocaine drops can confirm the presence of Horner's syndrome but cannot localize the lesion. Hydroxyamphetamine can distinguish the type of Horner syndrome as pre- or post-ganglionic. Hydroxyamphetamine causes norepinephrine release from intact nerve endings. In a pre-ganglionic lesion, the pupil will dilate, while in lesions distal to the superior sympathetic ganglion, the pupil will fail to dilate (Campbell , 2005).

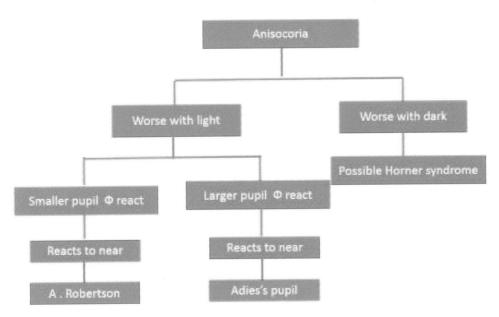

Figure 5: Anisocoria assessment.

2.5   Ophthalmoscopy

Fundoscopic examination will provide additional valuable information. The routine ophthalmoscopic examination in neurologic patients is generally done through an undilated pupil. The small aperture may minimize reflections from the cornea.

The ocular fundus is the only place in the body where blood vessels can be visualized directly. The disc, the macula and the arteries are the areas that should be evaluated. The disc is commonly round, and the nasal margin is normally blurred compared to the temporal (Campbell , 2005). It consists of a peripheral rim (axons from the retina entering the optic nerve) and a central cup, depressed due to underlying lamina cribosa. The central retinal artery and its branches emanate from the disc. The macula, thinner than other retinal areas, without blood vessels, lies temporal and below the disc, with a dark appearance (Campbell , 2005).

Our interest will focus on the aspect of the disc. It may be pallid, due to loss of the optic nerve fibers, which is the primary pathology leading to atrophy.

There are several pathological situations that can produce swelling of the disc, such as acute optic neuritis, retinal vein occlusion and raised intracranial pressure (Plant *et al.* 2009). Usually, this is called papilledema, an acquired optic nerve edema caused by elevated intracranial pressure (Cornblath, 2009).

2.6   Visual field testing

The visual fields are related to peripheral vision. The normal field is wider in the inferior and temporal quadrants than in the superior and nasal quadrants. Patient cooperation, good fixation, and adequate illumination are essential for visual field examination. Several methods are available for visual field examination. Even sophisticated confrontation assessment cannot reach the accuracy of formal field testing (Campbell, 2005).

As a screening technique, in cases of non-specific visual complaint, small amplitude finger movements in upper and lower quadrants in the far periphery, asking the patient to point to the finger that moves, can be appropriate.

More exacting techniques compare the patient and the examiner's field dimensions using various targets. One with high sensitivity is a small (ideally 5 mm) red pin. Each eye must be assessed in turn, with the target being moved slowly in from the periphery while asking the patient when the color red becomes detectable. They will initially see it as black at the periphery where there are no color sensitive cones. A red pin, by stimulating fewer cones than a white pin, detects more subtle defects (Cooper & Metcalfe, 2009).

Another simple, thorough examination can be done by finger counting in all four quadrants, coupled with hand comparison. This technique has the advantage of minimizing the dissociation between the visual perception of the object and the movement (Thurtell & Tomsak, 2012).

When confrontation tests are not adequate for clinical circumstances, formal field tests are done. These may include tangent screen examination, kinetic perimetry or computerized automated static perimetry (Campbell, 2005). Perimetry is the measurement of visual field on a curved surface while campimetry measures the visual fields on a flat surface. The tangent screen (standard method for campimetry) or the Amsler grid, are useful for central vision evaluation. For peripheral visual fields, a perimeter must be used. Perimetry may be static or kinetic depending on the use of a moving or static stimulus. For kinetic perimetry a test object moves along the different quadrants and it is noted when the object is detected. The Goldmann perimeter is the most commonly used kinetic perimeter.

Automatic perimetry using static stimuli has replaced manual perimetry because of the greater sensitivity for detecting visual field defects. The threshold for perception of various objects at various locations is measured and statistical analysis performed. The Humphrey Visual Field Analyzer is commonly used, with reliability indices included determined by the false-negative and false-positive responses (Campbell, 2005), with better sensitivity for glaucoma than for neuro-ophthalmic disorders.

For neurological purposes, visual field abnormalities can be divided into scotomas, hemianopias, altitudinal defects and concentric reduction of the fields. Scotomas are areas of impaired vision in the field, with normal surrounding vision. Hemianopia is defined as impaired vision in half of the visual field of each eye. It may be homonymous, with corresponding halves of each eye, or heteronymous, in opposite halves of each eye, usually bitemporal.

An altitudinal visual field defect involves the upper or lower half of vision, without crossing the horizontal meridian. Usually, it is caused by retinal vascular disease and is unilateral. Concentric reduction of the visual fields may affect one or all parts of the periphery. Symmetric constriction through all meridians is the most common. Optic atrophy secondary to papilledema, glaucoma or other retinal causes may be one of the main etiologies of visual fields contraction (Campbell, 2005).

3   Visual Loss Approaching

For practical purposes the differential diagnosis can be narrowed by attempting to localize the lesion along the visual pathway, as well as defining the time course of the visual loss. Neuro-ophthalmologic examination, previously described, will help achieve this. When thinking about visual loss, the more systematic the approach is, the more accurate the diagnosis will be.

The first question is whether the visual loss is unilateral or bilateral. Unilateral visual loss generally occurs from pre-chiasmal lesions: refractive error, media abnormalities (corneal, lens or vitreous opacity), retinal/macular lesions, optic neuropathy. Bilateral visual loss occurs with chiasmal or post-chiasmal lesions: optic tract, thalamic nuclei, optic radiation or occipital pathology, or with bilateral pre-chiasmal lesions. To confirm whether the loss is unilateral or bilateral, a patient must be asked to cover each eye to specifically check whether the loss is monocular or binocular. A patient with a homonymous hemianopia may say that the eye with the temporal field defect is the only eye affected (Cornblath, 2009).

The next question to address is to characterize the visual loss. If acuity is affected, the patient describes loss of detail, inability to read or blurred vision. Pre-chiasmal lesions: refractive error, corneal, lens or vitreous opacity, and macular or optic nerve lesion can all affect acuity. Homonymous hemianopia (post-chiasmal lesion) will only reduce acuity in bilateral cases. It is important to distinguish whether the problem is with distance, color vision or targets morphology.

In relation to distance, refractive problems have a distance-near difference. In uncorrected hyperopia or presbyopia, near vision is abnormal. The reverse is frequent with uncorrected myopia. Colors vision impairment can be described as red desaturation or faded or washed colors. Peripheral retinopathy and post-chiasmal lesions usually spare color vision, whereas optic neuropathy does affect it (Cornblath. 2009).

With regards to object morphology, metamorphopsia is defined as a phenomenon in which lines or edges appear curved or distorted. It is typically seen with macular disease, but in migraine cases or patients with visual field defects, such distortions can also be present (Kirshner, 2012).

Missing parts of vision must be tested. Hemianopia (missing parts vertically oriented) indicates a chiasmal or post-chiasmal process. Altitudinal field loss (horizontally oriented missing parts) is typically seen with ischemic optic neuropathy, but may be caused by some retinal conditions

The third useful approach is the temporal profile of visual loss. As a framework, it may be separated into four groups based on timing (Lueck, 2010): (1) Transient: patients return to normal almost immediately; (2) Acute: coming on over seconds to minutes; (3) Subacute: over days to weeks; (4) Chronic: over months to years.

3.1   Transient Visual Loss

In case of transient visual loss, we must establish if it is unilateral or bilateral. The most common cause of transient visual loss is temporary ischemia. The term "amaurosis fugax" is used to describe it, and may have a retinal or an occipital lobe cause. Typically the visual loss is complete, black, with a previous curtain coming down or up in some cases (Lueck, 2010). Vascular etiologies such as emboli from the carotids, aortic arch, or heart to the retinal circulation, must be excluded. In the elderly, a hyperviscosity syndrome secondary to giant cell arteritis

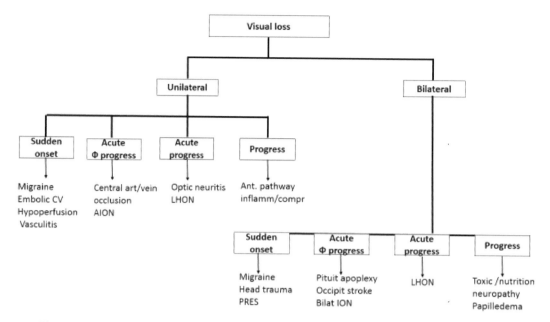

Figure 6: Visual loss framework. CV: cerebrovascular. AION: Anterior ischemic optic neuropathy. LHON: Leber hereditary optic neuropathy. PRES: posterior reversible encephalopathy syndrome. ION: ischemic optic neuropathy.

Embolic cerebrovascular disease
Migraine/vasospasm
Hypoperfusion (hypotension, hyperviscosity, hypercoagulability)
Ocular (glaucoma, optic disc edema, retinal venous stasis)
Vasculitis (giant cell arteritis)
Other: Uhthoff phenomenon

Table 1: Causes of transient monocular vision loss.

can be responsible, even without headache or other symptoms (Melson & Weyand, 2007). These attacks are of sudden onset, with duration of minutes (Thurtell & Tomsak, 2012; Tomsak, 1997).

In young patients retinal artery vasospasm called "retinal migraine" can be responsible, sometimes being misdiagnosed as migraine aura without headache. The latter diagnosis is associated with positive visual phenomena such as lights or flashing, and gradual spread across the visual field over minutes (Lueck, 2010). It is usually benign and responds to calcium channel blockers (Thurtell & Rucker, 2009; Tomsak, 1997).

Some patients with reduced blood supply to the eye, due to an internal carotid artery high-grade stenosis or occlusion, may report transient monocular vision loss in bright light or with postural changes, likely due to impaired regeneration of photopigments secondary to ocular ischemia (Kaiboriboon et al, 2001).

Transient monocular vision loss with increase in body temperature is known as the Uhthoff phenomenon. It may occur more commonly in optic neuritis associated with demyelinating disease, but also with other optic neuropathies. The phenomenon seems to be the result of a transient conduction block within the optic nerve. Vision returns to normal with temperature normalization (Thurtell & Tomsak, 2012).

In patients with papilledema, brief "obscurations" or "greyouts" are described, precipitated by postural changes or Valsalva-like maneuvers (Lueck, 2010). These transient episodes of visual loss are probably secondary to transient hypoperfusion of the edematous nerve head. Similar episodes can occur with systemic hypotension, giant cell arteritis or retinal venous stasis (Egan, 2009).

Simultaneous transient binocular visual loss is frequently due to transient dysfunction of the visual cortex. Visual migraine aura is the most common cause, especially in younger patients. Vasospasm or other causes of cerebral hypoperfusion (thromboembolism, systemic hypotension, hyperviscosity or vascular compression) can also cause this symptom (Thurtell & Rucker, 2009). Last but not least, head trauma in children and posterior reversible encephalopathy syndrome (PRES) (Hinchey et al., 1996) should also be excluded as causes of transient binocular blindness.

3.2 Sudden Monocular Visual Loss Without Progression.

Acute visual loss mostly suggests a vascular cause. In anterior ischemic optic neuropathy (AAION), a distinction must be established between arteritic and non-arteritic etiologies, because the early treatment of the former can prevent irreversible lesions. The major goal of therapy in AAION is to prevent contralateral visual loss. A pale fundus with systemic inflammatory markers will point to an arteritic cause (Lueck, 2010). Central retinal artery occlusions are usually caused by embolic or thrombotic events. In adults with vascular risk factors for atherosclerosis, venous thrombosis at the lamina cribrosa of the sclera may produce occlusion of the central retinal vein (Table 2) (Thurtell & Tomsak, 2012). It causes a central scotoma with sparing of peripheral vision.

Retrobulbar optic nerve infarction, also known as posterior ischemic optic neuropathy, is less common, but can result from perioperative hypotension (cardiac bypass surgery) or other causes of hemodynamic failure. No abnormal ophthalmologic signs are found other than an eventual optic atrophy (Lueck, 2010).

| Central retinal artery or vein occlusion |
| Anterior ischemic optic neuropathy |
| Posterior ischemic optic neuropathy |
| Traumatic optic neuropathy |
| Retinal detachment |
| Vitreous hemorrhage |

Table 2: Causes of sudden monocular visual loss without progression.

3.3 Sudden Binocular Vision Loss Without Progression.

Acute, permanent, binocular vision loss, if not caused by trauma, is commonly due to a stroke involving the post-chiasmal visual pathways. Lesions behind the lateral geniculate nuclei spare pupillary responses, helping topographic diagnosis (Lueck, 2010). Bilateral occipital vascular lesions can result in complete loss of vision in both eyes, known as cortical blindness.

This condition, when accompanied by a denial of the visual loss and confabulation, is referred to as Anton's syndrome (Thurtell & Tomsak, 2012).

Bilateral ischemic optic neuropathies and chiasmal compression, as happens in the case of pituitary apoplexy, can also be considered. Although other symptoms are usually present in pituitary apoplexy, such as headache, diplopia or confusion, subtle presentations have been described (Sibal *et al.*, 2004).

3.4   Sudden Visual Loss With Progression.

Acute, painful monocular visual loss that subsequently worsens can be due to optic nerve inflammation (optic neuritis). The visual loss develops over hours to days before stabilizing, preceded by pain that worsens with ocular movements. The association between optic neuritis and demyelinating diseases is known, with neuropathy sometimes being the first sign of disease (Thurtell & Tomsak, 2012). There may be papillitis or optic disc swelling, except in retrobulbar cases in which ophthalmoscopy is normal.

Leber hereditary optic neuropathy (LHON), a maternally transmitted disease resulting from mutations in the mitochondrial deoxyribonucleic acid (DNA) genes encoding subunits of respiratory chain complex I, can cause sudden visual loss with subsequent progression. Onset is initially monocular with bilateral involvement in approximately 6 months. It affects young adult men with acute or subacute painless central visual loss associated with RAPD (Lueck, 2010; Thurtell & Tomsak, 2012).

3.5   Progressive Visual Loss.

This is the hallmark of compressive lesions affecting afferent visual pathways.

Anterior visual pathway inflammation	Optic neuritis
	Sarcoidosis
	Meningitis
Anterior visual pathway compression	Tumors
	Aneurysms (specially supraclinoid internal carotid artery, junction between the carotid and ophthalmic artery)
	Thyroid-associated orbitopathy
Hereditary optic neuropathies	Toxic and nutritional optic neuropathies
	Chronic papilledema

Table 3: Causes of progressive visual loss.

Common compressive lesions such as pituitary tumors, craniopharyngiomas and meningiomas can affect the chiasm. Optic nerves may be altered due to granulomatous diseases like sarcoidosis or tuberculosis, or compression at the orbital apex from thyroid-associated orbitopathy with minimal motility disturbance. In all cases, the visual loss can be insidious and only discovered during a routine examination (Thurtell & Tomsak, 2012).

The hereditary optic neuropathies are bilateral and usually diagnosed during the first two decades of life. Characteristically, there are abnormal color vision and central scotomas with sparing of the peripheral fields. Optic discs are pallid temporally. The most common inherited optic neuropathy is the autosomal dominant variety, known as dominant optic atrophy (Yu-Wai-Man *et al.*, 2011).

Toxic and nutritional optic neuropathies are usually bilateral and progressive. Most cases of tobacco-alcohol amblyopia are probably related to vitamin B deficiencies. Bariatric surgery and ketogenic diet are other conditions that lead to nutritional deficiency. Etahmbutol, amiodarone, isoniazid, chloramphenicol and iodoquinol are medications toxic to the optic nerves. Vigabatrin, digitalis, chloroquine, hydroxychloroquine and phenothiazines are toxic to the retina. A gradual painless visual loss over weeks to months is frequent, as are dyschromatopsia, cecocentral scotomas and later, optic atrophy (Tomsak, 1997; Thurtell & Tomsak, 2012).

Chronic papilledema from any cause of intracranial hypertension can produce progressive optic neuropathy. Clinically, gray color optic discs and visual fields constriction, with initial nasal defects and spared central vision, are characteristic (Thurtell & Tomsak, 2012).

4   Pupillary Abnormalities

The pupil consists of a hole and its shape is regulated by the pupillo-constrictor and the pupillo-dilator muscles, with the former being innervated by the parasympathetic autonomic nervous system and the latter by the sympathetic autonomic nervous system (Wilhelm, 2007).

Pupillary abnormalities are caused by a myriad of mechanisms and the details of the clinical history and neuro-ophthalmic examination are essential to direct investigations and reveal the underlying dysfunction. Pupillary abnormalities can be classified into two different categories: disorders of the light reflex and disorders of the parasympathetic and sympathetic innervation to the eye (Bremner, 2008).

4.1   Abnormalities of the Light Reflex

- **Complete afferent pupillary defect**
  This is present when a lesion affects the anterior visual pathway of the eye and there is complete blindness. Neither the ipsilateral nor contralateral pupils will react to direct light reflex but the indirect reflex will be intact on the blind side.

- **Relative afferent pupillary defect or Marcus Gunn pupil**
  This defect is identified by the swinging light test: when the light is rapidly alternated between the two eyes and moved to the affected side, there may be a dilatation of both pupils. This finding reflects the fact that decreased light is being transmitted to the brainstem, indicating a lesion in the afferent optic eye, either in the optic nerve or retina. The most common cause is optic neuritis (*vide* optic nerve disease section).

- **Central lesions of the light reflex**
  - **Argyll Robertson Syndrome** - Typically occurs in tertiary syphilis and pupils are small, irregular and do not react to light but do react to accommodation.

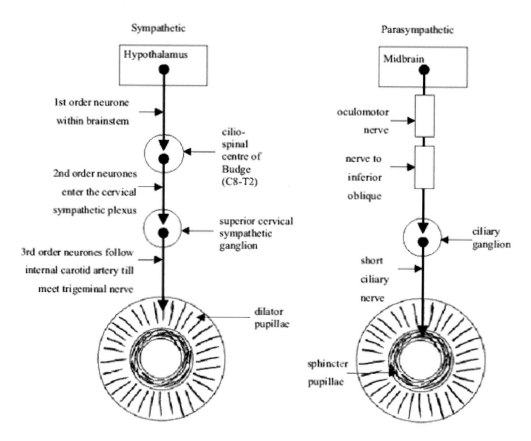

Figure 7: Autonomic pupil innervation systems.

○ **Parynaud Syndrome** – This is caused by a lesion in the dorsal midbrain, typically a pineal gland tumor. Other etiologies are also possible and include multiple sclerosis, hydrocephalus, angiomas, infections, stroke and metastasis. This syndrome is composed of four clinical signs: dilated pupils that do not react to light but do react to accommodation, supranuclear paralysis of upgaze, convergence retraction nystagmus and eyelid retraction (Collier's sign).

4.2 Diagnosis of Parasympathetic and Sympathetic Disorders

It is worth mentioning that the size of the pupil results from a balance between the parasympathetic tonus, which constricts the pupil, and the sympathetic tonus, which dilates it.

• **Parasympathetic disorders**

○ **Adie's pupil** - This is characterized by idiopathic damage to parasympathetic fibers. It presents with a mydriatic pupil that has an exaggerated tonic response to accommodation and a slow redilatation when returning to gaze into the distance. Because there is a sectorial denervation of the sphincter papillae, only portions of it will react to light. It typically affects young adults, with a female predominance. The diagnosis is clinical but it can be confirmed using a muscarinic agonist such as 0.1% pilocarpine which constricts Adie's pupil but not a normal or atropinised pupil. When there is an associated generalized areflexia, the expression Holmes-Adie syndrome is applied.

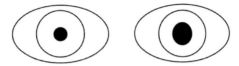

Figure 8: Adie's pupil. There is a mydriatic pupil on the left eye that has a tonic response to accommodation in addition to a slower redilatation.

- o **Atropinised pupil** – This is also a mydriatic pupil but the cause is usually iatrogenic. It may result from an adverse effect of ipratropium bromide nebulizers, hyoscine patches or anticholinergic creams.

- o **III cranial nerve palsy** –Here we see a mydriatic pupil unreactive to light and accommodation. There is an associated ptosis and ipsilateral limitation of eye movements. In the case of an incomplete III nerve palsy, pupil involvement implies an extrinsic compressive lesion and prompt imaging is recommended to exclude aneurysms. One rule of thumb for clinicians is that a pupil-sparing incomplete III nerve palsy needs careful monitoring to ensure that the pupil does not become involved.

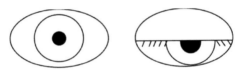

Figure 9: III cranial nerve palsy. Left mydriatic pupil (unreactive to light and accommodation) on top of ptosis and ipsilateral limitation of eye movements.

- **Sympathetic disorders Horner´s syndrome** – The presence of a unilateral partial ptosis (a result of loss of tone in Müller muscle) with an ipsilateral myosis, slight elevation of the lower lid (so called "upside-down ptosis"), anhidrosis and enophthalmus defines Horner's Syndrome. It is worth mentioning that it is most apparent in the dark and a redilatation lag may be present i.e. a slow redilatation after a brisk constriction to light.

It results from pre- or post-ganglionic lesions and the list of causes includes carotid dissections, lateral medullary syndrome, Pancoast tumors, birth trauma and cluster headache. Hence, imaging of head, neck and chest may be required although some cases remain idiopathic. In congenital cases, because an intact sympathetic supply is required for a normal coloration of iris, heterochromia is present. In children, the presence of Horner's syndrome requires urgent imaging to exclude neuroblastoma. Bilateral cases may be seen with diabetes and other autonomic neuropathies (e.g. amyloid), old age, opiate use, coma and tertiary syphilis.

To localize the lesion, hydroxyamphetamine is used as it dilates pre-ganglionically and does not influence post-ganglionic lesions.

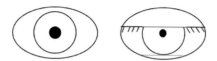

Figure 10: Horner's syndrome. Apart from a left myosis there is a partial ptosis, elevation of the lower lid, anhidrosis and enophthalmus.

4.3   Physiological Anisocoria

This is present in up to 20% of the population (Rucker *et al.*, 2004). It varies from day to day and can switch between eyes, but the essential characteristic is that the difference keeps constant in light and darkness. When examining these patients, pupillary reflexes are normal.

5   Optic Nerve Disease

Optic neuropathies are disorders that affect the optic nerve. The list of causes is broad, including inflammation, infection, vascular causes, compression, genetic and metabolic diseases, as well as trauma (Plant *et al.*, 2009). The classical features of an optic neuropathy are a central visual loss and a relative afferent pupillary defect detected on examination. In spite of the possibility of having a swollen or pale optic nerve, in retrobulbar neuritis the appearance is completely normal. Etiological clues include the age of patient, time of onset and progression, presence of pain or bilateral involvement, level and pattern of visual loss and finally, the appearance of the optic nerve.

5.1   Optic Neuritis

By far the most common cause of optic neuropathy is inflammation and, in this context, the term optic neuritis is applied. It is usually a subacute unilateral visual loss that typically affects young females. The deficit is characterized by decrease of visual acuity, contrast sensitivity, color perception and the appearance of a visual field defect (that may be central, altitudinal, arcuate or a generalized constriction). It is common to have associated pain, which is exacerbated by eye movements and often precedes the visual loss. One important feature to mention is that albeit prominent, pain does not interfere with sleep (if pain is so severe that interferes with sleep, alternative diagnoses should be considered). Approximately one third of individuals will also experience photopsias.

Optic neuritis may happen as a Clinical Isolated Syndrome (CIS), in the context of an established Multiple Sclerosis (MS), Neuromyelitis Optica (NMO) or Acute Disseminated Encephalomyelitis (ADEM). While the clinical presentation in CIS and MS is similar to the one already described, patients with NMO tend to have more aggressive episodes: they are often bilateral, chiasmitis is possible, and does carry a worse visual prognosis.

There are systemic immune-mediated conditions that are also responsible for the appearance of optic neuritis, such as sarcoidosis. Although optic neuritis is the commonest presenting feature, involvement of the optic nerve by a granuloma should be considered (it is usually visible on fundoscopy and associated with vitritis and periphlebitis). Systemic lupus erythematosus (SLE) is a further possible cause.

On examination, both color vision and pupil light reflex are impaired in a disproportionate manner comparing to the acuity loss. The swinging light manoeuvre is crucial as a relative afferent pupillary defect (RAPD) can be present but it is important not to forget that RAPD is absent in cases of bilateral involvement of the optic nerves. Because the inflammatory process in many cases only involves the posterior part of the optic nerve, the majority of patients have no fundoscopic abnormalities ("the patient sees nothing and the doctor sees nothing"). In spite of that, up to one third of patients may have disc edema.

Although the diagnosis is a clinical one, investigation plays an important role in establishing the etiology. In this context, cerebral MRI is crucial. Patients with cerebral demyelinating lesions identified will have a higher probability of developing multiple sclerosis. When NMO is suspected, MRI (cerebral and spinal) and the anti aquaporin 4 antibody test should be performed.

In the case of optic neuritis most patients recover spontaneously. Despite not affecting the final outcome, high dose steroids are usually given in order to speed up the recovery. IV steroids are more desirable than oral formulations as the latter may increase the risk of further episodes of optic neuritis (Beck *et al.*, 1992). A meta-analysis of 12 randomized controlled clinical trials of steroid treatment in optic neuritis and multiple sclerosis, confirmed the efficacy of high-dose intravenous treatment in short-term visual recovery, but without statistically significant benefits in long-term prognosis (Brusaferri & Candelise, 2000).

Feature	Possible Diagnosis
Sudden onset, no progression	Arteritic or non arteritic ischemic optic neuropathy
Optic atrophy and failure to clinical improvement	Compression (meningioma, aneurysm, metastasis)
Sequential (bilateral) and maternal inheritance	Leber's optic neuropathy
Chronic course, bilateral, family history	Autosomal dominant optic neuropathy, autosomal recessive optic neuropathy and Leber's optic neuropathy
Severe pain	Granulomatous optic neuropathy or sinus mucocele
Bilateral optic nerve involvement *ad initium*	Neuromyelitis optica, Leber's optic neuropathy, Herpes virus 6

Table 4: Red flags in the diagnosis of optic neuritis (adapted from Hickman S).

5.2   Chronic Relapsing Inflammatory Optic Neuropathy (CRION)

This is a condition with unknown etiology and whose outstanding feature is not only a favorable response to steroids but also a relapse when such therapy is suspended. The clinical presentation is similar to classical optic neuritis but pain is more severe and bilateral involvement may occur.

5.3   Ischemic Optic Neuropathies

Vascular neuropathies are divided according to etiology. When inflammation occurs it is classified as arteritic. When it is absent, the term non-arteritic is used.

- **Non-arteritic optic neuropathies**
  One possible classification of these disorders is according to the anatomic location. Thus, a division between anterior and posterior ischemic optic neuropathies is possible.

- **Anterior Ischemic Optic Neuropathies (AION)** – Ischemia at the level of the posterior short ciliary artery results in AION and the most common form is the non-arteritic process. It is associated with traditional risk factors including arterial hypertension, diabetes, ischemic heart disease (Salomon *et al.*, 1999) and obstructive sleep apnea syndrome, in addition to hypotension.

  It predominantly affects middle aged and elderly individuals and it is clinically characterized as a unilateral, acute and maximal at onset, painless visual loss. The visual field defect is commonly inferior and respects the horizontal meridian (lower altitudinal field defect) because the upper part of the disc is thought to be more vulnerable to hypoperfusion. While spontaneous recuperation is extremely infrequent, worsening after onset has been described.

  Edema of the disc is present in the acute phase and the disc itself is crowded and cupless. When chronicity develops, the upper pole of the disc becomes atrophic. Second eye involvement occurs in 20-40% of cases within months to years. No treatment is warranted but some authors recommend secondary prevention with aspirin (Cohen, 2009).

- **Posterior Ischemic Optic Neuropathies (PION)** – This diagnosis that should only be considered in the setting of hypotension and giant cell arteritis since compressive causes are far more frequent than PION (Costello, 2009).

- **Arteritic optic neuropathies**
  Giant cell arteritis (GC) is a well recognized cause of AION and less commonly of PION. There are some clinical features that might help to distinguish it from its non-arteritic counterparts: not only is the loss of vision more pronounced but there are also premonitory losses of vision; furthermore, the disc looks pale early in the course of the disease. Recognized associated symptoms include headache, jaw claudication, malaise, weight loss and proximal limb weakness.

  Palpation of the temporal, facial and occipital arteries is mandatory because they may feel tender, thickened and pulseless. On addition, the diagnosis workup includes a serologic search for elevated biomarkers of inflammation (elevated sedimentation rate and C-reactive protein), platelets and gamma GT, as well as temporal arterial biopsy. Once this diagnosis is identified, therapy with steroids and platelet anti-aggregants should be started promptly to prevent further visual loss. As mentioned, the goal of an early treatment is to avoid a contralateral involvement. Arteritic optic neuropathies can also occur in other diseases such as polyarteritis nodosa, systemic lupus erythematosus, Churg-Strauss syndrome and other ANCA positive vasculitis.

5.4   Idiopathic Intracranial Hypertension

This typically affects young overweight females and a highly suggestive feature is the presence of visual obscurations that are positionally provoked (e.g. on bending forward). On examination one can find papilledema, retinal hemorrhages and visual field defects (namely enlarged blind spot and inferonasal constriction). As this is a diagnosis of exclusion, causes of intracranial hypertension such as cerebral venous thrombosis, space occupying lesions and meningitis must first be considered.

5.5   Infectious Optic Neuropathies

The differential diagnosis is also broad and only the most frequent causes will be considered. The main characteristics can be consulted in Table 5.

	Agent	Optic Involvement	Other Particularities	Treatment
Bacteria	*Borrelia burgdorferi*	Optic neuropathy	Occurs in the context of Bannwart syndrome, usually associated with meningitis and intracranial hypertension	Ceftriaxone
	Treponema pallidum	Acute phase: AION and PION Chronic phase: Optic atrophy	Fundoscopy: disc pallor in chronic lesions; Syphilis	Penicillin
	Bartonella henselae	Neuroretinitis	Macular star on fundoscopy (exudates in a radial pattern around the macula)	Doxycicline
	Mycobacterium tuberculosis	Retrobulbar optic neuritis or granulomatous inflammation	In association to meningoencephalitis	Isoniazid, rifampin, pyrazinamide, ethambutol
	Mycoplasma pneumonia	Optic neuropathy	In the setting of pneumonia and meningoencephalitis	Macrolides, tetracycline, fluorquinolones
Viruses	HIV	Optic neuropathy	Uncommon	HAART
	CMV	Optic neuropathy and necrotizing retinitis	Common in AIDS; May coexist with CMV related ventriculitis and lumbosacral polyradiculitis	Ganciclovir, foscarnet
	EBV and VZV	Optic neuropathy	Rare	Acyclovir and corticosteroids
	Herpes virus 6	Optic neuropathy, occasionally bilateral	Rare Immunocompetent or AIDS	Foscarnet and corticosteroids
Parasites	*Toxoplasma gondii*	Granulomatous inflammation of optic nerve and neuroretinitis	More common in AIDS and encephalitis setting	Pyrimethamine with folinic acid and sulfadiazine
Fungi	*Cryptococcus neoformans*	Optic neuropathy	In setting of AIDS, meningitis and intracranial hypertension	Amphotericin B with flucytosine, fluconazole

Table 5: Infectious optic neuropathies.

5.6   Neoplastic and Paraneoplastic Optic Neuropathies

Neoplasms can interfere with optic nerve function in several ways, either by direct compression, infiltration, elevation of intracranial pressure or remote effects (paraneoplastic syndromes). These patients do not present with an acute deficit but with an insidious visual loss. Optic nerve atrophy is also possible and reflects retrograde axonal degeneration. Hence, whenever optic atrophy it is present, compression must be excluded.

On the one hand, there are primary neoplasms of the optic nerve. Albeit rare, low grade glioma is the most common infiltrative lesion of the optic nerve and most of them are juvenile pilocytic astrocytomas. It affects children and is frequently associated with neurofibromatosis type 1. High grade gliomas are also rare but occur more commonly in the adult population. One other possibility is the presence of primary optic nerve meningiomas, which predominantly affect middle-aged females and are generally unilateral. Patients may describe gaze-evoked amaurosis, diplopia, transient visual obscurations and slowly progressive loss of vision of the affected side. When multifocal, they are usually associated with neurofibromatosis type 2.

Within optic nerve secondary neoplasms, lymphoma (usually in the setting of a systemic or central nervous system process) and metastatic lesions, must be kept in mind.

Finally, when considering paraneoplastic syndromes, lung carcinoma is the typical example.

5.7   Genetic Optic Neuropathies

Autosomal dominant optic atrophy is caused by a mutation in the OPA1 gene located in the long arm of the chromosome 3. It starts early in life and is characterized by an insidious and bilateral visual loss, predominantly affecting the central vision. It may be associated with sensorineural hearing loss.

Leber's Hereditary Optic Neuropathy is a mitochondrial disorder with maternal inheritance that predominantly affects young males, in a sequential fashion. In the majority of individuals, bilateral involvement ultimately appears and the rate of visual loss is generally quicker than in the dominant hereditary example. The visual defect also presents as a central scotoma with preservation of the peripheral field.

5.8   Toxic And Deficiency Optic Neuropathies

Toxic and deficiency neuropathies tend to be bilateral, although one eye may be affected first. Examples include consumption of tobacco, alcohol, amiodarone, cyclosporine, digoxin and vitamin B12 deficiency. Radiation induced optic neuropathy usually appears after 1 or 2 years of exposure.

5.9   Trauma

Because the optic nerve is tightly fixed when it exits the orbit through the optic foramen, it is vulnerable to the effect of percussive forces transmitted in the context of head trauma.

6   Chiasmal And Retrochiasmal Disorders

6.1   Chiasmal lesions

According to the position of the pituitary gland, there are three possible positions of the chiasm:

1.   Pre-fixed: before the sellar region

2.   Directly above the pituitary gland (in 80% of cases)

3.   Post-fixed: after the sellar region

Lesions have different clinical manifestations depending on the location of the chiasm. Bitemporal hemianopia is the characteristic sign of chiasmal disease and in fact, in the first two positions the manifestation is a bitemporal hemianopsia. However, if lesions affect a post-fixed located chiasm, the result is a defect that resembles an optic neuropathy.

Chiasm involvement includes compressive and non-compressive causes. Causes of compression are legion but, in the adult patient, the most common are both tumors (such as pituitary tumors, meningiomas and craniopharyngiomas) and aneurysms (Schiefer & Hart, 2001). Other possible etiologies include inflammatory (namely adenohypophisitis) and infectious processes (such as pituitary abscesses). In order to determine the precise etiology, imaging should always be performed (preferably MRI).

Among the non-compressive causes, pituitary apoplexy should not be missed. This is a medical emergency that presents with sudden headache and visual loss; because it courses with endocrinological dysfunction it may be fatal if not promptly recognized and treated. There are some possible inflammatory causes such as sarcoidosis and neuromyelitis optica.

6.2   Retrochiasmal Lesions

Homonymous hemianopia is the hallmark of retrochiasmal lesions. Depending on the location of the lesion an incongruous (combination of crossed and uncrossed retinal axons) or congruous homonymous hemianopia may occur (Schiefer & Hart, 2001).

- Isolated lesions of the **o**ptic tract are rare and often result from suprasellar diseases (tumors such as craniopharyngioma, aneurysms, among others). There is no visual acuity loss and an incongruous homonymous field defect is found. When examining the patient, one should look for an afferent pupillary defect in the eye ipsilateral to the greater visual loss.

- Lesions affecting the lateral geniculate nucleus (LGN) are also uncommon and are often caused by vascular insults. They do not result in loss of visual acuity nor afferent papillary defect. The characteristic visual field defect is an incongruous homonymous hemianopia.

- Optic radiation lesions course with congruous homonymous hemianopia.

- Lesions in the occipital cortex are the most common cause of congruous homonymous hemianopia. They are mainly a result of a vascular disorder and their distinguishing feature is the presence of macular sparing.

When the primary visual cortex or visual association areas are disrupted by disorders such as degenerative diseases, tumors and vascular insults, visuospatial and visuoperceptual abnormalities can occur. These symptoms may have a huge impact on daily living activities: visuospatial abnormalities may result in road traffic accidents due to failure to judge distances and visuoperceptual problems lead to reading difficulty despite preserved single letter visual acuity. Several syndromes and focal signs have been described (Barton, 2005; Plant *et al.*, 2009):

- **Peduncular Hallucinosis** occurs when the lesion affects the thalamus and upper midbrain. Patients report vivid and well formed hallucinations.

- **Polyopia** manifests as a single target that is seen as multiple. It usually develops after a few seconds of fixation and does not resolve with a pinhole.

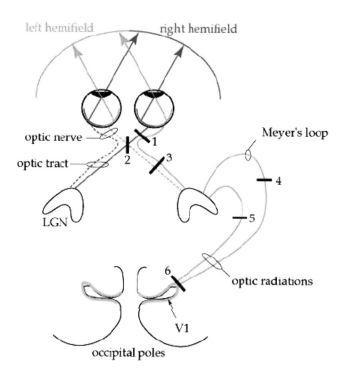

Figure 11: Visual pathway. 1: Pre-chiasmal lesion. 2: Chiasmal lesion. Retrochiasmal lesion: 3: Optic tract. 4: Meyer's loop. 5: LGN. 6: Occipital cortex.

- **Palinopsia** or visual perseveration is defined as a recurrence of an object after its removal that persists despite eye closure. The illusory image is well incorporated into the visual environment. It often results from non-dominant occipito-parietal lesions.

- **Metamorphopsias** are perceptual disturbances in which objects seem abnormally shaped or seem to have an abnormal size. They may occur in partial seizures and migraine attacks.

- **Agnosias** are the inability to recognize objects or spatiotemporal contexts although the primary perception is intact as well as motor function. The parietal lobes provide visuospatial information, the temporal lobes information about the recognition of colors, faces, objects and a pathway that integrates information.

- **Charles Bonnet Syndrome** consists of visual hallucinations (perception of external visual stimuli that are not present) in patients with visual acuity loss or visual field deficits. It is thought to be caused by disinhibition of the visual cortex in the setting of visual deprivation. The visual field defects are generally bilateral (Pelak, 2009).

- **Balint's Syndrome** is caused by bilateral parietal and/or occipitoparietal lobe lesions and consists of optic ataxia (misreaching under visual guidance), ocular apraxia (inability to make voluntary fast eye movements to a visual target) and simultagnosia (inability to perceive the global visual scene).

- **Anton's Syndrome** is seen in parietal temporal lesions of the non-dominant hemisphere and it is characterized by an inability to recognize the visual defect (visual anosognosia) (Zihl, 2007).

Authors

Ana Valverde
Hospital Fernando Fonseca, Portugal

Sara Machado
Hospital Fernando Fonseca, Portugal

References

Barton J et al. *The field defects of anterior temporal lobectomy: a quantitative reassessment of Meyer's loop. Brain 2005; 128(Pt 9):2123-33.*

Barton J, Caplan L. *Cerebral visual dysfunction. In: Bogousslavsky J, Caplan L. Stroke Syndromes, 2nd Edn. Cambridge: Cambridge University Press. 2000; p.87-110.*

Beck RW, Cleary PA, Anderson MM et al. *A randomized, controlled trial of corticosteroids in the treatment of acute optic neuritis. N Eng J Med 1992; 326: 581-88.*

Bremner FD. *Pupillary Disorders. In: Kidd DP, Newman NJ, Biousse V. Neuro-ophthalmology. Philadelphia: Butterworth-Heinemann Elsevier. 2008; p. 264-279.*

Brusaferri F, CandeliseL. *Steroids for multiple sclerosis and optic neuritis: a meta-analysis of randomized controlled clinical trials. J Neurol 2000; 247: 435-42.*

Campbell WW. *The optic nerve. In: De Jong's. The neurological examination. 6th Edn. Lippincott Williams &Wilkins. 2005; p 116-148.*

Cohen AB, Pless M. *Optic neuropathy with disc edema. Continuum Lifelong Learning Neurol. 2009; 15(4):22-46.*

Cooper SA. *Higher visual function: hats, wives and disconnections. Pract Neurol 2012; 12: 349-357.*

Cooper SA, Metcalfe RA. *Assess and interpret the visual fields at the bedside. Pract Neurol 2009; 9: 324-334.*

Cornblath WT. *Introduction to visual loss. Continuum Lifelong Learning Neurol 2009; 15(4):13-21.*

Costello F. *Retrobulbar optic neuropathies. Continuum Lifelong Learning Neurol. 2009; 15(4):47-67.*

Donders RC. *Clinical features of transient monocular blindness and the likelihood of atherosclerotic lesions of the internal carotid artery. J Neurol Neurosurg Psychiatry. 2001; 71(2):247-9.*

Egan RA. *Transient visual loss. Continuum Lifelong Learning Neurol. 2009; 15(4):85-92*

Hickman SJ. *The bare essentials Neuro-ophthalmology. Practical Neurol. 2011; 11:191-200.*

Hill et al. *Most cases labeled as "retinal migraine" are not migraine. J Neuroophthalmol. 2007; 27(1): 3-8.*

Hinchey J, Chaves C, Appignani B et al. *A reversible posterior leukoencephalopathy syndrome.N Eng J Med 1996 Feb (22); 334(8): 494-500*

Job OM, Schatz NJ, Glaser JS. *Visual loss with Langerhans cell histiocytosis: multifocal central nervous system involvement. J Neuroophthalmol. 1999; 19(1):49-53.*

Kaiboriboon K, Piriyawat P, Selhorst JB. *Light-induced amaurosis fugax. Am J Ophthalmol. 2001; 131(5):674-6.*

Kirshner HS. *The agnosias. In: Daroff RB, Fenichel GM, Jankovic J, Mazziota J, eds, Bradley's Neurology Clinical Practice, 6th Edn. Philadelphia: Elsevier. 2012; p.133-160.*

Lueck CJ. *Loss of vision. Practical Neurol. 2010; 10: 315-325.*

Lueck CJ, Gilmour DF, Mclwaine GG. *Neuro-ophthalmology: examination and investigation. J Neurol Neurosurg Psychiatry. 2004; 75(4):2-11.*

Melson MR, Weyand CM, Newman NJ et al. *The diagnosis of giant cell arteritis. Rev Neurol Dis 2007; 4: 128-42.*

Pelak V. *Visual hallucinations and higher cortical visual dysfunction. Continuum Lifelong Learning Neurol. 2009; 15(4):93-105.*

Plant G, Acheson J, Clarke C et al. *Neuro-Ophthalmology. In: Clarke C, Howard R, Rossor M, Shorvon S. Neurology a Queen Square textbook. Oxford: Wiley-Blackwell. 2009; p.489-532.*

Rucker JC, Biousse V, Newman NJ. *Ischemic optic neuropathies. Curr Opin Neurol. 2004; 17 (1):27-35.*

Salomon O, Huna-Baron R, Kurtz S et al. *Analysis of prothrombotic and vascular risk factors in patients with nonarteritic anterior ischemic optic neuropathy. Ophthalmology 1999; 106: 739-42.*

Schiefer U, Hart W. *Functional Anatomy of the Human Visual Pathway. In: U. Schiefer, Wilhelm H, Hart W. Clinical Neuro-ophthalmology: A practical guide. Heidelberg: Springer, 2007; p.19-28.*

Sibal L, Ball SG, Connolly V et al. *Pituitary apoplexy: a review of clinical presentation, management and outcome in 45 cases. Pituitary 2004; 7(3): 157-63*

Stark R. *Clinical testing of visual fields using a laser point and a wall. Pract Neurol 2013; 13: 258-259.*

Thayaparan K, Crossland MD, Rubin GS. *Clinical assessment of two new contrast sensitivity charts. Br J Ophthalmol 2007; 91: 749-752.*

Thurtell MJ, Tomsak RL. *Neuro-Ophthalmology: Afferent Visual System. In: Daroff RB, Fenichel GM, Jankovic J, Mazziota J, eds, Bradley's Neurology Clinical Practice, 6th Edn. Philadelphia: Elsevier. 2012; p.635-643.*

Thurtell MJ, Rucker JC. *Transient visual loss.Int Ophthalmol Clin 2009; 49(3): 147-66.*

Tomsak RL. *An approach to acquired visual loss in adults. J Ophthalm Nurs Techno 1997; 16(5): 229-34.*

Wilhelm H, Wilhelm B. *Diagnosis of Pupillary. In: U. Schiefer, Wilhelm H, Hart W. Clinical Neuro-ophthalmology: A practical guide. Heidelberg: Springer. 2007; p.55-69.*

Winterkorn et al. *Brief report: treatment of vasospastic amaurosis fugax with calcium-channel blockers. N Engl J Med 1993; 329(6):396-8.*

Yu-Wai-Man P, Griffiths PG, HudsonG et al. *Inherited mitochondrial optic neuropathies. Genet 2011; 48(4): 284.*

Zeki S, Ffytche DH. *The Riddoch syndrome: insights into the neurobiology of conscious vision. Brain. 1998; 121: 25-45.*

Zhang X, Kedar S, Lynn MJ, et al. *Homonymous hemianopsias: clinical anatomic correlations in 904 cases. Neurology 2006; 66(6):906–910.*

Zihl J, Schiefer U, Schiller J. *Central Disturbances of Vision. In U. Schiefer, Wilhelm H, Hart W. Clinical Neuro-ophthalmology: A practical guide. Springer, 2007: 185-194.*

Acanthamoeba Keratitis: An Update

Nadia Al Kharousi, Upender Wali and Sitara Azeem

1 Introduction

Acanthamoeba is one of the most commonly isolated amoebae in environmental samples due to its cosmopolitan distribution and can act as both an opportunistic and nonopportunistic pathogen. Genotype T4 is the most commonly found strain found in the environment and also responsible for Acanthamoeba keratitis (AK) (Di Cave *et al.*, 2009). AK is a painful, sight-threatening, and difficult-to-treat corneal infection. Clinically, AK often presents as a unilateral infection among contact lens wearers, with bilateral involvement found in only 2% to 15% of cases (Bacon *et al.*, 1993; Hargrave *et al.*, 1999; Wilhelmus *et al.*, 2008; Radford *et al.*, 1998). Acanthamoeba is a ubiquitous protozoan and a rare causative organism for keratitis, representing 0.15 per million cases of keratitis in the USA; 70% to 85% of cases of acanthamoeba keratitis are associated with contact lens use (Hutchinson & Apel, 2002). However, AK comprises only 5% of contact lens related microbial keratitis (Houang *et al.*, 2001; Butler *et al.*, 2005; Acharya *et al.*, 2007). Since 1973 acanthamoeba has been increasingly associated with potentially dangerous and sometimes blinding keratitis. This infection is more recognized in developed countries amongst contact lens wearers. The prevalence of AK has risen in the past 20 to 30 years, mainly due to the increase in number of contact lens wearers' worldwide (Lam *et al.*, 2002; Seal, 2003). A number of outbreaks since 2004 have made acanthamoeba infection a national epidemic of significant importance. Contact lens wear is not always the main risk factor for infection. In a recent epidemiological study from India only 0.9% of reported cases of AK were thought to be associated with contact lens wear (Lalitha *et al.*, 2012). In USA and UK, 3% to 15% of AK infections occur in non-contact lens users (Stehr-Green *et al.*, 1989; Radford *et al.*, 2002). The major risk factors were associations with eye trauma and poor water supply. There is an increased incidence of AK during summer, probably due to increased number of acanthamoeba organisms in a warmer and humid climate. All normal individuals mount a humoral immune response to the infection, which is effective in vascularised regions of the body. However, in the immunopriviliged cornea, the normal oxidative destruction of the organism by neutrophils is limited. Despite its invasive course into the cornea and its ability to penetrate Descemet membrane and endothelium, persistence of acanthamoeba in the anterior chamber and subsequent endophthalmitis in an otherwise healthy individual is presumed to be prevented by a strong immune response against the pathogen (based on animal models). This may be due to a strong neutrophilic response thereby reducing trophozoites to undetectable levels without encystment (Clarke *et al.*, 2005).

To date eight species of acanthamoeba are known to cause infections (differentiated on the basis of cyst morphology and antigenic composition). A. castellani and A.polyphaga are the most common strains to cause AK (Mathers *et al.*, 2000). Acanthamoeba, a free-living protozoan (unicellular eukaryocyte) thrives in dust, soil, fresh or brackish water reservoirs, sewers, insect vectors, public water supplies, over head water tanks, ponds, lakes, swimming pools, sea water, hot tubs, ventilation ducts, bottled water, eyewash stations and tainted contact lens solutions. It is also found as a commensal in upper respiratory tract. The cysts (metabolically dormant) are resistant to freezing, desiccation, alterations in osmolarity, chemical microbial agents and the levels of chlorine routinely used in municipal water supplies and swimming pools. In majority of cases there is a positive history of contact lens use and exposure to contaminated source with or without corneal trauma. The incidence of contact lens related AK may range from 40% to 93 (Mathers *et al.*, 2000). The infection rate of AK is 0.25 to 0.33 per 10,000 contact lens wearers' yearly (Lam *et al.*, 2002; Seal, 2003).

Risk factors: There are multiple risk factors which predispose contact lens wearers to develop microbial keratitis, including AK. Any break in the epithelium is an invitation for AK, especially if it is associated with prior swimming, use of contaminated solutions or poor hand hygiene. The annual incidence of microbial keratitis amongst overnight lens wear with hydrogel contact lenses is almost ten times more (19.5 cases per 10,000) compared to daily-wear hydrogel contact lenses(1.9 – 2.0 cases per 10,000). The reason for this increased risk is overnight collection of stagnant tear layer under the lenses, predisposing to trapping of microbes between the cornea and the lens (Stapleton *et al.*, 2008). Soft lenses carry a higher risk compared to daily wear rigid lenses. This is so because the movement of rigid lenses ensures better circulation of tears, thereby, reducing chances of piling up of organisms. It is also due to cumulative effect of corneal hypoxia induced microcystic epithelial lesions which, in turn, predispose to epithelial erosions, necrosis and peeling off of epithelium. In presence of risk factors like overnight use of contact lenses, such a break in the continuity of epithelium increases risk of infection by more than five times (Stapleton *et al.*, 1992). Wearers may be more prone to epithelial defects with Silicone hydrogel lenses, the reason may be as wearing time increases, the ingredients of the cleaning solution get washed out. AK is uncommon with daily disposable contact lenses.

Poor hygiene remains the major factor even amongst well-to-do users, probably because of lack of time or change in lifestyle. Poor handling of storage cases increases the risk of microbial keratitis by a factor of approximately 3.7. Biofilms are common in lens cases and can harbor resistant organisms. Such organisms can be easily transferred to contact lenses soaked in such cases. Simple washing of hands before handling lenses can decrease risk of microbial keratitis by 1.5 times (Dart *et al.*, 2008; Stapleton *et al.*, 2008).

Smoking triples the risk of microbial keratitis in contact lens wearers. The possible mechanisms could be effect of toxins on the ocular surface and changes in the immune system (Stapleton *et al.*, 2008).

Stapleton found that lenses purchased on line (internet) had a 4.8 times greater risk of developing microbial keratitis compared to patients who purchased their lenses at authorized centers. Lack of eye examination and inadequate or no education prior to use of contact lenses could be possible explanations. Also, first time users are more prone to microbial keratitis (Stapleton *et al.*, 2008).

A particular risk arises when contact lens solution is prepared from salt tablets dissolved in distilled water or tap water. Though saline tablets were taken off the US market in the 1980s, they still continue to be available in countries with low socio-economic status. Contact lens solutions have been coming under increasing scrutiny for sustaining acanthamoeba survival. Hiti et al found that all-in-one solutions were inferior to two-step cleaning regimes at eradicating encysted organisms of two separate pathogenic strains, raising concerns for the current recommended practice for contact lens hygiene (Hiti *et al.*, 2005). Peroxide based cleaning solutions are most effective against acanthamoeba. Use of orthokeratology in parts of the world is an additional risk factor (Xuguang *et al.*, 2003). Silicone hydrogel lenses are being increasingly prescribed and may be 'stickier' to acanthamoeba organisms (Hammersmith *et al.*, 2006). The adhering ability of the organism to hydrogel lenses is enhanced in presence of bacterial co-contamination, and enables it to adhere to an intact epithelium (Gorlin *et al.*, 1996; McLaughlin *et al.*, 1991; Niederkorn *et al.*, 1999). This adhering property is due to binding between glycoproteins and glycolipids in human corneal epithelial cells, and mannose binding protein in acanthamoeba cell walls (Clarke *et al.*, 2012).

The dormant double walled containing cellulose cyst (10 – 25 microns) of acanthamoeba is highly resilient and survives very harsh conditions. Under appropriate environment the cysts release motile trophozoites (15 – 45 microns) which produce enzymes that cause tissue destruction. The trophozoites feed on small algae, bacteria and other protozoans. The triad of corneal trauma, exposure to contaminated water or contact lens solution and contact lens wear forms a classical risk factor group. It appears children do not develop AK even though approximately 13% of children under 17 years old are contact lens wearers and there is popular use of colored lenses in this population. The most common symptoms include pain, photophobia, redness, tearing and decrease in visual acuity. Early diagnosis and modern treatment can restore visual acuity of 6/12 in 90% patients (Dart *et al.*, 2009; Wali *et al.*, 2012).

It has been observed that epithelial infection with acanthamoeba is augmented by bacterial or viral co-infection, with contact lenses providing a platform for both organisms to simultaneously infect the cornea (Badenoch *et al.*, 1990). AK characteristically presents as a localized corneal epithelial lesion in the form of diffuse punctuate epitheliopathy or dendritic epithelial lesion (Figure 1). These lesions are often misdiagnosed as herpetic keratitis and treated with antiviral agents with or without steroids. The epithelial defects may wax or wane during the course of the disease, regardless of whether the infection is responding to the medication. Single or multiple grayish-white nonsuppurative epithelial or stromal infiltrates, progressing to a paracentral ring infiltrate or an ulcer, indicate deeper involvement (Figure 2). Radial perineuritis (inflamed and enlarged corneal nerves) or keratoneuritis, limbiitis and scleritis may be other features. Perineural infiltrates are virtually pathognomonic for AK, being present in up to 63% of cases diagnosed within 6 weeks (Dart *et al.*, 2009). They occur due to accumulation of trophozoites around the nerves. Careful slit-lamp examination is necessary to identify perineuritis as only 1 or 2 nerves may be affected.

2   Diagnosis

The diagnosis of AK is broadly based on clinical features, supported by laboratory and confocal microscopy. The severity of the disease is related to duration of the infection, the depth of the lesion and any extra-corneal involvement. Table 1.

Laboratory: Smear Staining (Giemsa, periodic-acid-schiff, calcouflour white, acridine orange, 10% potassium hydroxide and Diff-Quik modified Romanowski stain), cultures (nonnutrient agar with E.coli or E.aerogenes overlay, blood agar, buffered charcoal-yeast extract agar), immunohistochemistry, and *in vivo* confocal microscopy continue to remain main methods of investigation in AK. Multiplex acanthamoeba beta-globin polymerase chain reaction (MAB-PCR) is a new method to diagnose AK. This real-time technique allows rapid diag-

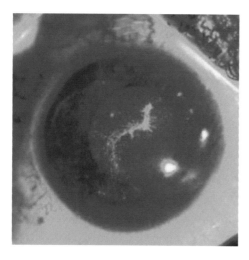

Figure 1: Pseudodendrit. Slit-lamp image of a typical epithelial dendritic lesion staining positive with fluoresceine stain in a patient with contact lens induced acanthamoeba keratitis. The lesion was positive for acanthamoeba on culture but confoscan was negative for cysts. The lesion responded to propamidine and biguanide (polyhexamethylene).

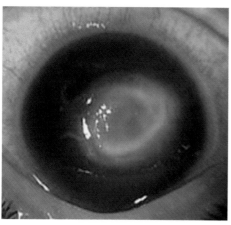

Figure 2: ring ulcer in AK. Figure 2: A classical ring infiltrate with an ulcer in a patient with confoscan positive acanthamoeba keratitis. The culture was negative.

Early disease (≤ 1 month): Mild	Mid-stage disease: Mild to moderate	Late disease (≥ 1 month): moderate	Late disease (≥ 1 month): severe
Epitheliopathy (punctate, epithelial or subepithelial infiltrates, pseudodendrites, limbiitis.	Pseudodendrites, perineural infiltrates (radial keratoneuritis).	Limbiitis, ring infiltrates, frank ulcers (Figure 2), sterile anterior uveitis with or without hypopyon, endothelial plaques, disciform reaction, decreased corneal sensation, corneal epithelial defect.	Large non-healing epithelial defects, Corneal abscess, corneal melt or perforation, hypopyon, scleritis, glaucoma, iris atrophy, cataract, posterior segment inflammation and ischemia.

Table 1: Duration and severity-related Clinical findings in AK.

nosis and prompt treatment in infectious keratitis (Maubon *et al.*, 2012). H1 nuclear magnetic resonance (NMR) spectroscopy has recently been used to identify acanthamoeba in vitro (Hauber *et al.*, 2011). Corneal epithelial and stromal biopsy may be indicated in difficult cases where diagnosis is not certain and treatment is not effective. Recently femtosecond-assisted diagnostic corneal biopsy (FAB) in infectious keratitis has provided adequate specimens without intra- or early post-operative complications (Yoo *et al.*, 2008).

Confocal microscopy has recently become a powerful tool for rapid diagnosis of the infection *in vivo*; however, it should not be a substitute for culture and microbiological analysis (Wali *et al.*, 2012). The obvious advantage of *in vivo* and *ex vivo* microscopy is that biopsy could be avoided and the diagnosis can be instantaneous in the hands of an experienced operator. The cysts may be seen as double layered structures (Figure 3) or appear as round hyperreflective lesions (Figure 4). Sometimes it may be difficult to differentiate acanthamoeba cysts from inflamed and enlarged keratocytes, and inflammatory cell aggregates. The sensitivity and specificity of confocal microscopy is too low to rely on it for a definitive diagnosis. New imaging models like Hiedelberg Retinal Tomography Rostok module give excellent resolution of cysts (Kobayashi *et al.*, 2008).

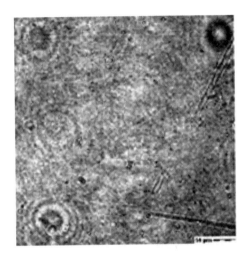

Figure 3: Double walled acanthamoeba cysts (arrows) in a patient who developed infection after undergoing refractive surgery.

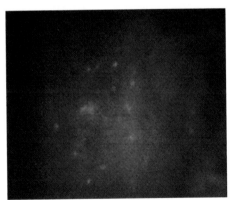

Figure 4: Confoscan (Nidek) image showing multiple refractile cysts.

Acanthamoeba keratitis is a challenge from the very beginning. The diagnosis, laboratory investigations and treatment may be frustrating and unpredictable. Any progressive, non-responding contact lens related microbial keratitis should always raise suspicion of AK. Failure to consider acanthamoeba as a cause of progressive, non-responding keratitis amounts to negligence.

3 Treatment

The first successful medical strategies for the treatment of AK came in 1985, and since then there have been novel developments in the antiamoebic agents and treatment protocols. Despite these advances, there are currently no licensed drugs for use in AK, and more than 15% of patients who are infected and treated still have severe loss of vision (Duguid *et al.*, 1997). There are no standardized algorithms for management of AK; treatment practices range from topical treatment (monotherapy or multiple topical therapeutic agents including oral antifungals) to aggressive surgical intervention like penetrating keratoplasty for severe infections. While acanthamoeba trophozoites are sensitive to a wide range of chemotherapeutic agents (antibiotics, antiseptics, antifungals, antiprotozoals including metronidazole, antivirals, and antineoplastic agents), very few of these are acanthamoebicidal. The number of cases of AK globally is not enough to organize a cohort trial to determine an effective strategy to treat this infection. Drugs which are effective in killing trophozoites in vitro at a specific concentration do not kill cysts, which need higher concentration. Also, the cysts are difficult to eradicate because they elude both the immune system and antiamebic agents. Successful treatments in AK have been reported by several investigators using a combination of antibiotics, antiparasitic, antiprotozoal, antifungal and antiviral drugs (Auran *et al.*, 1987). Since many patients of AK are not seen by expert ophthalmologists, the diagnosis is often missed or delayed in the initial critical period of 3-4 weeks. Treatment during this time period is very important for the eventual prognosis of visual acuity. Most cases in these weeks are treated with conventional antibiotics presuming the infection to be bacterial keratitis. Another factor that makes treatment of AK difficult and delayed is the poor access to anti-acanthamoeba medications. For example, propamidine isethionate is not approved for use in the United States, and ophthalmologists require off-label use of this medication (Vaddavalli *et al.*, 2011). Biguanides such as chlorhexidine and polyhexamethylene biguanide (PHMB) are not readily accessible at most pharmacies and are synthesized from industrial-grade components. The delays, and the tissue toxicity from such potential impurities compromise their effectiveness (Cavanagh, 2007).

So it is important to maintain a high level of index of suspicion for acanthamoeba infection in any patient who does not respond to antibiotics within 3 to 5 days.

The current treatment options in AK include antiamebic antimicrobials. Most of these agents are effective against free-living trophozoites but have reduced efficacy against cysts. The most successful therapeutic response has been found with a combination of biguanide (Chlorhexidine 0.02% or PHMB 0.02%) with a diamidine (propamidine isethionate 0.1% or hexamidine 0.1%). Chlorhexidine and PHMB have been found to have the best and most consistent amoebicidal and cysticidal activity in vitro, while hexamidine has faster amoebicidal effect than propamidine against both trophozoites and cysts in vitro (Elder *et al.*, 1994; Hay *et al.*, 1994; Perrine *et al.*, 1995). It seems monotherapy works well for superficial epithelial lesions while a combination works well for deeper stromal infections. Addition of propamidine-isethionate is case-dependent and some specialists encourage its use in patients who report later than 30 days and have painful ring lesions with perineuritis. Broadly, treatment can be divided into three categories (Table 2):

The major groups of drugs used against acanthamoeba include biguanides, diamidines, aminoglycosides and azoles. The pharmacotherapeutics of these drugs is given in Table 3. Other drugs which have been tried in AK include metronidazole 0.4% (Sun *et al.*, 2006), and dimethyl sulfoxide (which improves efficacy of propamidine)

Monotherapy	Dual Therapy	Triple therapy
Biguanides(PHMB and chorhexidine) as first line of treatment.	Biguanides and Diamidines (propamidine, hexamidine, pentamidine)#	Biguanides, Diamidines# and Neomycin (5%) or Metronidazole (1%)

Diamidines are not recommended for monotherapy due to the emergence of resistant strains.

Table 2: Modes of therapy in AK.

Chemical Group	Mechanism of Action	Drug agent	Concentration [ocular]
Cationic antiseptics (Steric Biguanides)	Inhibit cytoplasmic membrane function and respiratory enzymes. Structural and intracellular damage to trophozoites and cysts.	Chlorhexidine digluconate [1] Polyhexamethylene biguanide (PHMB, polyhexanide)[2]	0.02% to 0.2%[3](200 to 2000μg/ml) 0.02% to 0.06%[3] (200 to 600 μg/ml).
Aromatic diamidines	Structural membrane changes affecting cell permeability. Denaturation of cytoplasmic proteins and enzymes. Inhibit DNA synthesis.	Propamidine isethionate (Brolene)[4] Pentamidine isethionate[5] Hexamidine	0.1% (1000 μg/ml). 0.05% to 0.1% 0.1%
Aminoglycosides	Disrupt the plasmalemma of organism and facilitate the drug entry into cornea.	Neomycin Paromomycin	Not available as Neomycin only. Combined with polymyxin B and either bacitracin [ointment] or gramicidin [drops].
Triazoles / Imidazoles	Destabilize the cell walls. interrupt the synthesis of ergosterol, an integral component of fungal cell walls which has also been identified in the plasma membrane of Acanthamoeba species,	Clotrimazole[6] Voriconazole Fluconazole Ketoconazole Miconazole [7] Itraconazole	1% 1% 0.2% 5% 1% Not available

[1.] Chlorhexidine 1% can also be used to cauterize surface of non-healing ulcers.

[2.] PHMB can be used 6-24 times a day without any toxic effect to the corneal epithelium.

[3.] Concentrations used in resistant cases.

[4.] Also available as 0.15% dibrom-propamidine (Brolene ointment). Propamidine isethionate is available over-the–counter in United Kingdom.

[5.] Pentamidine isethionate powder can be mixed with artificial tears and applied topically.

[6.] The sterile powder of clotrimazole can be mixed with artificial tears to obtain 1% solution and applied topically every 2 hours.

[7.] The intravenous preparation of miconazole can be applied topically (1 drop every 2 hours).

Table 3: Pharmacotherapy of commonly used anti-acanthamoeba drugs.

A quick, easy and effective guideline for treatment of AK with propamidine and Neosporine has been laid down by Bausch and Lomb (Table 4). This applies to centers where Neosporin is still used in the treatment of AK.

Topical biguanides are the only effective therapy for the resistant encysted form of the organism in vitro, if not always *in vivo*. Initial approach may be a combination of either chlorhexidine or PHMB in combination with an imidazole or propamidine. Once the diagnosis has been confirmed, the frequency of drops is an important parameter in the treatment and therapeutic response in AK. (Table 5) Sometimes the response to drops may not be evident for as long as 10-14 days. Overall understanding is that drops should be continued for 3-6 months in epithelial lesions and 6-12 months in deeper stromal lesions.

Initial intensive therapy (6 days).	Early maintenance therapy	Late maintenance therapy	Follow up visits
First 3 days: 1 drop every 30 minutes around the clock	Week 1: every 2 hours while awake	Four times a day. Both drops are at each interval and spaced by 5 minutes.	Days: 1,2,3,5,7,14,21 and 28
Second 3 days: 1 drop every hour while awake and 1 drop every 2 hours	Week 2: every 3 hours while awake		Months: 2,3,4,6,7 and 12
	Weeks 3 and 4: every 2 hours while awake		

Table 4: Treatment protocol for Propamidine isethionate (Brolene) and Neosporine* (Bausch and Lomb study-unpublished). *Neomycin is ineffective against cysts in vitro and has a significant hypersensitivity rate. Use of neomycin and metronidazole (0.4%) is not widely accepted in the treatment of AK, and probably has no role in modern therapy.

First 48 hours	Next 72 hours:	Next 3-4 weeks	Next several weeks to 6 months
1 hourly day and night	1 hourly day time only.	2 hourly day time only.	Four times a day to tailor dose.

Table 5: Frequency of drops in AK.

Persistent corneal and scleral inflammations may be due to necrotic protozoa and walls of the cysts rather than active trophozoites. This may invite unwanted, excessively prolonged and intense antiamebic therapy; thereby increasing toxicity and morbidity of the disease (Yang *et al.*, 2001). Centers where laboratory facilities are not adequate usually start with a triple therapy of propamidine, chlorhexidine and PHMB. This combination works well when combined with an imidazole agent. Relapses are common when the dose is tapered, and it may be mandatory to start with the original dose again.

Repeat smears and cultures should be encouraged in case there is no symptomatic or morphological improvement after 7-10 days of treatment. Poor response to antiamoebic therapy may be due to following factors:

1. Inadequate intrastromal therapeutic level of the drug due to its binding to tissue components.

2. In vivo inactivation of the drug.

3. Organisms *in vivo* are more resistant than in vitro.

4. Possible bacterial or herpes coinfection.

In combined acanthamoeba and fungal infections (commonly fusarium) topical 0.02% PHMB, 0.1% propamidine, 1% clotrimazole and 5% natamycin work well. Double biguanide (PHMB and chlorhexidine) therapy may offer an additional advantage in cases that are resistant to standard therapy of biguanide-diamidine combination (Giulio *et al.*, 2011). A clinical trial comparing chlorhexidine monotherapy with PHMB monotherapy found similar efficacy in AK, with visual acuity improving in the majority of patients with each medication (Lim *et al.*, 2008). Chlorhexidine may have more serious side effects such as corneal necrosis, cataracts, and iris atrophy when used for a prolonged period (Murthy *et al.*, 2002; Ehlers *et al.*, 2004). The lack of randomized clinical trials comparing combination therapy with monotherapy for AK makes an evidenced-based decision difficult.

In case of epithelial toxicity, antiamoebics should be stopped for 3 to 7 days. If the toxicity disappears in the form of improvement in clinical signs and symptoms, restart the therapy where it was stopped. In case of persisting toxicity, propamidine should be stopped after two weeks. PHMB alone may be used.

Topical voriconazole(1%) is suggested to have good corneal penetration in the setting of active inflammation, and has been evaluated in patients with active epithelial disease (Vemulakonda *et al.*, 2008). It has been used as second line treatment for AK unresponsive to chlorhexidine and hexamidine. Intrastromal voriconazole (25µg/mL) has been used successfully in treating chlorhexidine- and hexamidine-resistant deep epithelial and stromal acanthamoeba infections (Bang *et al.*, 2010). In patients who had recurrent AK in the grafts following PKP, intracameral and intrastromal injections of voriconazole between each of the interrupted sutures (total dose 25µg/mL) has shown negative results for acanthamoeba. [50-Bang] Recalcitrant, chronic, deep stromal AK has been successfully treated with extended systemic voriconazole (200 mg twice daily for up to 6 months) with good preservation of vision. Voriconazole may also have steroid sparing function. Baseline and repeat liver function tests are recommended in patients on voriconazole. Voriconazole has shown good activity against acanthamoeba trophozoites and rapid suppression of acanthamoeba cysts in vitro (Elmer *et al.*, 2010; Schuster *et al.*, 2006). Extended or multiple courses of voriconazole may be required before sustained resolution of inflammation can be achieved. Recurrences can occur within 6 weeks of discontinuing voriconazole therapy.

Corticosteroids have always been debatable in the treatment of AK, some authors favoring their use while others condemning them, and both having adequate reasons and explanations. In majority of early cases, corticosteroids are unnecessary. Those who recommend believe steroids prevent the encystment of trophozoites in vitro and may therefore enhance the effectiveness of topical treatment (O'Day, 2000). Dexamethasone has been found to induce rapid excystment manifesting in 2 to 6 fold increase in the number of trophozoites. Also, dexamethasone had a profound stimulatory effect on trophozoite proliferation, as well as cytolytic effect on corneal epithelial cells. It appears corticosteroids have a potentially deleterious effect on AK by adversely affecting the host's immune apparatus. They may prolong the effective treatment time but have not been correlated with increased treatment failure rates (Park *et al.*, 1997). Late immunomodulatory responses after the amoebae have been killed may be reduced by corticosteroids. The long-term benefit of topical corticosteroids is uncertain and may contribute to persistence of viable cysts or potentiate mixed infections. Probably their role should be viewed with caution and limited to specific indications such as limbitis, indolent ulcers, anterior scleritis, anterior chamber inflammation, uveitis and posterior segment inflammation. Such conditions respond dramatically to low-potency topical steroids such as prednisolone acetate 0.5%, 4 times daily. This is commenced only after minimum 2 weeks of biguanide treatment. Acanthamoba sclerokeratitis may need systemic immunosuppression. Corticosteroids may be compatible with medical therapy only when used under cover of antiamebic antimicrobials. The biguanides and or diamidines should be continued for at least 4 weeks after steroids are withdrawn. Current thinking is that a topical steroid may be added once sterilization period of antimicrobial therapy of several weeks has been completed. Park *et al.* found no link between starting steroids (even before antiamoebal treatment) and worsened visual outcomes (Park *et al.* 1997).

Persistent culture-positive AK, in spite of full antiamoebic therapy needs to be differentiated from severe corneal and extracorneal inflammations, which may not be related to infection. Since neither confocal microscopy nor PCR can differentiate between viable and non viable acanthamoeba cysts, the only option left for consistent diagnosis in such cases is culture of corneal scrapes or biopsies. Following step wise guidelines have been laid for treating persistently culture-positive AK:

Step 1	Step 2	Step 3
Exclude co-infections (bacterial, viral, fungal)	A triad of topical biguanides, topical steroids and systemic immunosuppression	Switching amongst biguanides (PHMB 0.02% and chlorhexidine 0.02%) and diamidines (propamidine and hexamidine).

Step 4	Step 5
If above concentrations fail increase the concentration of PHMB to 0.06% or chlorhexidine to 0.2% for a trial period of 2 weeks.	If above measures fail, therapeutic keratoplasty is the last option.

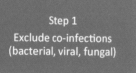
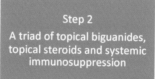

Treatment of acanthamoeba co-infections: Ten to 23% of AK patients may be polymicrobial (Sharma *et al.*, 2000; Sun *et al.*, 2006). All co-infections should be covered by antiameobic therapy. AK with bacterial infection should be treated with one of the fourth generation fluoroquinolones (moxifloxacin) while fungal co-infections respond to topical natamycin 5%. AK with herpetic infections should be treated with acyclovir or a co-drug.

Limbitis and scleritis may account for severe pain in AK. In most cases they respond to oral non-steroidal anti-inflammatory drugs like flurbiprofen. Scleritis is less common than limbitis, accounting for only 10% of cases in AK (Lee *et al.*, 2004), but can be severe and result in sclera necrosis and excruciating, uncontrollable pain. Systemic corticosteroids (prednisolone 1mg/kg/day) and ciclosporin (3 – 7.5mg/kg/day) are indicated in such cases for an average of 7 months (Lee *et al.*, 2004). Oral itraconazole 100 mg daily has been found to be effective in preventing the potential spread of trophozoites into adjacent tissues. This line of treatment in inflammatory complications of AK might also be useful in the management of severe ischemic posterior segment inflammation, if diagnosed early (Awwad *et al.*, 2007). It is possible that there may be no viable acanthamoeba in cornea in presence of limbitis and scleritis, and use of intensive topical antiamoebics with or without steroids may fail to control such inflammations. Immunosuppression is the only mode of therapy for controlling such inflammation and pain.

Persisting epithelial defect: This is a common manifestation and persisting inflammation is the most common reason for failure of re-epithelialization. Bacterial superinfection should always be excluded in such situations by repeating cultures. Persistent epithelial defects are managed as following:

1. Discontinue all topical therapy to reduce drug induced toxicity.

2. Prophylactic use of a low-frequency, non-preserved broad spectrum antibiotic for 5-7 days to prevent bacterial superinfection.

3. Reintroduce antiameobic therapy if there is improvement in clinical signs.

4. If above measures fail, perform lamellar keratectomy of necrotic tissue within the ulcer and send it for culture and histology. This procedure is both therapeutic and diagnostic.

5. Amniotic membrane grafting may speed up re-epithelialization.

4   Surgical Therapy

Epithelial debridement, combined with antiamoebic drugs, is most effective in early epithelial stages of infection (Auran *et al.*, 1987). Alcohol-assisted epithelial debridement facilitates detachment of full-thickness corneal epithelial layer in a controlled manner, unlike the fragile fragmented specimens obtained by mechanical scraping without alcohol, thereby preserving the tissue architecture. The debridement should be extensive and epithelial specimens sent for culture, histopathologic and electron microscopic examinations to reveal acanthamoeba organisms. Epithelial debridement with 20% alcohol did not prevent culturing of acanthamoeba. Debridement also facilitates topical absorption of drugs besides reducing the organism load. This simple procedure helps in removing mucin and biofilm substrates from corneal surface which hinder with drug penetration and reepithelialization. When combined with topical therapy and / or surface cauterization with chlorhexidine 1%, debridement is an useful adjunctive procedure in resistant cases (Brooks *et al.*, 1994).

Cryosurgery was used in eighties but has now largely been abandoned. In vitro studies had shown cryotherapy to kill trophozoites but not cysts (Brooks *et al.*, 1994).

Keratoplasty: Despite the availability of highly efficacious topical anti-acanthamoebal drugs, there remains a subset of patients who respond poorly to these and require surgical intervention. Penetrating keratoplasty (PKP) may be considered as a viable treatment modality for severe acanthamoeba keratitis, but only after medical treatment had failed. Since the availability of biguanides, PKP is no longer a therapeutic option (elimination of organisms) in AK (Awwad et al., 2007; Hammersmith, 2006). Therapeutic PKP is now reserved for following situations only:

1.   Corneal perforation that cannot be sealed by glue.

2.   Fulminant corneal abscess.

3.   Intumescent cataract.

Unlike grafts for other corneal infections which should be large enough to remove all contaminated tissue, the graft for AK should be kept to the minimum size required to excise all ulcerated and necrotic tissue only, retaining clinically healthy (which may be subclinically infected) tissue. This is because of higher risk of rejection with large grafts and repeat grafting may be needed in future in case of recurrence. The timing of performing penetrating keratoplasty in AK is debatable (Alizadeh et al., 2005). Anti-amoebic therapy should be used before surgery and be continued postoperatively using drugs and doses that will minimize or avoid signs of toxicity. PHMB 0.02% has low clinical toxicity profile comparable to either of the diamidines. PHMB 0.02%, 6 to 8 times daily immediately after surgery, with an adequate level of topical steroid to control inflammation is ideal in most cases. This should be continued for at least 3 weeks while results of culture of the host keratectomy specimen are available. If viable organisms are cultured, it is prudent to continue anti-amoebic therapy 4 to 8 times daily while high-doses of steroids are continued, usually for 6 months after surgery, as recurrent AK has occurred up to 3 months after an initially successful transplant (Dart et al., 2009). If culture of the excised host cornea is negative after 3 weeks, it can be assumed that most viable amoebae have been treated, and the topical anti-amoebic therapy is reduced to 4 times daily, and stopped after 1 month. Any relapse of limbitis or scleritis after graft surgery needs systemic immunosuppression.

Therapeutic keratoplasty retains a role in few, severe complications of AK but is not recommended for initial treatment. Cases showing signs of rapidly progressing severe stromal melting with impending perforation, or cases selected for visual rehabilitation are ideal candidates for this procedure. However, recurrence of infection is high even in apparently quite and treated eyes when PKP is performed within the first year after the onset of infection. Persistence of residual viable cysts probably within the limbus, compromised immunity and use of corticosteroids may contribute to such recurrence (Viswesvara & Stehr-Green, 1990). PKP should be done only after a full course of amebicidal therapy and a minimum of 3-6 months of disease-free follow-up. To improve the prognosis, some authors recommend not using corticosteroids in the early postoperative period of 2-3 weeks (Shi et al., 2009). Antiamoebic therapy can be tapered after PKP (Nguyen et al., 2010).

Complications of PKP in AK include graft rejection, stromal melting, wound leakage, glaucoma and cataract. Penetrating keratoplasty for visual restoration after acanthamoeba keratitis appears to have an excellent long-term prognosis, provided amoebic infection has resolved and concurrent glaucoma, if any, is controlled (Awwad et al., 2005). Transplantation does not always guarantee a complete cure, because 28% of transplanted grafts become reinfected, and most recurrences occur within 2 to 3 weeks (Shi *et al.*, 2009).

Deep anterior lamellar keratoplasty (DALK) has been performed successfully in AK unresponsive to intensive antimicrobial therapy (Parthasarathy & Tan, 2007). Total corneal stromal removal, down to Descemet membrane, combined with secondary amniotic membrane grafting has given a final visual acuity of 1.0 in few patients (Parthasarathy & Tan, 2007). Phototherapeutic keratectomy and DALK have also been reported to be effective in advanced cases of AK that fail to respond to medical therapy and corneal debridement (Taenaka *et al.*, 2007).

Corneal cross linking has given mixed reports about its success in AK. Using 0.1% riboflavin with 30-60 minute ultraviolet light A (UVA) irradiation, the results have been variable. It has been tried in animal corneal models infected with acanthamoeba organisms but did not prove effective in reducing the intensity and severity of the infection (Berra *et al.*, 2013; del Buey *et al.*, 2012). In cases with large ulcers associated with edema and corneal infiltration, UVA, as an adjunct to other antiamebic treatments has shown reasonable clinical improvement (Khan *et al.*, 2011). It is possible that the collagen stabilizing effect prevents further tissue damage and reproduction of the amoebae (Müller *et al.*, 2012). However, amebic infection occurring after treatment with cross-linking has also been reported (Pollhammer *et al.*, 2009; Zamora & Males, 2009; Pérez-Santonja *et al.*, 2009; Rama *et al.*, 2009). Total inactivation of amoebae requires higher ultraviolet doses and longer treatment periods but such therapy may have collateral effects. Patients may complain of considerable pain and photophobia within first 48 hours after application of the UVA/B2 treatment which usually disappears after 3 days. Second treatment of UVA/B2 irradiation may be applied if the ulcer size becomes static. Cross-linking may have a dual mechanism of action: the toxic action against pathogens and the marked increase in collagen resistance to bacterial digestive enzymes after irradiation (Iseli *et al.*, 2008; Morén *et al.*, 2010). Light-activated flavins interpose between base pairs of DNA, causing structural damage to these molecules and preventing replication of genome as well as trophozoites (Speck *et al.*, 1975). The free radicals generated by UVA irradiation of B2 cause oxidation of corneal collagen, inducing cross-linking and strengthening the collagen matrix. The stiffening effect of the treatment may induce the host immune system to control the corneal infection by avoiding the melting process. The oxidative injury from free radicals is also known to be cysticidal (Jackett *et al.*, 1978; Kilvington *et al.*, 1994). Corneal collagen crosslinking leads to dose-dependent keratocyte apoptosis (Wollensak *et al.*, 2004). Acanthamoeba is thought to feed on keratocytes, so cell depletion may create a hostile environment for the protozoan. Keratocyte apoptosis is induced due to DNA damage by this therapy. Fortunately keratocyte cell loss occurs only between 300 and 350μm of corneal depth (at UVA irradiance 3 mW/cm2; exposure 30 minutes). The keratocyte loss is temporary because of the regenerative ability of these cells, and repopulation is complete within 6 months (by which time the acanthamoebae are eradicated), thereby encompassing few complications (Mazzotta *et al.*, 2007). There may be transient stromal edema but no endothelial cell loss or changes to corneal or lens transparency have been observed. Although results from individual case reports seem promising, there are no formal clinical trials available so far to recommend its incorporation into standard practice. It is important to remember that ultraviolet light B and ultraviolet light C are highly damaging to DNA, and are not used in humans. Since no evidence based statements are available about the efficacy of the UVA and B2 as an independent treatment for AK, treating physicians are advised to continue the medical treatment concurrently. The UVA and B2 treatment is presumed to be safe for the corneal endothelium and central retina when the appropriate irradiance levels are used in corneas thicker than 400 µm (Wollensak *et al.*, 2003; Goldich *et al.*, 2010). Corneal opacification and deep infections may pose a hurdle to UVA transmission.

Methylene blue mediated photodynamic therapy has been studied to be effective against acanthamoeba in vitro and has synergistic effects with PHMB and amphotericin B, but not with voriconazole (Mito *et al.*, 2012).

In a case series of 4 patients with AK, Kandori et al have observed that phototherapeutic keratectomy is beneficial in lesions limited to one third of the corneal stromal layer, and not responding to chlorhexidine or polyhexamethylene biguanide. The therapy has direct effect on resistant amebic cysts ensuring better visual recovery (Kandori *et al.*, 2010).

5 Prognosis

Late diagnosis (>30 days), low initial visual acuity, corneal neovascularization, large infiltrates, corneal perforations and surgical interventions are associated with worse visual prognosis (Bouheraoua *et al.*, 2013).

6 Review of Literature

The treatment part of AK has seen lot of changes in recent years, aided by new methods of diagnosis and laboratory investigations. A variety of existing and new substances have been tried in AK. Though none of these have been approved yet, they offer a wide hope in the current management of AK. This part of review of literature in AK is mainly focused on its treatment part.

Low concentrations of benzalkonium chloride (BAK), previously demonstrated to concentrate and persist in ocular surface epithelium, exhibit significant antiacanthamoebal activity in vitro at or below concentrations found in commercially available ophthalmic solutions. Thus preservatives like BAK may potentiate the effect of antiamebic drops (Tu *et al.*, 2013).

Sodium salicylate has shown potential as a component of contact lens care solutions designed to reduce acanthamoebal attachment to contact lenses (Beattie *et al.*, 2011). "Bioclen FR One Step" is the only available povidone-iodine based system for the disinfection of silicone hydrogel lenses and soft contact lenses in the market. Bioclen FR has been proven to be highly effective against bacteria and fungi. In one study three clinical acanthamoeba isolates were found to be sensitive to this solution (Martin –Navarro *et al.*, 2010).

Recently the amebicidal activity of the family of cationic carbosilane dendrimers has been observed against Acanthamoeba castellanii trophozoites. Such agents could potentially become significant new amebicidal compounds for prevention and therapy of acanthamoeba infections (Heredero-Bermejo *et al.*, 2013).

Acriflavine neutral has shown a time- and dose-dependent amebicidal action on the trophozoites and cysts of A. castellanii, and A. hatchetti. As a result, Acriflavine could be proposed as a new agent for the treatment of acanthamoeba infections. It still needs to be evaluated by in-vivo tests to confirm the efficiency of its biological effect (Polat *et al.*, 2013).

Anti-acanthamoebic potential of resveratrol and curcuminoids (demethoxy curcumin) has been found to prevent adhesion of amoebae to cells, and reduce cytotoxicity to the host cells. However, neither resveratrol nor demethoxycurcumin had any effect on the proteolytic activities of Acanthamoeba castellanii (Aqeel *et al.*, 2012).

A study has evaluated the in vitro amoebicidal activity of methanolic extracts of Origanum syriacum and Origanum laevigatum and found the numbers of the viable Acanthamoeba castellanii trophozoites and cysts were decreased. Of the extracts tested, O. syriacum showed the stronger amoebicidal effect on the trophozoites and cysts (Degerli *et al.*, 2012).

Based on experimental keratitis, Neosporin with lower doses of Chlorhexidine may be beneficial to treat patients with AK (Polat *et al.*, 2012). Also based on AK in animal models, Miltefosine (a phospolipid, protein kinase B inhibitor) treatment yielded much higher cure scores than propamidine isethionate plus polyhexanide (Polat *et al.*, 2012).

Methanolic extract of Salvea staminea showed remarkable amoebicidal effect on A. castellanii and could be considered a new natural agent against acanthamoeba. The extract showed no cytotoxicity on corneal cells (Goze *et al.*, 2009).

Alexidine has been found to be effective in killing the trophozoites and acanthamoeba cysts comparable with chlorhexidine. Alexidine may be an effective therapeutic option because of its potency and low toxicity to the corneal tissues when applied topically *in vivo* (Alizadeh *et al.*, 2009).

Capsofungin has been found in vitro to inhibit trophozoites of three tested species of acanthamoeba. Furthermore, this drug was cysticidal against A. castellanii and A. culbertsoni. Caspofungin could represent a new anti-acanthamoeba agent if its efficacy is proved *in vivo* (Bouyer *et al.*, 2006).

7   The Future

Small interfering RNA (siRNA) is the most essential and best-known double-stranded RNA (dsRNA) that is used for RNA interference (RNAi). It is a gene silencer. It is usually not present in the cell and is incorporated artificially. Since it can be synthesized, it may be considered for use as a potent therapeutic agent. Small interfering RNAs act against the catalytic extracellular serine proteases and glycogen phosphorylases, produced by acanthamoeba. The silencing of proteases resulted in acanthamoeba failing to degrade human corneal cells, and silencing of glycogen phosphorylase caused amoebae to be unable to form mature cysts. This siRNA-based treatment dramatically affected the growth rate and cellular survival of the amoebae within less than 48 hours after the initiation of the treatment. The future use of the combination of these siRNAs is proposed to be a revolutionary and potential therapeutic approach against pathogenic strains of acanthamoeba (Lorenzo-Morales *et al.*, 2010).

8   Conclusions

As none of the above discussed methods of diagnosis and treatment of AK has become standardized, there is still need to find a guideline in this direction. Biguanides and diamidines still form the mainstay of treatment for straightforward cases, but evidence has shown that steroids may be used safely in cases with a significant inflammation and under specified indications. Oral steroids are preferred over topical steroids in severe inflammation as the later may prove dangerous in terms of secondary infections, corneal thinning or even perforation. Surgery has been necessary for resistant disease, and we have seen that DALK may provide good outcomes whilst maintaining the host endothelium. Laser photokeratectomy may become more important as we continue to explore its indications. Initial reports have shown cross linking as a handsome promise. It may be a useful adjunct to surgery or possibly even a treatment modality in its own; however, cross-linking needs further studies. With modern management, 90% of patients can expect to retain visual acuity of 6/12 or better and fewer than 2% become blind, although treatment may take 6 months or more (Dart et al., 2009). In spite of big achievements in diagnosis and management, AK may prove both frustrating and often, devastating. The success of medical treatment for AK depends on severity of disease at presentation and interval between the onset of symptoms and initiation of therapy (before encystations). The best outcome is expected when treatment is started within 18 days of the first symptom. The take home message for contact lens wearers remains simple: "Prevention is better than cure".

Authors

Nadia Al Kharousi
Ophthalmology, Sultan Qaboos University, Muscat, Oman

Upender Wali
Ophthalmology, Sultan Qaboos University Hospital, Muscat, Oman

Sitara Azeem
Ophthalmology, Sultan Qaboos University, Muscat, Oman

References

Acharya NR, Lietman TM, Margolis TP. Parasites on the rise: a new epidemic of Acanthamoeba keratitis. Am J Ophthalmol 2007;144:292–293.

Alizadeh H, Neelam S, Cavanagh HD. Amoebicidal acitivities of alexidine against 3 pathogenic strains of acanthamoeba .Eye Contact Lens.2009 Jan;35(1):1-5.

Alizadeh H, Niederkorn JY, McCulley JP: Acanthamoeba keratitis. In Krachmer JH, Mannis MJ, Holland EJ, editors: Cornea, Fundamentals, Diagnosis and Management, volume I, London, 2005, Elsevier Mosby, pp1115-1122.

Aqeel Y ,Iqbal J, Siddiqui R, Gilani AH ,Khan NA.Anti –Acanthameobic properties of reserveratrol and demethoxycurcumin. Exp Parasitol.2012 Dec;132(4):519-23.

Auran JD et al. Acanthamoeba keratitis. A review of the literature. Cornea. 1987; 6(1):2-26.

Awwad ST, Heilman M, Hogan RN, et al. Severe reactive ischemic posterior segment inflammation in Acanthamoeba keratitis: a new potentially blinding syndrome. Ophthalmology 2007;114:313–320.

Awwad ST, Parmar DN, Heilman M, Bowman RW, McCulley JP, Cavanagh HD.Results of penetrating keratoplasty for visual rehabilitation after Acanthamoeba keratitis.Am J Ophthalmol.2005 Dec;140(6):1080-1084.

Awwad ST, Petroll WM, McCulley JP, Cavanagh HD. Updates in Acanthamoeba keratitis. Eye Contact Lens 2007; 33:1– 8.

Bacon AS, Frazer DG, Dart JK, Matheson M, Ficker LA, Wright P. A review of 72 consecutive cases of Acanthamoeba keratitis, 1984–1992. Eye 1993;7:719 –725.

Badenoch PR, Johnson AM, Christy PE, Coster DJ. Pathogenicity of Acanthamoeba and a Corynebacterium in the rat cornea. Archives of Ophthalmology. 1990;108(1):107–112.

Bang S, Edell E, Eghrari AO, Gottsch JD.Treatment with voriconazole in 3 eyes with resistant Acanthamoeba keratitis. Am J Ophthalmol.2010 Jan ;149 (1) :66-9.

Beattie TK ,Tomlinson A, Seal DV, McFadyen AK .Salicylate inhibition of acanthamoebal attachment to contact lenses.Optom Vis Sci. 2011 Dec;88(12):1422-32.

Berra M, Galperin G, Boscaro G, Zarate J, Tau J, Chiradia P, Berra A .Treatment of Acanthamoeba keratitis by corneal cross – linking. Cornea .2013 Feb;32(2):174-8.

Bouheraoua N, Gaujoux T, Goldschmidt P, Chaumeil C, Laroche L, Borderie VM. Prognostic factors associated with the need for surgical treatments in acanthamoeba keratitis. Cornea.2013 Feb;32(2):130-6.

Bouyer S, Imbert C, Daniault G,Cateau E, Rodier MH. Effect of caspofungin on trophozoites and cysts of three species of Acan-thamoeba.J Antimicrob Chemother. 2007 Jan;59(1):122-4. Epub 2006 Oct 31.

Brooks JG, Coster DJ, Badenoch PR. Acanthamoeba Keratitis. Resolution after epithelial debridement. Cornea. 1994;13:186-9.

Butler TK, Males JJ, Robinson LP, et al. Six-year review of Acanthamoeba keratitis in New South Wales, Australia: 1997–2002. Clin Experiment Ophthalmol 2005;33:41– 46.

Cavanagh HD. Acanthamoeba keratitis: 2007: a train wreck in slow motion. Eye Contact Lens 2007;33:209.

Clarke B, Sinha A, Parmar DN, Sykakis E. Advances in the Diagnosis and Treatment of Acanthamoeba Keratitis. J Ophthalmol. 2012; 2012: 484892. Published online 2012 December 6. doi: 10.1155/2012/484892. PMCID: PMC3529450

Clarke DW, Alizadeh H, Niederkorn JY. Failure of Acanthamoeba castellanii to produce intraocular infections. Invest Ophthalmol Vis Sci 2005;46:2472–2478.

Dart JK, Radford CF, Minassian D, Verma S, Stapleton F. Risk factors for microbial keratitis with contemporary contact lenses: a case-control study. Ophthalmology. 2008 Oct;115(10):1647-54,1654.e1-3.

Dart JKG, Saw VPJ, Kilvington S. Acanthamoeba keratitis: Diagnosis and treatment update 2009. Am J Ophthalmol 2009;148:487-499.

Degerli S ,Tepe B, Celiksoz A, Berk S, Malatvali E .Invitro amoebicidal activity of Origanum syriacum and Origanum laeviga-tum on Acanthamoeba castellani cysts and trophozoites. Exp Parasitol.2012 May;131(1):20-4.

del Buey MA, Cristóbal JA, Casas P, Goñi P, Clavel A, Mínguez E, Lanchares E, García A, Calvo B. Evaluation of in vitro effica-cy of combined riboflavin and ultraviolet a for Acanthamoeba isolates. Am J Ophthalmol.2012 Mar;153(3):399-404.

Di Cave D, Monno R, Bottalico P, et al. Acanthamoeba T4 and T15 genotypes associated with keratitis infections in Italy. Euro-pean J Clin Microbiol Infect Dis 2009;28(6):607– 612.

Duguid IG, Dart JK, Morlet N, et al. Outcome of Acanthamoeba keratitis treated with polyhexamethyl biguanide and propami-dine. Ophthalmology 1997;104:1587–92.

Ehlers N, Hjortdal J. Are cataract and iris atrophy toxic complications of medical treatment of Acanthamoeba keratitis? Acta Ophthalmol Scand 2004;82:228 –31.

Elder MJ, Kilvington S, Dart JK. A clinicopathologic study of in vitro sensitivity testing and Acanthamoeba keratitis.Invest Oph-thalmol Vis Sci 1994;35:1059 –1064.

Elmer Y Tu ,Charlotte E Joslin and Megan E Shoff .Successful Treatment of Chronic Stromal Acanthamoeba Keratitis with Oral Voriconazole Monotherapy.Cornea. 2010 September; 29(9): 1066–1068.

Ferrari G, Matuska S and Rama P. Double –Biguanide Therapy for Resistant Acanthamoeba keratitis.Case Rep Ophthalmol. 2011 Sep-Dec; 2(3): 338–342.

Goldich Y, Marcovich AL, Barkana Y, et al. Safety of corneal collagen cross-linking with UV-A and riboflavin in progressive keratoconus. Cornea 2010;29:409 –11.

Gorlin AI, Gabriel MM, Wilson LA, Ahearn DG. Effect of adhered bacteria on the binding of acanthamoeba to hydrogel lenses. Arch Ophthalmol. 1996;114:576-80.

Goze I, Alim A, Dag S, Tepe B, Polat ZA.In vitro amoebicidal activity of Salvia staminea and Salvia caespitosa on acanthamoeba castellani and their cytotoxic potentials on corneal cells.J Ocul Pharmacol Ther.2009 Aug;25(4):293-8.

Hammersmith KM. Diagnosis and management of acanthamoba keratitis. Curr Opin Ophthalmol. 2006;17(4):327-31.

Hargrave SL, McCulley JP, Husseini Z. Results of a trial of combined propamidine isethionate and neomycin therapy for Acanthamoeba keratitis. Brolene Study Group. Ophthalmology 1999;106:952–957.

Hauber S, Parkes H, Siddiqui R, Khan NA. The use of high-resolution 1H nuclear magnetic resonance (NMR) spectroscopy in the clinical diagnosis of Acanthamoeba. Parasitology Research. 2011;109(6):1661–1669.

Hay J, Kirkness CM, Seal DV, Wright P. Drug resistance and Acanthamoeba keratitis: the quest for alternative antiprotozoal chemotherapy. Eye 1994;8:555–563.

Heredero-Bermejo I, Copa-Patiño JL, Soliveri J, García-Gallego S, Rasines B, Gómez R, de la Mata FJ, Pérez-Serrano J. Invitro evaluation of the effectiveness of new water –stable cationic carbosilane dendrimers against Acanthamoeba castellani UAH –T 17c 3 trophozoites.Parasitol Res2013 Mar;112(3):961-9.

Hiti K, Walochnik J, Faschinger C, Haller-Schober EM, Aspöck H. One- and two-step hydrogen peroxide contact lens disinfection solutions against Acanthamoeba: how effective are they? Eye. 2005;19(12):1301–1305.

Houang E, Lam D, Fan D, Seal D. Microbial keratitis in Hong Kong: relationship to climate, environment and contact- lens disinfection. Trans R Soc Trop Med Hyg 2001;95:361–367.

Hutchinson K, Apel A. Infectious keratitis in orthokeratology. Clin Experiment Ophthalmol. 2002;30(1):49–51.

Iseli HP, Thiel MA, Hafezi F, Kampmeier J, Seiler T. Ultraviolet A/riboflavin corneal cross-linking for infectious keratitis associated with corneal melts. Cornea 2008;27(5): 590–594.

Jackett PS, Aber VR, Lowrie DB. Virulence and resistance to superoxide, low pH and hydrogen peroxide among strains of Mycobacterium tuberculosis. J Gen Microbiol 1978;104:37– 45.

Kandori M, Inoue T, Shimabukuro M, Hayashi H, Hori Y, Maeda N, Tano Y.Four cases of Acanthamoeba keratitis treated with phototherapeutic keratectomy.Cornea.2010 Oct;29(10):1199-202.

Khan YA, Kashiwabuchi RT, Martins SA, et al. Riboflavin and ultraviolet light A therapy as an adjuvant treatment for medically refractive acanthamoeba keratitis report of 3 cases. Ophthalmology 2011;118(2):324 –331.

Kilvington S, White DG. Acanthamoeba: biology, ecology and human disease. Rev Med Microbiol 1994;5:12–20.

Kobayashi A, Ishibashi Y, Oikawa Y, Yokogawa H, Sugiyama K. In vivo and ex vivo laser confocal microscopy findings in patients with early-stage acanthamoeba keratitis. Cornea. 2008 May;27(4):439-45.

Lalitha P, Lin CC, Srinivasan M, et al. Acanthamoeba keratitis in South India: a longitudinal analysis of epidemics. Ophthalmic Epidemiology. 2012;19(2):111–115.

Lam DS, Houang E, Fan DS, et al. Hong Kong Microbial Keratitis Study Group. Incidence and risk factors for microbial keratitis in Hong Kong: comparison with Europe and North America. Eye 2002;16:608–18.

Lee GA, Gray TB, Dart JK, et al. Acanthamoeba sclerokeratitis:treatment with systemic immunosuppression. Ophthalmology. 2002;109:1178 –1182.

Lim N, Goh D, Bunce C, et al. Comparison of polyhexamethylene biguanide and chlorhexidine as monotherapy agents in the treatment of Acanthamoeba keratitis. Am J Ophthalmol. 2008;145:130–135.

Lorenzo-Morales J, Martin-Navarro C.M., Lopez-Arencibia A, Santana-Morales MA, Afonso-Lehmann RN, Maciver SK, Valladares B, and Martinez-Carretero E. Therapeutic Potential of a Combination of Two Gene –Specific Small Interfering RNAs against Clinical Strains of Acanthamoeba.Antimicrob Agents Chemother.2010 December;54(12):5151-5155.

Martin-Navarro CM, Lorenzo-Morales J, López-Arencibia A,Valladares B, Pinero JE.Acanthamoeba spp.:efficacy of Biolen FR One Step , a povidone-iodine based system for the disinfection of contactlenses.Exp Parasitol. 2010 Sep;126(1):109-12.

Mathers WD, Nelson SE, Lane J. Confirmation of confocal microscopy diagnosis of Acanthamoeba keratitis using polymerase chain reaction analysis. Arch Ophthalmol. 2000;118:178-83.

Maubon D, Dubosson M,Chiquet C,Yera H ,Brenier –Pinchart MP ,Cornet M, Savy O ,Renard E ,Pelloux H .A one –step multiplex PCR for acanthamoeba keratitis diagnosis and quality samples control.Invest Ophthalmol Vis Sci.2012 May 14;53(6):2866-72.doi:10.1167/iovs.11-8587.

Mazzotta C, Balestrazzi A, Traversi C, et al. Treatment of progressive keratoconus by riboflavin-UVA-induced crosslinking of corneal collagen: ultrastructural analysis by Heidelberg Retinal Tomograph II in vivo confocal microscopy in humans. Cornea 2007;26:390 –7.

McLaughlin GL, Stimac JE, Luke JM, et al. Development of Acanthamoeba-cornea coincubation assays. Reviews of Infectious Diseases. 1991;13(supplement 5):S397–S398.

Mito T, Suzuki T, Kobayashi T, Zheng X, Hayashi Y, Shiraishi A, Ohashi Y. *Effect of photodynamic therapy with methylene blue on Acanthamoeba in vitro.Invest Ophthalmol Visc Sci .2012 Sep 19;53(10):6305-13.*

Morén H, Malmsjö M, Mortensen J, Ohrström A. *Riboflavin and ultraviolet a collagen crosslinking of the cornea for the treatment of keratitis. Cornea 2010;29(1):102–104.*

Müller L, Thiel MA, Kipfer-Kauer AI, Kaufmann C. *Corneal cross-linking as supplementary treatment option in melting keratitis: a case series. Klinische Monatsblatter fur Augenheilkunde. 2012;229(4):411–415.*

Murthy S, Hawksworth NR, Cree I. *Progressive ulcerative keratitis related to the use of topical chlorhexidine gluconate (0.02%). Cornea 2002;21:237–9.*

Nguyen TH ,Weisenthal RW, Florakis GJ, Reidy JJ, Gaster RN, Tom D.*Penetrating keratoplasty in active Acanthamoeba keratitis.Cornea.2010 Sep;29(9):1000-4.*

Niederkorn JY, Alizadeh H, Leher H, McCulley JP. *The pathogenesis of Acanthamoeba keratitis. Microbes and Infection. 1999;1(6):437–443.*

O'Day DM, Head WS. *Advances in the management of keratomycosis and Acanthamoeba Keratitis. Cornea. 2000;19:681-7.*

Park DH, Palay DA, Daya SM, Stulting RD, Krachmer JH, Holland EJ. *The role of topical corticosteroids in the management of Acanthamoeba keratitis. Cornea. 1997;16(3):277–283.*

Parthasarathy A, Tan DTH. *Deep lamellar keratoplasty for Acanthamoeba keratitis. Cornea. 2007;26(8):1021–1023.*

Pérez-Santonja JJ, Artola A, Javaloy J, Alió JL, Abad JL. *Microbial keratitis after corneal collagen crosslinking. J Cataract Refract Surg 2009;35(6):1138 –1140.*

Perrine D, Chenu JP, Georges P, Lancelot JC, Saturnino C,Robba M. *Amoebicidal efficiencies of various diamidines against two strains of Acanthamoeba polyphaga. Antimicrob Agents Chemother 1995;39:339 –342.*

Polat ZA , Karakus G .*Cytotoxic effect of acriflavine against clinical isolates of Acanthamoeba spp.Parasitol Res.2013. Feb;112(2):529-33.*

Polat ZA , Obwaller A, Vural A , Walochnik J .*Efficacy of miltefosine for topical treatment of Acanthamoeba keratitis in Syrian hamsters.Parasitol Res.2012 Feb;110(2):515-20.*

Polat ZA, Vural A. *Effect of combined chlorhexidine gluconate and neosporin on experimental keratitis with two pathogenic strains of Acanthamoeba .Parasitol Res. 2012 May;110(5):1945-50.*

Pollhammer M, Cursiefen C. *Bacterial keratitis early after corneal crosslinking with riboflavin and ultraviolet-A. J Cataract Refract Surg 2009;35(3):588 –589.*

Radford CF, Lehmann OJ, Dart JK. *Acanthamoeba keratitis: multicentre survey in England 1992–6. National Acanthamoeba Keratitis Study Group. Br J Ophthalmol 1998;82: 1387–1392.*

Radford CF, Minassian DC, Dart JK. *Acanthamoeba keratitis in England and Wales: incidence, outcome, and risk factors. Br J Ophthalmol 2002;86:536 –542.*

Rama P, Di Matteo F, Matuska S, Paganoni G, Spinelli A. *Acanthamoeba keratitis with perforation after corneal crosslinking and bandage contact lens use. J Cataract Refract Surg 2009;35(4):788 –791.*

Schuster FL, Guglielmo BJ, Visvesvara GS. *In-vitro activity of miltefosine and voriconazole on clinical isolates of free-living amebas: Balamuthia mandrillaris, Acanthamoeba spp., and Naegleria fowleri. J Eukaryot Microbiol. 2006 Mar-Apr;53(2):121–126.*

Seal DV. *Acanthamoeba keratitis update-incidence, molecular epidemiology and new drugs for treatment. Eye 2003;17:893–905.*

Sharma S, Garg P, Rao GN. *Patient characteristics, diagnosis, and treatment of non-contact lens related Acanthamoeba keratitis. Br J Ophthalmol 2000;84:1103–1108.*

Shi W, Liu M, Gao H, Li S, Xie L. *Perioperative treatment and prognostic factors for penetrating keratoplasty in Acanthamoeba keratitis unresponsive to medical treatment. Graefes Arch Clin Exp Ophthalmol.2009 Oct;247(10):1383-8.*

Speck WT, Chen CC, Rosenkranz HS. *In vitro studies of effects of light and riboflavin on DNA and HeLa cells. Pediatr Res 1975;9:150 –3.*

Stapleton F, Dart J, Minassian D. *No-ulcerative complications of contact lens wear. Arch Ophthalmol. 1992;110:1601-6.*

Stapleton F, Keay L, Edwards K, et al. *The incidence of contact lens-related microbial keratitis in Australia. Ophthalmology. 2008 Oct;115(10):1655-62.*

Stehr-Green JK, Bailey TM, Visvesvara GS. The epidemiology of Acanthamoeba keratitis in the United States. Am J Ophthalmol 1989;107:331–336.

Sun X ,Zhang Y,Li R, Wang Z, Luo S ,Gao M,De ng S,Chen W, Jin X.Acanthamoeba keratitis :clinical characteristrics and management .Ophthalmology.2006 Mar ; 113 (3) : 412-6.

Taenaka N, Fukuda M,Hibino T, Kato Y , Arimura E, Ishii Y, Shimomura Y. Surgical therapies for Acanthamoeba keratitis by phototherapeutic keratectomy and deep lamellar keratoplasty.Cornea.2007 Aug;26(7):876-9.

Tu EY, Shoff ME, Gao W, Joslin CE .Effect of Low Concentrations of Benzalkonium Chloride on Acanthamoebal Survival and Its Potential Impact on Empirical Therapy of Infectious Keratitis.Jama Ophthalmol.2013 Mar 21:16.

Vaddavalli PK, Garg P, Sharma S, Sangwan VS, Rao GN, Thomas R. Role of confocal microscopy in the diagnosis of fungal and Acanthamoeba keratitis. Ophthalmology. 2011;118(1):29–35.

Vemulakonda GA, Hariprasad SM, Mieler WF, Prince RA, Shah GK, Van Gelder RN. Aqueous and vitreous concentrations following topical administration of 1% voriconazole in humans. Arch Ophthalmol. 2008 Jan;126(1):18–22.

Viswesvara GS, Stehr-Green JK. Epidemiology of free-living ameba infections, J Protocol 37(4):25S-33S,1990.

Wali UK, Al Kharousi N. Confoscan: An ideal therapeutic aid and screening tool in acanthamoeba keratitis. Middle East Afr J Ophthalmol 2012;19:422-5.

Wilhelmus KR, Jones DB, Matoba AY, Hamill MB, Pflugfelder SC, Weikert MP. Bilateral acanthamoeba keratitis. Am J Ophthalmol 2008;145:193–197.

Wollensak G, Spoerl E, Wilsch M, Seiler T. Endothelial cell damage after riboflavin-ultraviolet-A treatment in the rabbit. J Cataract Refract Surg 2003;29:1786 –90.

Wollensak G, Spoerl E, Wilsch M, Seiler T. Keratocyte apoptosis after corneal collagen cross-linking using riboflavin/UVA treatment. Cornea 2004;23(1):43– 49.

Xuguang S, Lin C, Yan Z, et al. Acanthamoeba keratitis as a complication of orthokeratology. Am J Ophthalmol 2003;136:1159–61.

Yang YF, Matheson M, Dart JK. Persistence of Acanthamoeba antigen following Acanthamoeba keratitis. Br J Ophthalmol. 2001;85:277-80.

Yoo SH, Kymionis GD, O Brien TP, Ide T, Culbertson W, Alfonso EC. Femtosecond –assisted diagnostic corneal biopsy (FAB) in keratitis. Graefes Arch Clin Exp Ophthalmol.2008 May ;246(5) :759-62.

Zamora KV, Males JJ. Polymicrobial keratitis after a collagen cross-linking procedure with postoperative use of a contact lens: a case report. Cornea 2009;28(4):474-476.

Fibrotic Diseases of the Eye: Potential Therapeutic Targets

Sarbani Hazra and Aditya Konar

1   Introduction

To enable photo transduction, light must pass through all the clear surfaces and media of the anterior segment of the eye i.e. cornea, aqueous humor, lens, vitreous humor and reach the retina. This natural physiology warrants maintaining this highly organized organ in perfect homeostasis.

During life time the eye may be subjected to various insults in the form of chemical and physical injury, inflammation, and infections etc which culminate into fibrosis. Fibrosis is a consequence of excess production and deposition of fibrous connective tissue in an organ. TGF beta is a major cytokine that regulates various physiological and pathological processes in the body, it spearheads the various events during wound healing i.e. cell migration and proliferation, protein synthesis and tissue repair. It also induces a large number of growth factors. Numerous studies have revealed distinct physiological functions of TGF beta and its isoforms in embryonic tissue development, but post natal it is established that over expression of TGF beta is the underlying cause of wound healing associated fibrotic disorders (Saika 2006). Traditionally it is thought that TGF beta activate fibroblasts which proliferate and produce excessive connective tissue in fibrosis. But recent literature suggests that the epithelial cells also contribute to the event by generation of fibroblast in a process called epithelial mesenchymal transition.

In this chapter we shall highlight the TGF beta pathway for epithelial mesenchymal transition (EMT) and its implications in the various eye tissues where it leads to fibrosis and vision impairment.

2   Epithelial Mesenchymal Transition (EMT)

EMT is a biological phenomenon during which, epithelial cells that are normally polarized, immotile and adhered to the basement membrane, are subjected to series of biochemical changes enabling them to acquire a mesenchymal cell phenotype, characterized by loss of polarity, acquisition of spindle shaped configuration, invasiveness, resistance to apoptosis, enhanced capacity to migrate and increased production of extracellular matrix.

A series of molecular events that trigger and lead to completion of EMT process include activation of transcription factor, expression of specific cell surface protein, reorganization and expression of cell cytoskeleton proteins, enhanced expression of matrix degrading proteins and changes in expression of some specific micro-RNAs.

The term transition in EMT reflects the reversibility of the process and plasticity of the cells to revert back into epithelial cells through mesenchymal epithelial transition (MET), though very little is known about this process. Evidence of cellular plasticity and reversal between EMT and MET are best reported during embryogenesis and organ formation (Lee *et al.*, 2006).

Epithelial mesenchymal transition has been classified as three distinct types in biological settings (Kalluri and Weinberg, 2009). EMT Type 1 is witnessed during implantation, embryo formation and organogenesis, it neither leads to fibrotic nor invasive cell types; moreover, reversal to mesenchymal cells is a physiological event here. Type 2 EMT is associated with inflammation, wound healing, tissue regeneration and organ fibrosis. Type 3 EMT is typically a feature of neoplastic cells that have been subjected to genetic or epigenetic changes; these cells have changes that affect their oncogenes and tumor suppressor genes and are thereby capable of invasion, metastasis, leading to life threatening consequences of cancer progression.

3   Inflammation and Fibrosis

Fibrosis of organs is an irreversible progressive change arising due to acute or chronic inflammatory conditions leading to excess deposition of extracellular matrix of which collagen 1 is a major constituent. This leads to loss of normal architecture and function of the organ and eventually results into organ failure. Fibrosis of vital organs like lung, kidney and liver are among the leading cause of death even in developed countries; fibrosis in eye is vision threatening and in extreme cases, blinding.

Fibroblasts, the most important contributor to fibrosis are a class of cells distinctly different from epithelial, endothelial and hematopoietic cells, distributed throughout the mesenchymal tissues, synthesize extracellular matrix to form the structural framework for tissue support. Fibroblasts play a major role in the healing process following injury; in the reparative phase, fibroblasts are activated to form the new ECM to support re-epithelialization. Dysregulated activity of fibroblasts and their excess proliferation and survival leads to overproduction of ECM and arrest of re-epithelialization, resulting into tissue fibrosis. A subset of fibroblast, the myofibroblast which express alpha SMA, produce huge amount of collagen 1, are the key players in organ fibrosis. Traditionally, origin of myofibroblasts was considered as conversion from tissue resident fibroblasts. Further studies have identified the other sources of myofibroblasts (Hinz *et al.*, 2007) which include, the bone marrow derived fibroblasts, they are recruited into the tissues by chemokine receptors (Keeley *et al.*, 2011) and convert into myofibroblasts; blood vessel wall smooth muscle cells are also considered progenitors of myofibroblasts. Transition of epithelial cells into mesenchymal type (EMT) is a significant event in fibrotic pathology (Kalluri and Neilson 2003).

Among inflammatory cells that regulate fibrotic events, macrophages the key players are recruited from either inflammatory monocytes or resident monocytes. In the fibrotic tissue the macrophages resemble the alternatively activated M2 cells than the classically activated cells M1. M2 cells express immunosuppressive protein IL-10, Arginase 1 and suppress the induction of Th1 cells; on the other hand M1 cells express cytokines like IL-1, IL-12, IL-23 and recruit the Th1 cells.

Fibrosis that follows inflammation is orchestrated by a number of inflammatory mediators, the various pro inflammatory factors constitute of plasma components, platelet derived factors and cytokines released from injured cells and infiltrating leucocytes.TGF beta is the major cytokine that contributes significantly in conversion of fibroblast to myofibroblast and epithelial to myofibroblast transition, and up regulates the genes for ECM deposition, thereby enhances fibrotic changes.

4   TGF Beta Signaling Pathway

The aqueous humor in the eye hosts a large number of cytokines and growth factors. TGF beta is a predominant cytokine present in the aqueous humor. It is normally released from the ciliary epithelium and the epithelium of the lens capsule in a latent form. Under various clinical conditions like inflammation, increased intraocular pressure etc the concentration of active TGF beta increases profoundly. TGF beta upon secretion by various cell types binds to TGF beta type-II receptor on the cell surface this in turn recruit and phosphorylate a TGF beta type-I receptor. These transmembrane serine–threonine kinase receptors phosphorylate R-SMAD proteins (SMAD1, SMAD2, SMAD3, SMAD5, and SMAD9). The activated R-SMAD has a high affinity for CoSMAD (SMAD4), they form a RSMAD/CoSMAD complex that enter the nucleus and cause gene transcription. Inhibitory SMADS (SMAD 6 and SMAD 7) prevent phosphorylation of SMAD 2 and SMAD 3 and inhibit the process.

In some cells TGF beta can also activate different arms of mitogen-activated kinase (MAPK) pathway and other stress kinases (ie, c-Jun-N-terminal kinase, JNK), p38MAPK pathway, RhoA-related signals, phosphatase2A, (Petritsch *et al.*, 2000) or PI3-kinase/ AKT (Gotzmann *et al.*,2002, Bhowmick *et al.*, 2001a).

Recent literature shows that p38MAPK activate phosphorylation of Smad3 in the middle linker region, a site distinctly different from the C terminal site phosphorylated by TGF beta (Vadlamudi *et al.*, 1999, Mori *et al.*, 2000). This also enhances Smad3/4 complex formation and nuclear translocation (Furukawa *et al.*, 2003), nuclear localization of Smad3/4 complex enhances expression of matrix components. TGF beta is the major cytokine responsible for pathogenesis of fibrosis in the eye (Saika *et al.*, 2009); although bone morphogenic proteins (BMPs), a member of the TGF beta superfamilly, EGF, FGF and IGF also make important contribution. Apart from induction of genes responsible for matrix production, TGF beta also induces expression of alpha smooth muscle actin in fibroblast that changes the morphogenic signature of fibroblast to myofibroblast (Evans *et al.*, 2003, Roberts *et al.*, 2003, Yang and Liu 2001, Dugina *et al.*, 1998, Zeisberg *et al.*, 2000, Serini and Gabbiani 1999). Fibroblast, the major cellular component in fibrotic tissue are accumulated in the wound area via proliferation, recruitment from bone marrow derived fibroblasts and also generated by epithelial mesenchymal transition (EMT) of the epithelial cells under stress (Iwano *et al.*, 2002). Individual contribution of these processes towards fibroblast generation has not been determined for fibrogenesis in eye tissues. Although it is highly probable that it will vary in different organ, in renal fibrogenesis 14-15% come from bone marrow, 36% from EMT and rest from local proliferation (Iwano *et al.*, 2002). EMT is a process in which epithelial cells under stress lose their morphogenic cues become fibroblast. In this process, epithelial cells are disaggregated from the basement membrane, lose polarity, tight junction, adheren junction, develop stress fibers, lamelopodia, filopodia and acquire motility. TGF beta plays most important role in the EMT. It assist basement membrane degradation through expression of MMP2 and MMP9 (Strutz *et al.*, 2002) and orchestrate the event through Smad3 dependent transcription as well as Smad independent p38MAP kinase activation (Zeisberg *et al.*, 2003) and GTPase-mediated signaling (Bhowmick *et al.*, 2001b, Boyer *et al.*, 1999, Yu *et al.*, 2002). Thus, irrespective of the process of development, TGF beta plays a vital role in fibrosis.

TGF beta receptors have been identified in various tissues of the eye (Saika 2006). In the following section we will discuss fibrosis in different tissues of eye and their implication in vision.

5   Cornea

Cornea the major refractive surface of eye is avascular and transparent. The transparency of cornea is a prerequisite for optimum vision and is maintained by the intricate arrangement of the structural components of the cornea.

The various layers of the cornea comprise of the outer most layer of epithelial cells, the middle stromal layer made up of collagen rich extracellular matrix and keratocytes and the inner most endothelial layer.

The unique composition of the cells, extracellular matrix and arrangement of collagen fibrils contribute to the transparency of the cornea. The crystalline protein content of the keratocytes which is similar to that found in lens epithelial cells plays a pivotal role in preventing light scattering and absorption of UV rays. The intricate size and spacing of the collegen fibrils i.e. 32nm size and 64 nm distance respectively in the stroma allows light transmittance (Maurice 1957, Goldman and Benedek 1967, Benedek 1971). The keratocytes are normally quiescent and maintain the high level of essential proteoglycans in the extracellular matrix, i.e. keratocan, lumican which help maintain transparency.

However following injury these cells become active again. After any injury involving the stromal layer, keratocytes undergo apoptosis; the epithelial cells adjacent to the wound defect lose their attachment and start sliding downwards towards the exposed stroma. The remaining viable keratocytes start proliferating with low ECM production, which contain keratocan, lumican and keratan sulphate chains. Alternatively under the influence of major cytokine TGF beta and other growth factors these cells may convert into myofibroblasts expressing alpha smooth muscle actin which produce collagen and other ECM components, hyaluronan, biglycan and low levels of keratan sulphate proteoglycans to form a disorganized opaque ECM (Hassell and Birk 2010). Interestingly Jester *et al.*, (1996) have shown that in differentiated myofibroblasts there is a marked increase in cell volume and dilution of corneal crystallins which is associated with light scattering. Therefore myofibroblast formation leads to alternation of extracellular matrix and dilution of corneal crystalline proteins, all culminating into loss of transparency and vision impairement.

There are several cell types that produce growth factors in the cornea but it is only the quiescent keratocytes which respond to these growth factors and produce ECM for stromal wound repair. In vitro studies, triggering keratocytes with different growth factors i.e. FGF-2, IGF-I, IGF-II and TGF beta all stimulated proteoglycan synthesis, but TGF beta also stimulated hyaluronan, fibronectin and biglycan synthesis, which are constituents of a fibrotic ECM and induced the appearance of a smooth muscle actin within the cells. Therefore TGF beta can solely cause keratocytes to become myofibroblasts (Jester 1996, Jester and Ho-Chang, 2003).

Recent studies show extracellular matrix components osteopontin and tenascin-C which are ligands of α9 integrin, play roles in corneal wound fibrosis and neovascularization. Although loss of osteopontin reduces macrophage invasion and myofibroblast differentiation in the healing stroma by suppression of fibrogenic gene expression in response to injury, it impairs closure of incisional wounds in the mouse cornea (Saika *et al.*, 2013).

Several clinical situations like trauma, infections, surgery and chemical injury lead to corneal scarring which is the third leading cause of blindness globally (Whitcher *et al.*, 2001).

Several studies have reported different approaches for prevention of corneal fibrosis. These therapeutic strategies include selectively killing the myofibroblasts (Schipper *et al.*, 1997, Azar and Jain 2001, Gupta *et al.*, 2011), gene targeting to silence TGF beta 1 with BMP 7 (Tandon *et al.*, 2013), triple combination targeting of TGF beta1, TGF betaR2,CTGF (Sriram *et al.*, 2013), vimentin inhibition (Das *et al.*,2014), histone deacetylase inhibitors (Sharma *et al.*, 2009, Tandon *et al.*, 2012), peroxisome proliferator-activated receptor-gamma (PPARgamma) agonist (Pan et a. 2009, Huxlin *et al.*, 2013, Uchiyama *et al.*, 2013), rapamycin (Milani 2013), infiximab (Ferrari *et al.*, 2013) and also novel approaches by pharmaceutical inhibition of TGF beta 1 (Chowdhury *et al.*, 2013). A volume of knowledge has been gained from several studies on the understanding of pathobiology of EMT, fibrosis and corneal opacity, but still remains to be understood when and why wound fibroblasts decide to become myofibroblasts and identifying such mechanism may help in reversing EMT. This will perhaps give hope for not just prevention but also treatment of established corneal fibrosis.

6   Effect of Fibrosis in Glaucoma Pathology

Glaucoma is the second leading cause of blindness worldwide. Degeneration of neuronal tracts due to progressive loss of ganglion cells prevents transmission of efferent signals from retina to visual cortex. Increase in intraocular pressure, resulting from either excessive production or resistance to aqueous out flow by the trabecular meshwork, is the main causative factor for degeneration of optic nerve head. It has been established through several studies that TGF beta is involved in laying the disproportionate extra cellular matrix, both in terms of quantity and quality, in the trabecular mesh work leading to hindrance in the outflow of aqueous humor which results into rise in intraocular pressure (Lu¨tjen-Drecoll, 2005, Fleenor *et al.*, 2006). In patients with progressive open angle glaucoma (POGA) significantly higher level of TGF beta is observed (Tripathi *et al.*, 1994, Picht *et al.*, 2001, Inatani *et al.*, 2001, Ochiai and Ochiai 2002). The role of TGF beta in excessive production of matrix protein is also supported by the fact that it induces increased production of fibronectin and other matrix protein from cultured human trabecular meshwork cells (Fuchshofer *et al.*, 2007, Li *et al.*, 2000, Zhao *et al.*, 2004, Zhao and Russell, 2005). It is also reported to cross link fibronectin via induction of tissue transglutaminase (Welge-Lussen *et al.*, 2000, Tovar-Vidales *et al.*, 2008) and simulate the synthesis and secretion of lysyl oxidases, enzymes that cross-link ECM collagen and elastin fibers (Sethi *et al.*, 2011). Therefore in glaucoma TGF β induces excessive production as well as cross linking of the matrix protein, at the same time it diminishes matrix turnover by suppression of MMP activity (Fuchshofer *et al.*, 2003). However the factors that modulate TGF beta in the trabecular meshwork are still not clear. Increased expression of Thrombospondin-1 observed in POGA patients are thought to be involved in activation of TGF beta from its latent form (Flu¨gel-Koch *et al.*, 2004). Connective tissue growth factor, a regulator of TGF beta, is also induced in trabecular meshwork following TGF beta treatment (Chudgar *et al.*, 2006). Bone morphogenic proteins are implicated in regulation of multiple functions in ocular tissues (Wordinger and Clark, 2007); BMP4 and BMP7 block induction of

ECM proteins e.g. fibronectin-1, collagens IV and VI, TSP-1, and PAI-1 through inhibition of TGF beta 2 (Wordinger *et al.*, 2007, Fuchshofer *et al.*, 2007). Expression of several members of the bone morphogenetic protein (BMP) family, including BMP ligands (BMP2, BMP4, BMP5, and BMP7), receptors (BMPR1a, BMPR1b, and BMPR2), and BMP antagonists gremlin, noggin, and follistatin (Wordinger *et al.*, 2002, Fuchshofer *et al.*, 2009, Wordinger and Clark 2007) has been observed in trabecular meshwork cells. Elevated gremlin inhibits BMP4 antagonism of TGF beta that increases IOP, thus a balance of BMPs and their inhibitors may play a vital role in POGA (Wordinger *et al.*, 2007). A recent literature shows increased expression of follistatin in glaucomatous trabecular meshwork cells compared to its normal counterpart (Fitzgerald *et al.*, 2012). Modulation of BMP 7 by pharmacological means might be a potential strategy for prevention of POGA (Fuchshofer *et al.*, 2007). Further research initiative can divulge the complex relationship among TGF beta, BMPs and BMP inhibitors and can provide insight regarding possible target for prevention of POGA.

7 Fibrosis in Glaucoma Filtration Surgery

The most important determinant of optimum intraocular pressure following glaucoma filtration surgery is the wound healing response. Scar formation following any surgery is an established phenomenon. Major cause of bleb failure is the fibrosis that occurs under the influence of profibrotic factors that are released as a result of inflammatory response to surgery. TGF beta is a significant contributory cytokine identified in this pathology. Cytotoxic antimetabolites like 5-flurouracil, mitomycin C has increased the success of surgery but risk of toxicity associated complication remains. Use of TGF beta inhibitors (Cordeiro *et al.*, 1999, Mead *et al.*, 2003, Mietz *et al.*, 1998) fibrinolytic agents (WuDunn,1997, Azuara-Blanco and Wilson, 1998), anti-inflammatory agents (Migdal and Hitchings, 1983), MMP inhibitors (Daniels *et al.*, 2003) and anti metabolites (Chen 1983, The Fluorouracil Filtering Surgery Study Group 1989, Khaw *et al.*, 1993) have provided variable degree of success. However even with highest doses of antifibrotic and other adjunct therapy, surgery fails in many individuals, this warrants for further research towards development of new therapeutics.

8 Anterior Sub Capsular Cataract

The lens is unique in structure and function; it is avascular and transparent comprising of lens capsule which encloses within it the lens protein and lens fibres. The anterior and not the posterior capsule are lined by epithelial cells which contribute to lens fibre formation throughout the lifetime. The unique arrangement of the lens fibres as well as the epithelial cells and protein present therein, prevent light scatter and maintains transparency. Any loss in transparency of the lens or its capsule is termed as cataract.

Anterior sub capsular cataract is a primary cataract resulting due loss of normal morphology of lens epithelial cells, leading to formation of fibrotic opaque plaques below the lens capsule and vision impairment. The result of numerous studies conducted to uncover the pathogenesis of this condition have identified this as fibrotic disorder resulting from either trauma, inflammation, or even associated with some disease i.e. atopic dermatitis. TGF beta has been identified as the major cytokine that triggers epithelial mesenchymal transition in the lens epithelial cells (Lovicu *et al.*, 2002). The epithelial cells initially lose their cell-cell adhesion due to reduced expression of adhesion protein E-cadherin, presumably increased activity of the MMPs and MMP 9 in particular has been identified as the predominant player there (Nathu *et al.*, 2009). The cells actively proliferate to form multilayers and undergo transdifferentiation leading to plaque formation. Surgery is the only solution for anterior sub capsular cataract. Researchers are trying to find out methods that can reverse the process and inhibition of MMP activity by its inhibitors has shown promise (Dwivedi *et al.*, 2006).

9   Posterior Capsular Opacification (PCO)

Cataract is the leading cause of global blindness and posterior capsular opacification remains a major complication following cataract surgery (Apple *et al.*, 1992; Spalton, 1999; Pandey *et al.*, 2004) effecting significant vision loss (Ashwin *et al.*, 2009; Roh *et al.*, 2010). The incidence of PCO is still 8~34.3% in adults, and nearly 100% in children (Vasavada *et al.*, 2006; Vasavada and Nihalani 2006; Rönbeck *et al.*, 2009. The cytokines and growth factors released following surgery (Meacock *et al.*, 2000; Nishi, 1999; Wallentin *et al.*,1998) induce proliferation of the remaining lens epithelial cells of the anterior capsule. These epithelial cells under the influence of TGF beta undergo epithelial mesenchymal transition and transform into myofibroblasts. These myofibroblast, having the ability to move, migrate to the posterior capsule where they secrete increased amount of matrix protein (McDonnell *et al.*, 1983; Cobo *et al.*, 1984; Wormstone 2002). The deposition of excessive matrix protein as well as resulting contraction of the posterior capsule leads to the opacification of the posterior capsule. This fibrotic condition leads to vision impairment and blindness. TFG beta is the major cytokine that determines the pathophysiology of PCO (Saika *et al.*, 2004). Understanding of the pathophysiology of posterior capsular opacification formation and pathobiology of TGF beta in this process has enabled to design various strategies for PCO prevention. Selective killing of the remaining lens epithelial cells using various cytotoxic drugs e.g. daunarubicin, mitomycin C, 5-flurouracil, cyclosporine (Sternberg *et al.*, 2010, Haus and Galand, 1996, Totan *et al.*, 2008, Sharma and Panwar 2013) has successfully prevented PCO but the toxicity to the healthy intraocular tissues has restricted their clinical use. Improvisation of this technique by using a sealed capsule to deliver cytotoxic drug into the capsular bag during surgery has reduced the intraocular toxicity (Abdelwahab*et al.*, 2006, Duncan *et al.*, 2007), but the brief exposure of the drug eventually compromises with its therapeutic efficacy (Rękas *et al.*, 2013, Kim *et al.*, 2007). However, nanoparticle mediated delivery of doxorubicin has successfully prevented PCO without compromising with the safety of the intra ocular structures (Guha *et al.*, 2013). Inhibition of Akt phosphorylation using inhibitor AR-12 (Chandler *et al.*, 2010), silencing NF-kB pathway (Park *et al.*, 2010, Jia *et al.*, 2011), suppression of TGF beta expression by inhibition of DNA methylation using Zebularine (Zhou, 2012), use of cytoskeletal drugs (Sureshkumar, 2012) has shown promising results. Celecoxib and roficoxib has also prevented PCO formation by inhibition of cyclooxygenase -2, a protein associated with EMT in PCO formation (Chandler *et al.*, 2007). Suppression of matrix metalloproteinase has been reported as a potent approach towards PCO prevention (Wong *et al.*, 2004, Nishi *et al.*, 1996, Inan *et al.*, 2001, Awasthi *et al.*, 2008, Hazra *et al.*, 2012). Silencing of epidermal growth factor receptor using siRNA in human lens epithelial cells (Huang, 2011) and gene therapy using adeno virus mediated delivery of gene to over express proapoptotic molecules like bax or caspase 3 (Malecaze, 2006) has been exciting. Despite the tremendous efforts directed towards prevention of PCO, the solution still remain elusive.

10   Fibrotic Diseases at the Back of the Eye

The posterior segment of the eye starts with the vitreous humor, which is a gel like shock absorber for the retina is made up of water, collagen and hyaluronic acid. This also acts as a scaffold for cells i.e. retinal pigmented epithelium (RPE) or the glial cells migrating from the retina at the time of injury, hypoxia or break in the blood retinal barrier. The retina is multilayered consisting of neurons, blood vessels, extracellular matrix, resident cells and recruited cells like glial cells and monocytes.

A major cause of vision loss in developed country is pathologies associated with retinal or choroidal vasculature. Major blinding disorders like diabetic retinopathy (DR), proliferative vitreoretinopathy (PVR), age related macular degeneration (AMD), retinopathy of prematurity (ROP) are identified by characteristic features like vitreous/retinal hemorrhage, macular edema, neovascularization and fibrovascular scarring. It is interesting to note that in all of the diseases mentioned, the retina responds to insults by chronic healing process, which eventually culminates into fibrosis and impaired vision.

11   Proliferative Vitreoretinopathy

PVR is a fibrotic disorder, it occurs in 8-10% (Morescalchi *et al.*, 2013) of patients with primary retinal detachment, however the incidence is alarming as it develops in 75% patients as post surgical complication of retinal reattachment surgery (Pastor, 1998) and it continues to remain a major post operative challenge. It occurs in 40-60% patients with open globe injury (Colyer *et al.*, 2008).

Understanding the etiopathogenesis of the diseases has ushered different approaches for preventing or treating the condition. The presence of immune cells into the vitreous cavity following injury incites the production of growth factors and cytokines that interact with the retinal pigmented epithelium (RPE) cells and the muller cells. The major cytokines and growth factors involved are TGF beta, PDGF, TNF alpha, bFGF, they promote epithelial mesenchymal transition and migration of the RPE and Muller cells into the vitreous, thereby leading to a cascade of events resulting into expansion of the extracellular matrix in the retina. The subsequent contraction and wrinkling of this scaffold attached to the retina leads to retinal tear and detachment resulting into PVR. Understanding the molecular basis of the disease now enables to target two major events for preventing the disease progression i.e. arresting the epithelial mesenchymal transition of the RPE cells or Muller cell gliosis and subsequently the epiretinal membrane formation.

Anti-inflammatory drugs have been successful in prevention of PVR, intravitreal treatment with triamcinolone and methylprednisolone has significantly reduced the incidence of PVR in animal models (Hui *et al.*, 1993, Tano *et al.*, 1980, Rubsamen and Cousins, 1997), however the results failed to extrapolate in the same degree in human clinical trials (Koerner *et al.*, 1982, Hui and Hu, 1999, Jonas *et al.*, 2000, Bali *et al.*, 2010).

Anti proliferative compounds has been extensively investigated, for their efficacy in arresting the proliferation of the cells responsible for profibrotic changes. 5-fluorouracil (5-FU) has been widely used for prevention of PVR, sustained release of the drug at high concentration was 100% effective in prevention of retinal detachment (Borhani, *et al.*, 1995). Results from the human clinical trial with 5-Flurouracil (Asaria *et al.*, 2001, Wickham *et al.*, 2007) and adjuvant therapy with 5-Flurouracil and low molecular weight heparin (Sundaram *et al.*, 2010) were contradictory, in the former PVR was prevented, whereas the results of the latter study failed to show any improvement.

Effect of daunorubicin treatment following vitrectomy remains controversial; Wiedemann *et al.*, 1995, treated clinical patients with daunorubicin and found no improvement in visual acuity as compared to untreated control, whereas in another similar study significant improvement in visual acuity was reported (Kumar *et al.*, 2002).

Other pharmacological agents including colchicines (Lemor *et al.*, 1986) taxol (van Bockxmeer *et al.*, 1985), retinoic acid (Campochiaro *et al.*, 1991), glucosamine (Chesnokov *et al.*, 2009) are reported to prevent cell proliferation and migration but chimeric ribosome targeting the PCNA antigens failed to prevent recurrence of PVR in human clinical trial (Schiff *et al.*, 2007).

Growth factors being identified as major contributors towards the pathogenesis of the disease, appropriate inhibitors have been evaluated to prevent PVR. Kinase inhibitor Hypericin (Tahara *et al.*, 1999, Machado *et al.*, 2009), Herbimycin A (Imai *et al.*, 2000), Alkylphosphocholine (Eibl *et al.*, 2007), PDGFR kinase inhibitor AG1295 have all proven effective in preventing retinal detachment (Zheng *et al.*, 2003).

As TGF beta contributes significantly to the pathogenesis of PVR, use of TGF beta inhibitors to prevent the disease progression seems a logical approach. In this context it is worth mentioning that translisat which is normally used as antiallergic drug is also a potent inhibitor of TFG beta and intravitreal use of translisat in rabbit eye effectively prevented the severity of the disease without causing any side effects. Likewise gene therapy to suppress the TGF beta expression by intravitreal injection of adenovirus vector encoding soluble TGF beta receptor was developed by Oshima *et al.*, (2002), the receptor thus produced sequesters the local TGF beta and inhibits its action in the surrounding tissues thereby prevents the progression of PVR.

Other pathological processes involved in development of PVR have also been addressed as preventive strategies. Augmented intracellular reactive oxygen species (ROS) during PVR progression is capable of activating PDGFR and aggravating the disease process, intravitreal use of antioxidant *N*-acetylcysteine (NAC) in rabbit eye successfully protected from developing PVR (Lei *et al.*, 2010). Matrix metalloproteinase are essential components of wound remodelling, they cause degradation of extracellular matrix; thereby facilitate cell detachment and movement. Use of MMP inhibitor prinomastat, with the objective to prevent movement of RPE and gial cells into the vitreous has shown promise in inhibiting post traumatic PVR (Ozerdem *et al.*, 2001).

12   Subretinal Fibrosis

A classic example of subretinal fibrosis is age related macular edema (ARMD). This condition affects 12-15 million Americans over the age of 65. A big number of these patients experience permanent loss of vision due to choroidal neovascularization and fibrosis. The disease initiates with loss of function of the RPE cells either due ageing process or any form of disease. The RPE cells are inadvertently related to proper functioning and scavenging of the apoptotic photoreceptor cells (Bok, 1993). Inadequate functioning of the RPE cells lead to deposition of lipids and damaged proteins in the subretinal space termed as drusen (Crabb *et al.*, 2002). This results in fibrosis and thickening of the bruchs membrane and the circulation to the photoreceptors is compromised. This leads to formation of abnormal choroidal neovascularization and as they enter into the subretinal space, this often results into haemorrhage. The retina responds by inciting physiological healing processes which eventually culminate as fibrosis. Ultimately compromised photoreceptor, RPE and choroidal functions lead to macular dysfunction and results into blindness.

Therapeutic approach to prevent or treat this disease has met with limited success. Unfortunately, majority of the drugs in clinical use to treat ARMD are targeted to inhibit the choroidal neovascularization i.e. anti VEGF therapy and do not address the underlying pathology i.e. ischemia and inflammation. Very recent studies on cell based therapies to rescue retinal damage are exciting but much remains to be investigated and established (Friedlander 2007). Early therapeutic intervention with the aim to reduce inflammation and local hypoxia may prevent the photoreceptor death and maintain vision in future.

13   Epiretinal Fibrosis Involvement in Diabetic Retinopathy

Diabetic retinopathy is a significant cause of global blindness and more alarming as it affects the working population. The underlying pathology in diabetic retinopathy is again hypoxia leading to abnormal neovascularization. Classical changes in retinal vasculature in a diabetic eye includes microaneurysms, pericytic cell death, altered vascular permeability all leading to compromised circulation and hypoxia that acts as a trigger for neovascularization. Neovascularization can result in haemorrhage in the retina, subhyaloid space or in the vitreous body. These vessels continue to proliferate and are accompanied by fibrosis due to proliferation of glial cells (Gliosis), as they invade the vitreous humor and contract; there is traction on the retina, resulting in retinal detachment. (Friedlander, 2007)

Not much success has been attained in rehabilitating these eyes back to normalcy. Surgery and laser ablation of the peripheral vessels in order to reduce the metabolic demand of the retina are current modalities treatment in clinical practice, but demonstrate limited success.

14   Future strategies to prevent fibrotic eye diseases

14.1   Gene Therapy

Enhanced research and insight into understanding the mechanisms of fibrosis in various compartments of the eye resulted in indentifying signature genes, modulation of which may arrest fibrotic changes. Focus is put on the roles of myofibroblast and signals activated by the fibrogenic cytokine, transforming growth factor beta. Modulation of signal transduction molecules, e.g., Smad and mitogen-activated protein kinases, by gene transfer and other technology is beneficial and can be an important treatment regiment to overcome these diseases (Saika *et al.*, 2008).

In the cornea, TGF beta and its signal transduction have been major targets for prevention of fibrosis. Enhanced expression of decorin, (a member of the small leucine-rich proteoglycan family, is expressed in the corneal stroma and plays an important role in wound healing and structural support in the cornea) by gene therapy has significantly reduced TGF beta driven EMT (Mohan *et al.*, 2011).

In vitro studies with Smad2, Smad3, Smad4, and Smad7 siRNA to examine whether TGFβ in human corneal fibroblast cells relays its signal via the Smad pathway has shown that TGFβ-mediated keratocyte transdifferentiation to myofibroblasts occurs via Smad signaling and that Smad7 is an attractive target to prevent myofibroblast formation. Nanoparticle-mediated soluble extracellular domain of the transforming growth factor-β type II receptor (sTGFβRII) gene therapy has been used to reduce myofibroblasts and fibrosis in the cornea using an in vitro model(Sharma *et al.*, 2012).

Galiacy *et al.*, (2011) used gene therapy strategies to hinder excessive collagen deposition in corneal scar development. Using a recombinant AAV-based vector (AAV2/8) the researchers over expressed a specific fibril collagenase, matrix metalloproteinase (MMP) 14, to prevent collagen deposition and subsequent scarring following incisional injury to the cornea in mice.

In a study using adenovirus(Ad)-mediated gene transfer, proapoptotic molecules p53, procaspase 3, Bax, and TRAIL were over expressed to induce therapeutic programmed cell death of residual lens cells to prevent PCO, showed successful prevention of PCO in vitro as well as in vivo system (Malecaze *et al.*, 2006).

Over expression of platelet derived growth factor plays a significant role in development of proliferative vitreoretinopathy (PVR), Gene therapy with a retrovirus used to express a dominant negative alpha PDGFR has shown to attenuate PVR in a rabbit model of the disease (Ikuno and Kazlauskas 2002).

14.2   Cell based Therapy

Cell therapy to treat ocular fibrosis has best been demonstrated in cornea for pathology involving limbal stem cell deficiency. The limbus is the niche for stem cells that replace the corneal epithelial cells every 3-10 days. Loss of limbal stem cells can arise owing to chemical or thermal injuries, ultraviolet and ionizing radiation, Stevens-Johnson syndrome, multiple surgeries or cryotherapies, contact lens wear, extensive microbial infection, advanced ocular cicatricial pemphigoid, and aniridia. In addition, some LSCD cases are idiopathic. In LSCD, the conjunctival epithelium migrates onto the cornea (a process called conjunctivalization), resulting in a thickened, irregular, unstable corneal surface that is prone to defects, ulceration, corneal scarring, vascularization, and opacity. Corneal scarring and fibrosis originating from LSCD are currently best amenable to limbal stem cell transplant. Various clinical means of achieving this are, conjunctival-limbal autologous (CLAU) transplantation; living-related conjunctival-limbal allogeneic (lr-CLAL) transplantation; keratolimbal allogeneic (KLAL) transplantation; and ex vivo expansion of limbal stem cells transplantation (Ont Health Technol Assess Ser. 2008).

Cell based therapy for posterior segment fibrotic conditions stems from specific etiology. Fibrovascular conditions like diabetic retinopathy originating from ischemia could benefit by therapy with endothelial cells and their progenitors (Friedlander, 2007). Fibrotic pathologies like Age related macular degeneration (ARMD) where RPE loss, damage or atrophy are hallmark of disease pathology, may be reversible by replacement with RPE cells, though the therapy is still in laboratory stage of development.

14.3   Bionic eye

Eyes with irreversible vision impairment, refractory to any form of therapy may still hope to see with latest innovations like the bionic eye. FDA has given approval to begin U.S. trials of a retinal implant system that gives blind people a limited degree of vision. The Argus II Retinal Prosthesis System can provide sight - the detection of light to people who have gone blind from degenerative eye diseases like macular degeneration and retinitis pigmentosa. It consists of retinal implant with an array of 60 electrodes on a chip measuring 1 mm by 1 mm, which will replace the photoreceptors.

Component of eye	Cells involved	Clinical manifestation
Cornea	Corneal epithelial cells, keratocytes, resident fibroblasts, recruited fibroblasts.	Corneal scarring, loss of transparency and blindness
Trabecular meshwork	Epithelial cells of trabecular meshwork	Increased intraocular pressure, Glaucoma
Anterior lens capsule	Lens epithelial cells	Anterior subcapsular cataract
Posterior lens capsule	Lens epithelial cells	Posterior capsular opacification
Vitreous humor	RPE, Fibroblasts, gial cells	Proliferative Vitreoretinopathy, retinal detachment
Retina	RPE cell loss	AMD, Age related macular edema, blindness
Retina	Vascular endothelial cells	Diabetic retinopathy, neovascularization in retina, blindness

Table 1: Different components of eye that undergo fibrosis, the cells that undergo EMT and their clinical manifestation.

15   Conclusion

Tissue injury results into a cascade of events which is characterized by angiogenesis, cell proliferation, epithelial mesenchymal transition, deposition of extracellular matrix and wound contraction, all of which are physiological events resulting to healing. In the eye however these events have detrimental outcome on functional efficiency, these fibrotic scars hamper the transparency of the optical media or obscure light from reaching the retina, thereby results to compromise visual acuity. Excellent knowledge has been gained over the years on the pathogenesis of fibrosis in organs and their molecular pathways. Various approaches to address this phenomenon by intervening in the different pathways leading to fibrosis are being explored as part of healing by substitution. Focus is also on regenerative therapies to prevent scaring by replacing equivalent specialized cells. The near future should witness healing without scarring as a panacea for various diseases.

Authors

Sarbani Hazra
Department of Veterinary Surgery & Radiology, West Bengal University of Animal & Fishery Sciences, Kolkata, India

Aditya Konar
CSIR-Indian Institute of Chemical Biology, Jadavpur, Kolkata, India

References

Abdelwahab MT, Kugelberg M, Kugelberg U, Zetterstrom C. After-cataract evaluation after using balanced salt solution, distilled deionized water, and 5-fluorouracil with a sealed-capsule irrigation device in the eyes of 4-week-old rabbits. J. Cataract Refract. Surg. 2006; 32:1955-1960.

Apple DJ, Solomon KD, Tetz MR et al., Posterior capsule opacification. Surv Ophthalmol. 1992; 37(2):73-116.

Asaria RH, Kon CH, Bunce C, et al., Adjuvant 5-fluorouracil and heparin prevents proliferative vitreoretinopathy: results from a randomized, double-blind, controlled clinical trial. Ophthalmology. 2001; 108(7): 1179–1183.

Ashwin PT, Shah S, Wolffsohn JS. Advances in cataract surgery. Clin Exp Optom. 2009; 92:333-42.

Awasthi N, Wang-Su ST, Wagner BJ. Downregulation of MMP-2 and -9 by proteasome inhibition: a possible mechanism to decrease LEC migration and prevent posterior capsular opacification. Invest Ophthalmol Vis Sci. 2008; 49(5):1998-2003. doi: 10.1167/iovs.07-0624.

Azar DT, Jain S. Topical MMC for subepithelial fibrosis after refractive corneal surgery. Ophthalmology. 2001; 108(2):239-40.

Azuara-Blanco A, Wilson RP. Intraocular and extraocular bleeding after intracameral injection of tissue plasminogen activator. BrJ Ophthalmol.1998; 82:1345-1346.

Bali E, Feron EJ, Peperkamp E, Veckeneer M, Mulder PG, van Meurs JC. The effect of a preoperative subconjuntival injection of dexamethasone on blood-retinal barrier breakdown following scleral buckling retinal detachment surgery: a prospective randomized placebo-controlled double blind clinical trial. Graefes Arch Clin Exp Ophthalmol. 2010; 7:957-962.

Benedek G. Theory of the transparency of the eye. Appl Optics 1971; 10:459

Bhowmick NA, Zent R, Ghiassi M, McDonnell M, Moses HL. Integrin beta 1 signaling is necessary for transforming growth factor-beta activation of p38MAPK and epithelial plasticity. J. Biol. Chem. 2001a; 276:46707-46713.

Bhowmick NA, Ghiassi M, Bakin A, et al., Transforming growth factor-b1 mediates epithelial to mesenchymal transdifferentiation through a RhoA-dependent mechanism. Mol Biol Cell 2001b; 12:27–36.

Bok D. The retinal pigment epithelium: a versatile partner in vision. J. Cell Sci. Suppl. 1993; 17:189–195.

Borhani H, Peyman GA, Rahimy MH, Thompson H. Suppression of experimental proliferative vitreoretinopathy by sustained intraocular delivery of 5-FU. Int Ophthalmol. 1995; 19(1):43–49.

Boyer AS, Erickson CP, Runyan RB. Epithelial-mesenchymal transformation in the embryonic heart is mediated through distinct pertussis toxin-sensitive and TGFb signal transduction mechanisms. Dev. Dyn. 1999; 214:81–91.

Campochiaro PA, Hackett SF, Conway BP. Retinoic acid promotes density-dependent growth arrest in human retinal pigment epithelial cells. Invest Ophthalmol Vis Sci. 1991; 32(1):65–72.

Chandler HL, Webb TR, Barden CA, Thangavelu M, Kulp SK, Chen C-S, Colitz CMH The effect of phosphorylated Akt inhibition on posterior capsule opacification in an ex vivo canine model Mol Vis. 2010; 16: 2202–2214.

Chandler HL, Webb TR, Barden CA, Thangavelu M, Kulp SK, Chen C-S, Colitz CMH.Chandler HL, Barden CA, Lu P, Kusewitt DF, Colitz CM. Prevention of posterior capsular opacification through cyclooxygenase-2 inhibition. Mol Vis. 2007; 13:677-91.

Chen CW. Enhanced intraocular pressure controlling effectiveness of trabeculectomy by localapplication of mitomycin C. Trans Asia Pacif Acad Ophthalmol. 1983; 9:172-177.

Chesnokov V, Sun C, Itakura K. Glucosamine suppresses proliferation of human prostate carcinoma DU145 cells through inhibition of STAT3 signaling. Cancer Cell Int. 2009; 9:25.

Chowdhury S, Guha R, Trivedi R, Kompella UB, Konar A, Hazra S. Pirfenidone Nanoparticles Improve Corneal Wound Healing and Prevent Scarring Following Alkali Burn. Plos ONE 2013, 8(8): e70528. DOI: 10.1371/journal.pone.0070528

Chudgar SM, Deng P, Maddala R, et al.,: Regulation of connective tissue growth factor expression in the aqueous humor outflow pathway. Mol Vis 2006; 12:1117-26.

Cobo LM, Ohsawa E, Chandler D, Arguello R, George G. Pathogenesis of capsular opacification after extracapsular cataract extraction: an animal model. Ophthalmology. 1984; 91(7):857-863.

Colyer MH, Chun DW, Bower KS, Dick JSB, and Weichel ED. Perforating globe injuries during operation Iraqi freedom. Ophthalmology 2008; 115(11): 2087-2093.

Cordeiro MF, Gay JA, Khaw PT. Human anti-transforming growth factor-beta2 antibody: a new glaucoma anti-scarring agent. Invest Ophthalmol Vis Sci. 1999; 40:2225-2234.

Crabb JW et al., Drusen proteome analysis:an approach to the etiology of age-related macular degeneration. Proc. Natl. Acad. Sci. U. S. A. 2002; 99:14682-14687.

Daniels JT, Cambrey AD, Occleston NL, et al., Matrix metalloproteinase inhibition modulates fibroblast-mediated matrix contraction and collagen production in vitro. Invest Ophthalmol Vis Sci.2003; 44:1104-1110.

Das SK, Gupta I, Cho YK, Zhang X, Uehara H, Muddana SK, Bernhisel AA, Archer B, Ambati BK. Vimentin knockdown decreases corneal opacity. Invest Ophthalmol Vis Sci. 2014 May 22. pii: IOVS-13-13494. doi: 10.1167/iovs.13-13494.

Dugina V, Alexandrova A, Chaponnier C, Vasiliev J, Gabbiani G. Rat fibroblasts cultured from various organs exhibit differences in alpha-smooth muscle actin expression, cytoskeletal pattern, and adhesive structure organization. Exp. Cell. Res. 1998; 238:481–490.

Duncan G, Wang L, Neilson GJ, Wormstone IM. Lens cell survival after exposure to stress in the closed capsular bag. Invest. Ophthalmol.Vis. Sci. 2007; 48: 2701–2707.

Dwivedi DJ, Pino G, Banh A, Nathu Z, Howchin D, Margetts P, Sivak JG, West-Mays JA. Matrix Metalloproteinase Inhibitors Suppress Transforming Growth Factor--Induced Subcapsular Cataract Formation. Am J Pathol 2006; 168: 69-79. DOI: 10.2353/ajpath.2006.04108

Eibl KH, Lewis GP, Betts K, et al., The effect of alkylphosphocholines on intraretinal proliferation initiated by experimental retinal detachment. Invest Ophthalmol Vis Sci. 2007; 48(3):1305–1311.

Evans RA, Tian YC, Steadman R, et al., TGF-b1-mediated fibroblast–myofibroblast terminal differentiation-the role of Smad proteins. Exp Cell Res 2003; 282:90–100.

Ferrari G, Bignami F, Giacomini C, Franchini S, Rama P.Safety and efficacy of topical infliximab in a mouse model of ocular surface scarring. Invest Ophthalmol Vis Sci. 2013; 54(3):1680-8. doi: 10.1167/iovs.12-10782.

Fitzgerald AM, Benz C, Clark AF, Wordinger RJ. The Effects of Transforming Growth Factor-b2 on the Expression of Follistatin and Activin A in Normal and Glaucomatous Human Trabecular Meshwork Cells and Tissues. Invest Ophthalmol Vis Sci. 2012; 53 (11): 7358-7369.

Fleenor DL, Shepard AR, Hellberg PE, Jacobson N, Pang I-H, Clark AF. TGFβ2-Induced Changes in Human Trabecular Meshwork: Implications for Intraocular Pressure. Investigative Ophthalmology & Visual Science, 2006; 47(1): 226-234.

Flu¨gel-Koch C, Ohlmann A, Fuchshofer R, et al., Thrombo- spondin-1 in the trabecular meshwork: localization in normal and glaucomatous eyes, and induction by TGF-beta1and dexamethasone in vitro. Exp Eye Res 2004; 79:649-63.

Friedlander M. Fibrosis and diseases of the eye. J. Clin. Invest. 2007; 117:576–586. doi:10.1172/JCI31030.

Fuchshofer R, Stephan DA, Russell P, Tamm ER. Gene expression profiling of TGFbeta2- and/or BMP7-treated trabecular meshwork cells: identification of Smad7 as a critical inhibitor of TGF-beta2 signaling. Exp Eye Res. 2009; 88:1020–1032.

Fuchshofer R, Welge-Lussen U, Lu¨tjen-Drecoll E. The effect of TGF-beta2 on human trabecular meshwork extracellular proteolytic system. Exp Eye Res 2003; 77:757-65.

Fuchshofer R, Yu AH, Welge-Lussen U, Tamm ER. Bone morphogenetic protein-7 is an antagonist of transforming growth factor-beta2 in human trabecular meshwork cells. Invest Ophthalmol Vis Sci. 2007; 48:715–726.

Furukawa F, Matsuzaki K, Mori S, et al., *p38 MAPK mediates fibrogenic signal through Smad3 phosphorylation in rat myofibroblasts. Hepatology 2003; 38: 879–889.*

Galiacy SD, Fournié P, Massoudi D, Ancèle E, Quintyn JC, Erraud A, Raymond-Letron I, Rolling F, Malecaze F. *Matrix metalloproteinase 14 overexpression reduces corneal scarring. Gene Ther. 2011; 18:462–468.*

Goldman JN, Benedek GB. *The relationship between morphology and transparency in the nonswelling corneal stroma of the shark. Invest Ophthalmol Vis Sci 1967; 6:574.*

Gotzmann J, Huber H, Thallinger C, et al., *Hepatocytes convert to a fibroblastoid phenotype through the cooperation of TGF-b1 and Ha-Ras: steps towards invasiveness. J Cell Sci 2002;115:1189–1202.*

Guha R, Chowdhury S, Palui H, Mishra A, Basak S, Mandal TK, Hazra S, Konar A. *Doxorubicin-loaded MePEG-PCL nanoparticles for prevention of posterior capsular opacification. Nanomedicine (Lond). 2013; 8(9): 1415-1428.*

Gupta R, Yarnall BW, Giuliano EA, Kanwar JR, Buss DG, Mohan RR. *Mitomycin C: a promising agent for the treatment of canine corneal scarring. Vet Ophthalmol. 2011; 14(5):304-312. doi: 10.1111/j.1463-5224.2011.00877.x. Epub 2011 Apr 18.*

Hassell JR, Birk DE. *The molecular basis of corneal transparency. Experimental Eye Research 2010; 91: 326-335.*

Haus CM, Garland AL. *Mitomycin against posterior capsular opacification: An experimental study in rabbits. Br J Ophthalmol. 1996; 80:1087-91.*

Hazra S, Guha R, Jongkey G, Palui H, Mishra A, Vemuganti GK, Basak SK, Mandal TK, Konar A. *Modulation of matrix metalloproteinase activity by EDTA prevents posterior capsular opacification. Molecular Vision, 2012; 18:1701-1711.*

Hinz B, Phan SH, Thannickal VJ, Galli A, Bochaton-Piallat ML, Gabbiani G. *The myofibroblast: one function, multiple origins. Am. J. Pathol. 2007; 170, 1807–1816.*

Huang JC, Ishida M, Hersh P, Sugino IK, Zarbin MA. *Preparation and transplantation of photoreceptor sheets. Curr. Eye Res. 1998; 17:573–585.*

Huang Wan-Rong, Fan Xing-Xing, Tang Xin. *SiRNA targeting EGFR effectively prevents posterior capsular opacification after cataract surgery. Molecular Vision 2011; 17:2349-2355.*

Hui YN, Hu D. *Prevention of experimental proliferative vitreoretinopathy with daunomycin and triamcinolone based on the time course of the disease. Graefes Arch Clin Exp Ophthalmol. 1999; 237(7):601–605.*

Hui YN, Liang HC, Cai YS, Kirchhof B, Heimann K. *Corticosteroids and daunomycin in the prevention of experimental proliferative vitreoretinopathy induced by macrophages. Graefes Arch Clin Exp Ophthalmol. 1993; 231(2):109–114.*

Huxlin KR, Hindman HB, Jeon KI, Bühren J, MacRae S, DeMagistris M, Ciufo D, Sime PJ, Phipps RP. *Topical rosiglitazone is an effective anti-scarring agent in the cornea. PLoS One. 2013; 8(8):e70785. doi: 10.1371/journal.pone.0070785.*

Ikuno Y, Kazlauskas A. *An in vivo gene therapy approach for experimental proliferative vitreoretinopathy using the truncated platelet-derived growth factor alpha receptor. Invest Ophthalmol Vis Sci. 2002; 43(7):2406-11.*

Imai K, Loewenstein A, Koroma B, Grebe R, de Juan E Jr. *Herbimycin A in the treatment of experimental proliferative vitreoretinopathy: toxicity and efficacy study. Graefes Arch Clin Exp Ophthalmol. 2000; 238(5): 440-447.*

Inan UU, Ozturk F, Kaynak S, Ilker SS et al., *Prevention of posterior capsule opacification by retinoic acid and mitomycin. Graefes Arch Clin Exp Ophthalmol 2001; 239:693-697.*

Inatani M, Tanihara H, Katsuta H, Honjo M, Kido N, Honda Y. *Transforming growth factor-β2 levels in aqueous humor of glaucomatous eyes. Graefes Arch Clin Exp Ophthalmol. 2001; 239: 109–113.*

Ishida M, Lui GM, Yamani A, Sugino IK, Zarbin MA. *Culture of human retinal pigment epithelial cells from peripheral scleral flap biopsies. Curr. Eye Res. 1998; 17:392–402.*

Ito S, Sakamoto T, Tahara Y, et al., *The effect of tranilast on experimental proliferative vitreoretinopathy. Graefes Arch Clin Exp Ophthalmol. 1999; 237(8):691–696.*

Iwano M, et al., *Evidence that fibroblasts derive from epithelium during tissue fibrosis. J. Clin. Invest. 2002; 110:341–350. doi:10.1172/JCI200215518.*

Jester JV, Barry-Lane PA, Cavanagh HD. Petroll WM. *Induction of alphasmoothmuscle actin expression and myofibroblast transformation in cultured corneal keratocytes. Cornea 1996; 15: 505-516.*

Jester JV, Ho-Chang J. Modulation of cultured corneal keratocyte phenotype by growth factors/cytokines control in vitro contractility and extracellular matrix contraction. Exp Eye Res 2003; 77:581. [PubMed: 14550400]

Jia Z, Song Z, Zhao Y, Wang X, Liu P. Grape seed proanthocyanidin extract protects human lens epithelial cells from oxidative stress via reducing NF-κB and MAPK protein expression. Molecular Vision. 2011; 17:210-217.

Jonas JB, Hayler JK, Panda-Jonas S. Intravitreal injection of crystalline cortisone as adjunctive treatment of proliferative vitreoretinopathy. Br J Ophthalmol. 2000; 84(9):1064–1067.

Kalluri R, Weinberg RA. The basics of epithelial-mesenchymal transition. J. Clin. Invest. 2009; 119:1420–1428. doi:10.1172/JCI39101

Kalluri R, and Neilson EG. Epithelial-mesenchymal transition and its implications for fibrosis. J. Clin. Invest. 2003; 112: 1776–1784.

Keeley EC, Mehrad B, Strieter RM. The role of fibrocytes in fibrotic diseases of the lungs and heart. Fibrogenesis Tissue Repair 2011; 4: 2.

Khaw PT, Doyle JW, Sherwood MB, et al., Effects of intraoperative 5-fluorouracil or mitomycin C onglaucoma filtration surgery in the rabbit. Ophthalmology. 1993; 100:367-372.

Kim SY, Kim JH, Choi JS, Joo CK. Comparison of posterior capsule opacification in rabbits receiving either mitomycin-C or distilled water for sealed-capsule irrigation during cataract surgery. Clin Experiment Ophthalmol 2007; 35: 755–758.

Koerner F, Merz A, Gloor B, Wagner E. Postoperative retinal fibrosis – a controlled clinical study of systemic steroid therapy. Graefes Arch Clin Exp Ophthalmol. 1982; 219(6):268–271.

Kumar A, Nainiwal S, Choudhary I, Tewari HK, Verma LK. Role of daunorubicin in inhibiting proliferative vitreoretinopathy after retinal detachment surgery. Clin Experiment Ophthalmol. 2002; 30(5): 348–351.

Lee JM, Dedhar S, Kalluri R, Thompson EW. The epithelial-mesenchymal transition: new insights in signaling, development, and disease. J.Cell Biol. 2006; 172:973–981.

Lei H, Velez G, Cui J, et al., N-acetylcysteine suppresses retinal detachment in an experimental model of proliferative vitreoretinopathy. Am J Pathol. 2010; 177(1):132–140.

Lemor M, de Bustros S, Glaser BM. Low-dose colchicine inhibits astrocyte, fibroblast, and retinal pigment epithelial cell migration and proliferation. Arch Ophthalmol. 1986; 104(8):1223-1225.

Li J, Tripathi BJ, Tripathi RC: Modulation of pre-mRNA splicing and protein production of fibronectin by TGF-beta2 in porcine trabecular cells. Invest Ophthalmol Vis Sci. 2000; 41:3437-43.

Lovicu FJ, Schulz MW, Hales AM, Vincent LS, Overbeek PA, Chamberlain CG, McAvoy JW. TGFb induces morphological and molecular changes similar to human anterior subcapsular cataract. Br J Ophthalmol 2002; 86:220–226.

Lu¨tjen-Drecoll E. Morphological changes in glaucomatous eyes and the role of TGF_2 for the pathogenesis of the disease. Exp Eye Res. 2005; 81:1– 4.

Machado RA, Casella AM, Malaguido MR, Oguido AP. Experimental study of vitreoretinal proliferation inhibition by the use of hypericin. Arq Bras Oftalmol. 2009; 72(5):650–654.

Malecaze F, Decha A, Serre B, Penary M, Duboue M, Berg D, Levade T, Lubsen NH, Kremer EJ, Couderc B. Prevention of posterior capsule opacification by the induction of therapeutic apoptosis of residual lens cells. Gene Ther. 2006; 13(5):440-448.

Maurice DM. The structure and transparency of the cornea. J Physiol 1957; 136:263.

McDonnell PJ, Zarbin MA, Green WR. Posterior capsule opacification in pseudophakic eyes. Ophthalmology. 1983; 90(12):1548-1553.

Meacock WR, Spalton DJ, Stanford MR. Role of cytokines in the pathogenesis of posterior capsule opacification. Br J Ophthalmol. 2000; 84(3):332-336.

Mead AL, Wong TTL, Cordiero MF, et al., Anti-Transforming Growth Factor–b2 antibody: a new postoperative anti-scarring agent in glaucoma surgery. Invest Ophthalmol Vis Sci. 2003; 44:3394-3401.

Mietz H, Chevez-Barrios P, Feldman RM, Lieberman MW. Suramin inhibits wound healing following filtering procedures for glaucoma. Br J Ophthalmol 1998; 82:816-820.

Migdal C, Hitchings R. *The developing bleb: Effect of topical antiprostaglandins on the outcome of glaucoma fistulizing surgery.* Br J Ophthalmol. 1983; 67:655-660.

Milani BY, Milani FY, Park DW, Namavari A, Shah J, Amirjamshidi H, Ying H, Djalilian AR. *Rapamycin inhibits the production of myofibroblasts and reduces corneal scarring after photorefractive keratectomy. Invest Ophthalmol Vis Sci.* 2013; 54(12):7424-30. doi: 10.1167/iovs.13-12674.

Mohan RR, Tandon A, Sharma A, Cowden JW, Tovey JC. *Significant Inhibition of Corneal Scarring In Vivo With Tissue-Selective Targeted AAV5 Decorin Gene Therapy. Invest Ophthalmol Vis Sci.* 2011; 52(7):4833-4841.

Morescalchi F, Duse S, Gambicorti E, Romano MR, Costagliola C, and Semeraro F. *Proliferative Vitreoretinopathy after Eye Injuries: An Overexpression of Growth Factors and Cytokines Leading to a Retinal Keloid. Mediators of Inflammation* 2013; Article ID 269787, 12 pages http://dx.doi.org/10.1155/2013/269787

Mori S, Matsuzaki K, Yoshida K, et al., *TGF-b and HGF transmit the signals through JNK-dependent Smad2/3 phosphorylation at the linker regions. Oncogene* 2000; 23:7416–7429.

Nathu Z, Dwivedi DJ, Reddan JR, Sheardown H, West-Mays JA. *Temporal Changes in MMP mRNA Expression in the Lens Epithelium during Anterior Subcapsular Cataract Formation. Exp Eye Res.* 2009; 88(2): 323-330. doi:10.1016/j.exer.2008.08.014

Nishi O, Nishi K, Saitoh I, Sakanishi K *Inhibition of migrating lens epithelial cells by sustained release of ethylenediaminetetraacetic acid. J Cataract Refract Surg* 1996; 22 Suppl 1:863.

Nishi O. *Posterior capsule opacification, part 1: experimental investigations. J Cataract Refract Surg.* 1999; 25(1):106-117.

Ochiai Y, Ochiai H. *Higher concentration of transforming growth factor- in aqueous humor of glaucomatous eyes and diabetic eyes. Jpn J Ophthalmol.* 2002; 46:249–253.

Ont Health Technol Assess Ser. *Limbal stem cell transplantation: an evidence-based analysis.Health Quality Ontario. Ont Health Technol Assess Ser.* 2008; 8(7):1-58.

Oshima Y, Sakamoto T, Hisatomi T, Tsutsumi C, Ueno H, Ishibashi T. *Gene transfer of soluble TGF-beta type II receptor inhibits experimental proliferative vitreoretinopathy. Gene Ther.* 2002; 9(18):1214–1220.

Ozerdem U. · Mach- Hofacre B. · Keefe K. · Pham T. · Soules K. · Appelt K. · Freeman W.R.

The Effect of Prinomastat (AG3340), a Synthetic Inhibitor of Matrix Metalloproteinases, on Posttraumatic Proliferative Vitreoretinopathy Ophthalmic Res 2001; 33:20–23 (DOI:10.1159/000055636)

Pan H, Chen J, Xu J, Chen M, Ma R. *Antifibrotic effect by activation of peroxisome proliferator-activated receptor-gamma in corneal fibroblasts. Mol Vis.* 2009 Nov 10;15:2279-86.

Pandey SK, Apple DJ, Werner L, Maloof AJ, Milverton EJ. *Posterior capsule opacification: a review of the aetiopathogenesis, experimental and clinical studies and factors for prevention. Indian J Ophthalmol.* 2004; 52(2):99-112.

Park H-Y L, Kim I-T, Lin K-M, Choi J-S, Park M-O, Joo C-K. *Effects of Nuclear Factor-κB Small Interfering RNA on Posterior Capsule Opacification Invest Ophthalmol Vis Sci.* 2010; 51(9): 4707-4715.

Pastor JC. *Proliferative vitreoretinopathy: an overview. Surv Ophthalmol.* 1998; 43(1):3–18.

Petritsch C, Beug H, Balmain A, et al., *TGF-b inhibits p70 S6 kinase via protein phosphatase 2A to induce G (1) arrest. Genes Dev* 2000; 14:3093–3101.

Picht G, Welge-Luessen U, Grehn F, Lu¨tjen-Drecoll E. *Transforming growth factor-β2 levels in the aqueous humor in different types of glaucoma and the relation to filtering bleb development. Graefes Arch Clin Exp Ophthalmol.* 2001; 239:199–207.

Rękas M, Kluś A, Kosatka M. *Sealed-capsule irrigation with distilled deionized water to prevent posterior capsule opacification--prospective, randomized clinical trial. Curr Eye Res.* 2013; 38(3):363-70. doi: 10.3109/02713683.2012.748079.

Roberts AB, Russo A, Felici A, et al., *Smad3: a key player in pathogenetic mechanisms dependent on TGF-b. Ann NY Acad Sci* 2003; 995:1–10.

Roh JH, Sohn HJ, Lee DY, Shyn KH, Nam DH. *Comparison of posterior capsular opacification between a combined procedure and a sequential procedure of pars plana vitrectomy and cataract surgery. Ophthalmologica.* 2010; 224:42-6.

Rönbeck M, Zetterstrom C, Wejde G, Kugelberg M. *Comparison of posterior capsule opacification development with 3 intraocular lens types: five-year prospective study. J Cataract Refract Surg.* 2009; 35:1935-40.

Rubsamen PE, Cousins SW. Therapeutic effect of periocular corticosteroids in experimental proliferative vitreoretinopathy. Retina. 1997; 17(1): 44-50.

Saika et al., Fibrotic disorders in the eye: targets of gene therapy. Prog Retin Eye Res. 2008; 27. 177-196.

Saika S, Kono-Saika S, Ohnishi Y, et al., Smad3 signaling is required for epithelial– mesenchymal transition of lens epithelium after injury. Am J Pathol 2004; 16:651-663.

Saika S, Yamanaka O, Okada Y, Tanaka S, Miyamoto T, Sumioka T, Kitano A, Shirai K, Ikeda K. TGF beta in fibroproliferative diseases in the eye. Front Biosci (Schol Ed). 2009; 1:376-90.

Saika S, Sumioka T, Okada Y, Yamanaka O, Kitano A, Miyamoto T, Shirai K, Kokado H. Wakayama symposium: modulation of wound healing response in the corneal stroma by osteopontin andtenascin-C. Ocul Surf. 2013; 11(1):12-5.

Saika S. TGFb pathobiology in the eye. Laboratory Investigation 2006; 86, 106-115.

Schiff WM, Hwang JC, Ober MD, et al., Safety and efficacy assessment of chimeric ribozyme to proliferating cell nuclear antigen to prevent recurrence of proliferative vitreoretinopathy. Arch Ophthalmol. 2007; 125(9):1161-1167.

Schipper I, Suppelt C, Gebbers JO. Mitomycin C reduces scar formation after excimer laser (193 nm) photorefractive keratectomy in rabbits Eye (Lond). 1997; 11 (Pt 5):649-55.

Serini G, Gabbiani G. Mechanisms of myofibroblast activity and phenotypic modulation. Exp. Cell Res. 1999; 250:273–283.

Sethi A, Mao W, Wordinger RJ, Clark AF. Transforming growth factor-beta induces extracellular matrix protein cross-linking lysyl oxidase (LOX) genes in human trabecular meshwork cells. Invest Ophthalmol Vis Sci. 2011; 52:5240–5250.

Sharma A, Rodier JT, Tandon A, Klibanov AM, Mohan RR. Attenuation of corneal myofibroblast development through nanoparticle-mediated soluble transforming growth factor-β type II receptor (sTGFβRII) gene transfer. Mol Vis. 2012; 18:2598-607.

Sharma P, Panwar M. Trypan blue injection into the capsular bag during phacoemulsification: initial postoperative posterior capsule opacification results. J Cataract Refract Surg. 2013; 39(5):699-704. doi: 10.1016/j.jcrs.2012.11.025.

Spalton DJ. Posterior capsular opacification after cataract surgery. Eye. 1999; 13(pt 3b):489-492.

Sriram S, Robinson P, Pi L, Lewin AS, Schultz G Triple combination of siRNAs targeting TGFβ1, TGFβR2, and CTGF enhances reduction of collagen I and smooth muscle actin in corneal fibroblasts. Invest Ophthalmol Vis Sci. 2013; 54(13):8214-23. doi: 10.1167/iovs.13-12758.

Sternberg K, Terwee T, Stachs O, Guthoff R, Löbler M, Schmitz K-P. Drug-Induced Secondary Cataract Prevention: Experimental ex vivo and in vivo Results with Disulfiram, Methotrexate and Actinomycin D. Ophthalmic Res 2010; 44:225-236.

Strutz F, et al., Role of basic fibroblast growth factor-2 in epithelial-mesenchymal transformation. Kidney Int. 2002; 61:1714–1728.

Sundaram V, Barsam A, Virgili G. Intravitreal low molecular weight heparin and 5-fluorouracil for the prevention of proliferative vitreoretinopathy following retinal reattachment surgery. Cochrane Database Syst Rev. 2010; 7:CD006421. doi: 10.1002/14651858.

Sureshkumar J, Haripriya A, Muthukkaruppam V, Kaufman PL, Tian B. Cytoskeletal drugs prevent posterior capsular opacification in human lens capsule in vitro. Graefes Arch Clin Exp Ophthalmol. 2012; 250(4):507-514. doi: 10.1007/s00417-011-1869-4.

Tahara YR, Sakamoto TR, Oshima YR, et al., The antidepressant hypericin inhibits progression of experimental proliferative vitreoretinopathy. Curr Eye Res. 1999; 19(4):323–329.

Tandon A, Tovey JC, Waggoner MR, Sharma A, Cowden JW, Gibson DJ, Liu Y, Schultz GS, Mohan RR. Vorinostat: a potent agent to prevent and treat laser-induced corneal haze. J Refract Surg. 2012 Apr; 28(4):285-90. doi: 10.3928/1081597X-20120210-01.

Tandon A, Sharma A, Rodier JT, Klibanov AM, Rieger FG, Mohan RR. BMP7 Gene Transfer via Gold Nanoparticles into Stroma Inhibits Corneal Fibrosis In Vivo. PLOS ONE. 2013; 8(6):e66434.

Tano Y, Chandler D, Machemer R. Treatment of intraocular proliferation with intravitreal injection of triamcinolone acetonide. Am J Ophthalmol. 1980; 90(6):810-816.

Totan Yüksel, Yag̃cı Ramazan, Erdurmus Mesut, Bayrak Reyhan, Hepsen Ibrahim Feyzi. Cyclosporin effectively inhibits posterior capsule opacification after hacoemulsification in rabbits: a preliminary study. Clinical and Experimental Ophthalmology 2008; 36: 62–66 doi: 10.1111/j.1442-9071.2007.01653.x

The Fluorouracil Filtering Surgery Study Group. Fluorouracil filtering surgery study one-year follow-up. Am J Ophthalmol. 1989; 108:625-635.

Tovar-Vidales T, Roque R, Clark AF, Wordinger RJ. Tissue transglutaminase expression and activity in normal and glaucomatous human trabecular meshwork cells and tissues. Invest Ophthalmol Vis Sci. 2008; 49:622–628.

Tripathi RC, Li J, Chan WFA, Tripathi BJ. Aqueous humor in glaucomatous eyes contains an increased level of TGF-β2. Exp Eye Res. 1994; 58:723–727.

Uchiyama M, Shimizu A, Masuda Y, Nagasaka S, Fukuda Y, Takahashi H. An ophthalmic solution of a peroxisome proliferator-activated receptor gamma agonist prevents cornealinflammation in a rat alkali burn model. Mol Vis. 2013; 19:2135-50.

Vadlamudi R, Adam L, Talukder A, et al., Serine phosphorylation of paxillin by heregulin-1: role of p38 mitogen activated protein kinase. Oncogene 1999; 18:7253-7264.

van Bockxmeer FM, Martin CE, Thompson DE, Constable IJ. Taxol for the treatment of proliferative vitreoretinopathy. Invest Ophthalmol Vis Sci. 1985; 26(8):1140-1147.

Vasavada AR, Dholakia SA, Raj SM, Singh R. Effect of cortical cleaving hydrodissection on posterior capsule opacification in age-related nuclear cataract. J Cataract Refract Surg. 2006; 32:1196–200.

Vasavada AR, Nihalani BR. Pediatric cataract surgery. Curr Opin Ophthalmol. 2006; 17:54-61.

Wallentin N, Wickström K, Lundberg C. Effect of cataract surgery on aqueous TGF-β and lens epithelial cell proliferation. Invest Ophthalmol Vis Sci. 1998; 39(8):1410-1418.

Welge-Lussen U, May CA, Lutjen-Drecoll E. Induction of tissue transglutaminase in the trabecular meshwork by TGF-beta1 and TGF-beta2. Invest Ophthalmol Vis Sci. 2000; 41:2229-2238. [PubMed]

Whitcher JP, Srinivasan M, Upadhyay MP. Corneal Blindness: a global perspective. Bull W H O. 2001; 79: 214–221.

Wickham L, Bunce C, Wong D, McGurn D, Charteris DG. Randomized controlled trial of combined 5-fluorouracil and low-molecular-weight heparin in the management of unselected rhegmatogenous retinal detachments undergoing primary vitrectomy. Ophthalmology. 2007; 114(4):698-704.

Wiedemann P, Hilgers RD, Bauer P, Heimann K. Adjunctive daunorubicin in the treatment of proliferative vitreoretinopathy: results of a multicenter clinical trial. Daunomycin Study Group. Am J Ophthalmol. 1998; 126(4):550–559.

Wong TT, Daniels JT, Crowston JG, Khaw PT MMP inhibition prevents human lens epithelial cell migration and contraction of the lens capsule. Br J Ophthalmol. 2004; 88(7):868.

Wordinger RJ, Agarwal R, Talati M, Fuller J, Lambert W, Clark AF. Expression of bone morphogenetic proteins (BMP), BMP receptors, and BMP associated proteins in human trabecular meshwork and optic nerve head cells and tissues. Mol Vis. 2002; 8:241–250.

Wordinger RJ, Clark AF. Bone morphogenetic proteins and their receptors in the eye. Exp Biol Med (Maywood). 2007; 232:979–992.

Wordinger RJ, Fleenor DL, Hellberg PE, Pang IH, Tovar TO, Zode GS, Fuller JA, Clark AF. Effects of TGF-beta2, BMP-4, and gremlin in the trabecular meshwork: implications for glaucoma. Journal Invest Ophthalmol Vis Sci. 2007; 48(3):1191-200.

Wormstone IM. Posterior capsule opacification: a cell biological perspective. Exp Eye Res. 2002; 74(3):337-347.

WuDunn D. Intracameral urokinase for dissolution of fibrin or blood clots after glaucoma surgery. Am J Ophthalmol. 1997; 124:693-695.

Yang, J., and Liu, Y. Dissection of key events in tubular epithelial to myofibroblast transition and its implications in renal interstitial fibrosis. Am. J. Pathol. 2001; 159:1465-1475.

Yu L, Hebert MC, Zhang YE. TGF-beta receptor-activated p38 MAP kinase mediates Smad-independent TGF-beta responses. EMBO J. 2002; 21:3749–3759.

Zeisberg M, et al., BMP-7 counteracts TGF-beta1-induced epithelial- to-mesenchymal transition and reverses chronic renal injury. Nat.Med. 2003; 9:964–968.

Zeisberg M, Strutz F, Muller GA. Role of fibroblast activation in inducing interstitial fibrosis. J. Nephrol. 2000; 13(Suppl. 3):111-120.

Zhao X, Ramsey KE, Stephan DA, et al., Gene and protein expression changes in human trabecular meshwork cells treated with transforming growth factor-beta Invest Ophthalmol Vis Sci. 2004; 45:4023-34.

Zhao X, Russell P. Versican splice variants in human trabecular meshwork and ciliary muscle. Mol Vis. 2005; 11:603-8.

Zheng Y, Ikuno Y, Ohj M, et al., Platelet-derived growth factor receptor kinase inhibitor AG1295 and inhibition of experimental proliferative vitreoretinopathy. Jpn J Ophthalmol. 2003; 47(2):158–165

Zhou P, Lu Y, Sun XH. Effects of a novel DNA methyltransferase inhibitor Zebularine on human lens epithelial cells. Mol Vis. 2012; 18:22-8.

Morphine Causing a Delay in the Development of the Rat Embryo's Visual System and Other Parts of its Central Nervous System through Affecting the Placenta

Masoomeh Kazemi, Hedayat Sahraei, Elaheh Tekieh and Hamed Aliyari

1   Introduction

Opioids have been used for treatment of pain for thousands of years. Ancient Egyptian papyrus records reported the use of opium for pain relief (Andrea *et al.*, 2008; Pert & Snyder, 1973). In 1973, Candace Pert used radioactive morphine to evaluate the location of the morphine action site, and found, surprisingly, that the drug attached to very specific areas of the brain, dubbed "morphine receptors" (John *et al.*, 2012; Pert & Snyder, 1973). The majority of the clinically relevant opioids have their primary activity at the initial "morphine receptor" or "mu receptors" and are therefore considered "mu agonists." There are opioid receptors within the CNS as well as throughout the peripheral tissues. These receptors are normally stimulated by endogenous peptides (endorphins, enkephalins, and dynorphins) produced in response to toxic stimulation (Andrea *et al.*, 2008; Ek *et al.*, 2010; John *et al.*, 2012; Marion *et al.*, 2011). The non- alkalized form of morphine crosses the BBB easier and blood alkalization increases the fraction of non-ionized morphine. It is interesting to note that respiratory acidosis increases morphine concentrations of the brain due to increased cerebral blood flow secondary to higher carbon dioxide tension and facilitated delivery of the non-ionized form to the blood-brain barrier (BBB) (Doverty *et al.*, 2001; Ek *et al.*, 2010; Sara *et al.*, 2009). Widespread abuse of narcotic drugs and their side effects, especially on the nervous system of pregnant women's fetus, has led to numerous research works in this field. Previous studies showed that morphine consumption during pregnancy could set back the normal development of placenta (James *et al.*, 2004; Nestler, 2001; Wittwer & Steven, 2006). According to research carried out on pregnant women's fetus, most of the opioid-related disorders are caused by defects in the normal development of fetus central nervous system (CNS). Increasing dependence and addiction to these drugs and the importance of the resulted anomalies has prompted most researchers to carry out their research in this field in recent years (Anthony *et al.*, 2008; Joann *et al.*, 2012; Nestler, 2001). This article is a review of the studies conducted on the role of morphine in developing different parts of fetal nervous system including the cerebral ventricles, choroid plexus, spinal cord, and sight and taste senses (Kazemi *et al.*, 2012c; Sahraei *et al.*, 2011; Niknam *et al.*, 2013; Ramazani *et al.*, 2011; Ramazani 2010; Sadraei *et al.*, 2007; Sahraei *et al.*, 2013). The result of this review shows that opioid abuse by pregnant mothers delays the normal development of various fetal nervous systems. Today, with the increasing rate of drug addiction in the world, these drugs are one of the main problems that threaten human health and family integrity (David, 2004; Sara *et al.*, 2009; Wittwer & Steven, 2006). On the other hand, a group of opioid consumers are pregnant women, thus the side effects of drug abuse are not only limited to mother and her entourage, but also influences the next generation. Histopathologically, morphine crosses the placental barrier and has several effects on the fetus. In addition, the drug crosses the blood-brain barrier (BBB) and results in lots of abnormalities in fetus CNS (Kazemi *et al.*, 2014; Fowden, 2008; Sara *et al.*, 2009). The main objective of this paper is to study the fetal disorders resulted from morphine consumption by pregnant women and the role of consumption in the development of different parts of the fetus central nervous system.

1.1   The Role of Morphine in the Development of Placenta and Embryo Cavities in Pregnant Rats

Placenta is the main source of supply of food and hormones required for fetal development, including progesterone and estrogen, etc., especially in the second half of pregnancy. It is demonstrated that morphine can easily transfer across the placenta, and its retention in placenta prolongs fetal exposure to morphine. Furthermore, the existence of μ, κ, and δ type opioid receptors is confirmed in fetal tissues and placenta villi (Behravan *et al.*, 2007; Chahl, 1996; Collins *et al.*, 2005). However, oral morphine consumption causes difficulties in the formation of placental blood pools in pregnant Wistar rats. According to the studies, prescription of oral morphine during the pregnancy period increases the concentration of blood plasma corticosterone, and this phenomenon, in turn, enhances the morphine's function in postponing the placental development (Behravan *et al.*, 2007; Chahl, 1996; Fowden, 2008; James *et al.*, 2004). Our studies also showed that oral morphine consumption by pregnant women abnormally increases corticosterone levels. Morphine is a small lipophilic molecule that can easily cross the chorionic villi and delay the differentiation of embryonic and maternal layers of the placenta. Morphine consumption in pregnant women also reduces blood pools of the embryonic layers (Fowden, 2008; Kazemi *et al.*, 2011a; Kazemi *et al.*, 2011b). Further research using radioactive C14-Morphine to identify the highest density of morphine effect on the pregnant rat placenta showed that radioactive morphine was mostly detected in the opioid receptors of chorionic villi, particularly in its fetal part. Any disruption in the blood supply network of the placenta to fetus can cause defects such as hypoxia and other abnormalities (Kazemi *et al.*, 2012a; Kazemi *et al.*, 2014; Dehghani *et al.*, 2013; Kazemi *et al.*, 2010b). Further research on the side effects of time-dependent oral morphine consumption by pregnant rats showed that delay in the normal development of cytotrophoblastand syncytiotrophoblast cells of rat placental layers will increase based on the consumption duration. Embryonic cavities (amniotic and chorionic) are the base for fetus normal development. Amniotic cavity is filled with amniotic fluid, part of which originates from amniotic cells and the rest from mother's blood. Moreover, normal development of embryo kidneys increases the liquid every day. Abnormal increase in amniotic fluid results in hydramnious and its abnormal decrease results in oligohydramnious. Studies showed that morphine consumption during pregnancy delays the normal development of the embryonic cavities and this abnormality significantly decreases amniotic cavity which in turn disturbs the normal development of the embryo bed (Kazemi *et al.*, 2011a; Kazemi *et al.*, 2011b; Kazemi *et al.*, 2012a). This defect can also cause abnormal development and dysfunction of kidneys in newborns of addicted mothers. Existence of opioid receptors in chorionic villi allows the opioid, including morphine, to cross the placental barrier toward the fetus (Doerr & Kristal, 1991; Fowden, 2008; Kazemi *et al.*, 2011).

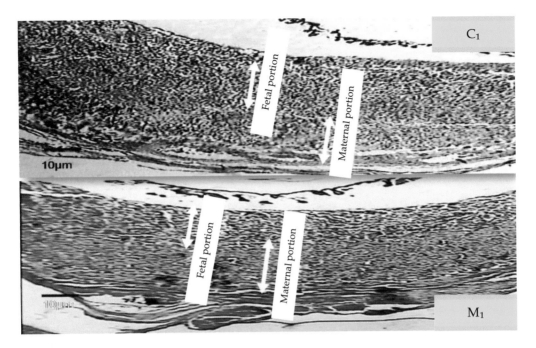

Figure 1: The maternal and fetal portion of placenta development in treated and untreated groups. Thickness reduction is clearly visible in morphine–treated embryo part (Dehghani *et al.*, 2013) in pregnancy 14th- day. Experiment (M1) and control (C1) groups.

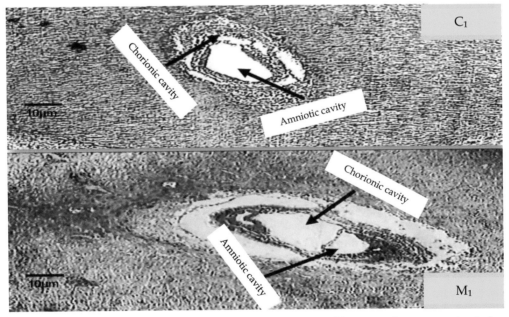

Figure 2-2: Surface reduction of amniotic cavity in morphine-treated versus untreated groups (Kazemi *et al.*, 2011a) in pregnancy 9th day. Experiment (M1-2) and control (C1-2) groups.

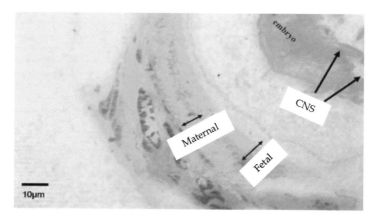

Figure 3-3: Expression of maximum density of morphine simultaneously on the placenta and embryo in consumer mothers by radioactive C14-Morphine in 14th- day of pregnancy. Note morphine effect site on the placental blood vessels, especially in the embryonic as well as on nervous system that was shown by arrows (Kazemi *et al.*, 2014).

1.2   The Role of Morphine in the Development of Neural Plate and Neural Tube of Rat Embryo

Precordial notochord and mesoderm induce the overlaying ectoderm to thicken and also form the neural plate. Early stages of embryonic development of the nervous system are more susceptible to damage caused by consuming drugs such as opioids, which have the greatest impact on development of the neural ectodermic cells (Nasiraei-Moghadam *et al.*, 2009; Nasiraei-Moghadam *et al.*, 2010). Previous research on oral morphine consumption by pregnant women showed that it delays the development of embryonic layers (ectoderm, mesoderm, and endoderm). Following a defect in ectoderm layer, formation of neural plate and neural tube in the ninth day of pregnancy is impaired (Maggi *et al.*, 2013). Subsequent investigations revealed that mothers' addiction to morphine, particularly during early pregnancy, may cause neurological abnormalities including delay in neural tube development. In this regard, it has been shown that opioid administration during pregnancy causes delay in embryonic development, reduces birth weight and neural tube defects such as spinabifida (Harris & Juriloff, 2010; Mesquita *et al.*, 2007; Nasiraei-Moghadama *et al.*, 2005). The disorder severity of developmental delay is more visible at 0.01 ng/ml dose. The effect of morphine on embryos' length and weight was dose-dependent and this may indicate that morphine acts on specific targets of embryonic tissues for induction of its effects. However, the effect of morphine on the thickness of neuroectoderm layer was not dose-dependent. It may be concluded that morphine might activate the mechanism (s) responsible for all the doses used. In addition, morphine may act on its receptors, located on embryonic cells and probably delay embryonic cell growth. Morphine also may influence the receptors located on the notocord. This embryonic structure serves as the neuroectoderm development coordinator (Juriloff & Harris, 2000; Momb *et al.*, 2012). Studies showed that following administration of morphine to rats during neural tube formation, morphine binds to opioid receptors in the central nervous system and results in severe anomalies such as exencephalycranioschisis, brachycephaly, and problems in neural tube closure (Misra *et al.*, 2003).

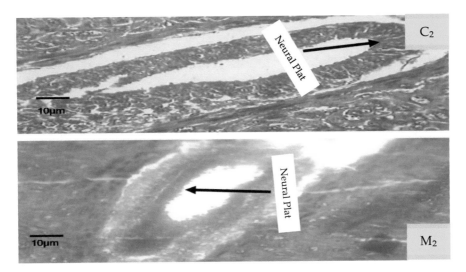

Figure 2: Delay in neural plate development in morphine-treated versus untreated groups (Nasiraei-Moghadam *et al.*, 2009) in pregnancy 19th day. Experiment (M_2) and control (C_2) groups.

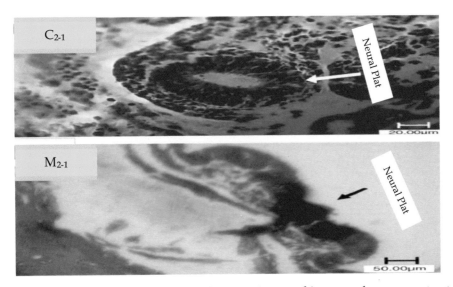

Figure 2-1: Delay in neural tube development in morphine-treated versus untreated groups (Nasiraei-Moghadama *et al.*, 2005)) in pregnancy 19th day. Experiment (M_{2-1}) and control (C_{2-1}) groups.

1.3   The Role of Morphine in the Development of Spinal Cord, Ependymal Duct, and Brain Vesicles of Rat Embryo

The nervous system develops initially as a neural tube with a narrow part called spinal cord and a wide cephalic part called brain vesicles. Spinal cord acts as a mediator between muscles and organizing center of the body and has a major role in transmission of motor and sensory messages. Based on previous studies, morphine consumption by pregnant women disrupts the normal development of spinal cord in both parts of white and gray matter (Kazemi &

Sahraei 2011; Nabiuni *et al.*, 2012; Niknam *et al.*, 2013). The ependymal canal is surrounded by primary nerve cells or neuroblasts which have high division potency. Accumulation of neuroblasts around ependymal canal leads to the formation of gray matter of the spinal cord. The white matter of spinal cord is formed from its outermost layer containing neuroblast nerve fibers. Any disruption in the development and function of the spinal cord leads to disturbance in perception of sensory messages sent from organs and in transmission of motor messages to muscles (Dziegielewska *et al.*, 2012; Mao *et al.*, 2002). This can cause major sensory and motor abnormalities in infants born from morphine-dependent mothers. Research has shown that morphine reduces the ependymal canal surface in fetal brain of morphine-addicted mothers. Considering that cerebral cavities and canals are responsible for transferring cerebro spinal fluid (CSF) and for feeding neurons, defect in the development of ependymal canal leads to defects in innerve cells development. Thereby, morphine consumption severely reduces the surface of primary brain vesicles (prosencephalon and rhombencephalon) and increases the brain cortex thickness. Normal development of the neural tube continues by formation of three prominences at cephalic end of the neural tube as prosencephalon, mesencephalon, and rhombencephalon, called primary brain vesicles (Kazemi & Sahraei, 2012; Yuan *et al.*, 2012). Research has shown that the development of neural tube in rat embryo is accomplished on the ninth day and that of primary brain vesicles on the tenth day of pregnancy. Since the central canal and cavities are the transferring pathways of nutrients (CSF) of the nervous system, they play a major role in the development and functioning of neural cells. Any deficiency in the development of the primary cavities due to morphine consumption, like that of prosencephal, will lead to a delay in the development of other parts of the nervous system growing from this part. Developmental deficiencies in the visual system are caused by deficiency in prosencephal development. In addition, deficiency in rhombencephalon development will lead to in visual center analyzing disorders (Dziegielewska *et al.*, 2012; Kazemi & Sahraei, 2012; Kazemi & Sahraei, 2011).

1.4   The Role of Morphine in the Development of Brain Ventricles, Choroid Plexus, and Ependymal Cells of Rat Embryo

Previous studies on the role of oral morphine consumption in the development of cerebral ventricles of the fetus of pregnant rats showed that morphine reduces the surface of lateral ventricles and the third ventricle in 17-day-old embryos (Kazemi *et al.*, 2009). Further investigations revealed that oral morphine decreases the surface of the fourth ventricle in 14-day-old embryos (Kazemi *et al.*, 2010c).

Cerebrospinal fluid flows from lateral ventricles into the third ventricle and then the fourth ventricle and ultimately enters the central canal. Thus, any factor disturbing the normal transmission of CSF within the cavities and central canal is considered as an interferer in the development of nerve cells (Mashayekhi *et al.*, 2009; Sahraei *et al.*, 2013). Decrease in ventricles and the central canal surfaces can be attributed to reduction of the cerebrospinal fluid volume that may result in irreparable anomalies in the functioning of the nervous system. Choroid plexus (CP) which feeds the nerve cells is formed of ependymal cells covered by vascular mesenchymal (Kazemi *et al.*, 2010a; Kazemi *et al.*, 2011c; Sahraei *et al.*, 2013). To accomplish the task of generating sufficient CSF, choroid plexus tissue receives a large blood supply relative to its size. In addition to CSF production, the CP acts as a filtration system, removing metabolic waste, foreign substances, and excess neurotransmitters from the CSF (Mashayekhi *et al.*, 2002;

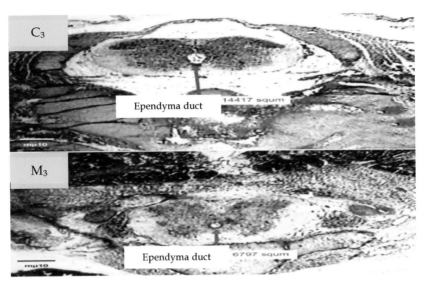

Figure 3: The development of spinal cord and ependymal duct. Reduced the ependymal canal and gray matter surface in morphine-treated groups (Kazemi *et al.*, 2011c) in pregnancy 17th day. (Experimental (M₃) and control (C₃) groups.

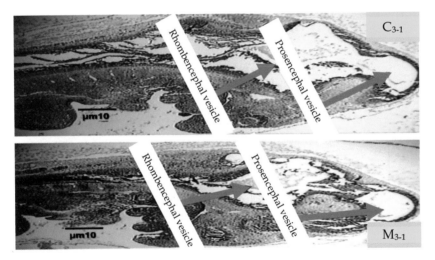

Figure 3-1: Brain cavities development. The surface reduction of primary brain vesicles (Prosencephalon and rhombencephalon) in morphine-treated group (Sahraei *et al.*, 2013) inpregnancy 10th day.Experimental (M₃₋₁) and control (C₃₋₁) groups.

Song & Zhao, 2001). Cerebrospinal fluid is synthesized, absorbed, and secreted by choroid plexus to the nervous system. Based on previous studies, oral consumption of morphine by pregnant rats can delay the normal development of fetal choroid plexus (Bachy *et al.*, 2008; Hassanzadeh *et al.*, 2011). Any disruption in the performance of this blood network, in terms of cerebrospinal fluid absorption and secretion, may cause nervous system malformations. For instance, abnormal increase of cerebrospinal fluid secretion leads to hydrocephalus which results in increment of brain ventricles surface and decrement of brain tissue thickness (Lara-Ramírez *et al.*, 2013; Marion *et al.*, 2011; Mashayekhi *et al.*, 2002). Abnormal decrease of cerebrospinal fluid results in ventricles surface and central canal decrease. Morphine, as an interferer of the normal development of the choroid plexus ependymal cells, abnormally increases the number of cells (Kazemi *et al.*, 2010a; Martin, 2006; Sargeant *et al.*, 2008). Studies using radioactive C14-Morphine have shown that the highest concentration of morphine effect is on the endothelial membrane of blood cells, where opioid receptors (μ, κ, and δ) are located. Therefore, destructive effects of morphine function are high in hyperemic parts. Since the function of choroid plexus is crucial for the development and supply of brain cells, its morphine-induced abnormalities play a major role in developmental defects of the nervous system cells (Hao Zhang 2010; Manchikanti *et al.*, 2010; Sahraei *et al.*, 2013). Oral morphine consumption will lead to disorders in the natural development of ependymal cells in the choroid plexus and also disorders in the nutritional performance of the choroid plexus. These abnormalities will lead to a delay in the development of neuroblast cells, including retinal cells of the visual system (Kazemi *et al.*, 2012b; Sahraei *et al.*, 2013).

1.5   The Role of Morphine in the Development of Olfaction and Sense of Taste in Rat Embryo

The olfactory system differentiation is dependent on epithelial-mesenchymal interaction. These interactions take place between the cells of the neural crest and ectoderm of frontonasal prominence to form the olfactory fossa. Olfactory bulb is also formed between crest cells and telencephalon floor (Christopher *et al.*, 2012; Sandra *et al.*, 2011). The olfactory tract is located behind the ethmoid bone of the skull. The olfactory nerve fibers pass through this bone and enter the olfactory bulb and end at glomerulus surface. The layer contains mitral and tufted cells the axons of which make the cranial nerve in mice (Dumas & Pollack, 2008; Sandra *et al.*, 2011). The nerve ends at primary olfactory cortex and other areas of the brain. Formation of different cells of olfactory bulb shows a precise and regular temporal pattern. The first neurons found in this area are mitral cells formed on days 14 to 16 of fetal life.

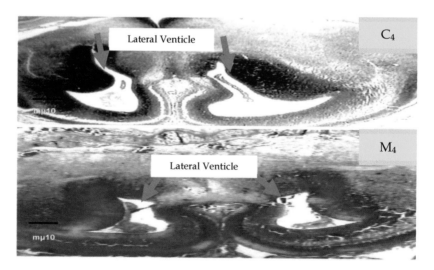

Figure 4: Development of brain ventricles and choroid plexus in Rat embryo. Decrement in brain ventricle surface and increment in choroid plexus surface are clearly visible in the morphine-treated group compared with the untreated group (Kazemi *et al.*, 2011c) in pregnancy 17th- day. Experiment (M_4) and control (C_4) groups.

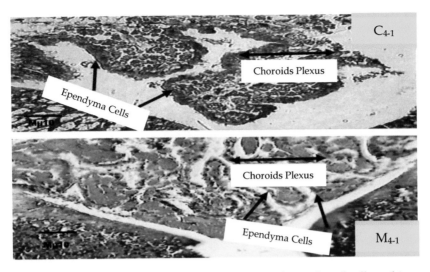

Figure 4-1: Ependymal cells in rat embryo. The number of ependymal cells and intracellular space has increased in morphine-treated groups (Sahraei *et al.*, 2013) in pregnancy 17th-day. Experiment (M$_{4-1}$) and control (C$_{4-2}$) groups.

Olfactory bulb, as the concentration center of olfactory information, is of great importance to the animal (Dumas & Pollack, 2008; Dziegielewska *et al.*, 2012). Studies have shown that oral administration of morphine to pregnant rats reduces the anteroposterior length and the weight of embryos. Microscopic observations have shown that morphine impairs the normal development of the olfactory bulb. Three different cells are detected in olfactory bulb layers called spherical, dark, and pyramidal cells but their types are not known since their developmental stages are not yet completed. During the olfactory bulb development, morphine induces cell transformation and the number of cells, and also increases the intercellular space (Dumas & Pollack, 2008; Kazemi *et al.*, 2012; Ramazani *et al.*, 2011). Morphometric observations have shown that the thickness of the outer and middle layers increases and that of the inner layer decreases. Defects in the development of olfactory bulb impair the transmission of olfactory messages to olfactory cortex. The olfactory cortex participates in the most important functions of the brain for survival through circuits that are created after birth. This area of the brain plays a significant role in creating and sustaining cognition and cognitive behaviors (Christopher *et al.*, 2012; Sandra *et al.*, 2011). Studies have shown that morphine delays the development of three layers of neuronal cells of the olfactory cortex and reduces the density of neurons and neurons projections. Together, these results demonstrated that acute olfactory impairment could attenuate already established addiction-related behaviors and expression of c-Fos in drug addiction-related brain regions, perhaps by affecting the coordination between reward and motivational systems in the brain. Olfactory system disorders caused by oral morphine consumption by pregnant women, showed that deficiencies in the development of the olfactory bulb in the prosencephal area lead to disorders in the correspondence between vision and olfaction (Christopher *et al.*, 2012; Dumas & Pollack, 2008; Niu *et al.*, 2013).

Taste system communicates with other sensory systems, especially with the sense of smell, as well as with trigeminal nerve and plays an important role in survival of an organism. Meanwhile, the tongue plays a particular role in the proper functioning of this sense due to its taste receptors (Ramazani *et al.*, 2010; Ramazani *et al.*, 2011). Exposure of the fetus to abnormal foreign material during tongue development may delay or impair its development resulting in abnormal functioning of the gustatory system. Mother's dependence on morphine reduces the large diameter of the tongue, increases the number of cells, and reduces cells size. Disorders in the natural development of the sense of taste cells due to morphine consumption, might lead to confusion in understanding the relations and the accurate analyzing of the senses of vision and taste (Temugin *et al.*, 2012).

1.6   The Role of Morphine in the Development of Visual System of Rat Embryo

Development and formation of visual system begins from diencephalon of forebrain as optic vesicles. During early development of the vertebrate embryo, a longitudinal groove on the neural plate gradually deepens and the ridges on either side of the groove (the neural folds) become elevated, and ultimately meet, transforming the groove into a closed tube, the ecto-derm wall which forms the rudiment of the nervous system. This tube initially differentiates into three vesicles (pockets): the prosencephalon at the front, the mesencephalon, and, be-tween the mesencephalon and the spinal cord, the rhombencephalon. [By six weeks in the human embryo the prosencephalon then divides further into telencephalon and diencephalon; and the rhombencephalon divides in to metencephalon and myelencephalon (Edward & Kaufman, 2003; Sengpiel & Kind, 2002).

As a vertebrate grows, these vesicles differentiate further still. The telencephalon differ-entiates in to the striatum, the hippocampus and the neocortex, among other things, and its cavity becomes the first and second ventricles. Diencephalon elaborations include the subthal-amus, hypothalamus, thalamus, and epithalamus, and their cavities form the third ventricle. The tectum, pretectum, cerebral peduncle, and other structures develop out of the mesenceph-alon the cavity of which grows into the mesencephalic duct (cerebral aqueduct). The meten-cephalon becomes, among other things, the pons and the cerebellum, the myelencephalon forms the medulla oblongata, and their cavities develop into the fourth ventricle. During the development of visual system, particularly retinal axons extend from the eye to the optic chi-asm at the ventral surface of the diencephalon (Puig-Domingo & Vila, 2013). Eye is a complex biological device. The functioning of a camera is often compared with the operation of the eye, mostly since both focus light from external objects in the field of view onto a light-sensitive medium. In the case of the camera, this medium is film or an electronic sensor; in the case of the eye, it is an array of visual receptors. With this simple geometrical similarity, based on the laws of optics, the eye functions as a transducer, as does a CCD camera. Light entering the eye is refracted as it passes through the cornea. It then passes through the pupil (controlled by the iris) and is further refracted by the lens. The cornea and lens act together as a compound lens to project an inverted image onto the retina (Lopez-Colome & Lopez, 2003; Mansour *et al.*, 1981; Qu *et al.*, 2002). Retina is the neural part of the eye and its proper development has a ma-jor role in visual system functioning (Temugin *et al.*, 2012). It consists of a large number of photoreceptor cells which contain particular protein molecules called opsins. Retinal thickness reduction, retinal layers not getting formed, and delay in retinal cells differentiation are some effects of oral morphine consumption by pregnant women on visual system functioning (Soleimani *et al.*, 2005; Tekieh *et al.*, 2010). Moreover, the overall size of fovea region and its central thickness that is connected to the optic nerve reduces (Ramazany *et al.*, 2009). In addi-tion, morphine administration during pregnancy impairs fetal normal development of the lens

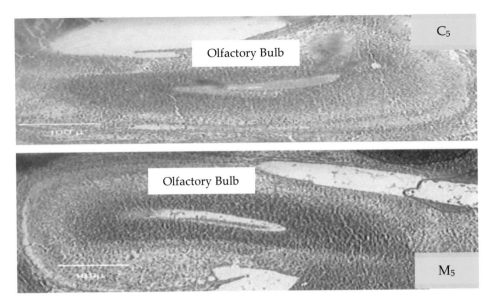

Figure 5: Olfactory bulb development. Morphine impairs the normal development of the olfactory bulb compared with untreated groups (Saeedabadi *et al.*, 2001) in pregnancy 19th day. Experiment (M5) and control (C5) groups.

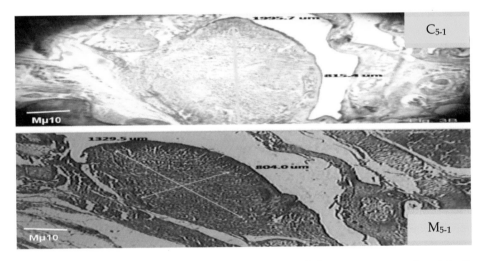

Figure 5-1: Tongue development. The large diameter of the tongue was reduced in the morphine-treated group (Ramazani *et al.*, 2011) in pregnancy 19th day. Experiment (M5-1) and control (C5-1) groups.

Which is composed of two cell types, epithelial and fiber cells, encased in a collagenous basement membrane (the capsule). The lens capsule forms the outermost layer of the lens and the lens fibers form the bulk of the interior of the lens. The cells of the lens epithelium, located between the lens capsule and the outermost layer of lens fibers, are found only on the anterior side of the lens. The lens itself lacks nerves, blood vessels, or connective tissues. The lens, by changing shape, functions to change the focal distance of the eye so that it can focus on objects at various distances, and thus allows a sharp real image of the object of interest to form on the retina (Anamaria *et al.*, 2007; Zachariou *et al.*, 2006). This is visible as a decrease in the lens length and an increase in the eyelid thickness. Morphine also causes a delay in migration of lens cells from around the center. Regarding morphine-induced increase of plasma corticosterone, the anomalies of visual system development resulted from morphine administration can be attributed to corticosterone intervention. Corticosterone has a very broad impact on development, proliferation, and migration of cells. Corticosterone causes excessive cellular proliferation, impaired development, and delay in cell migration during embryo development (Kazemi *et al.*, 2012b; Maggi *et al.*, 2013).

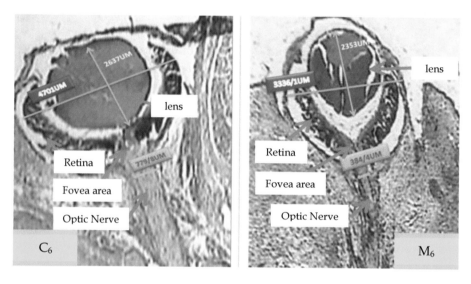

Figure 6: Eye development. A decrement in the lens length and an increment in the eyelid thickness were visible in morphine-treated groups (Kazemi *et al.*, 2012b) in pregnancy 17th day. Experiment (M6) and control (C6) groups.

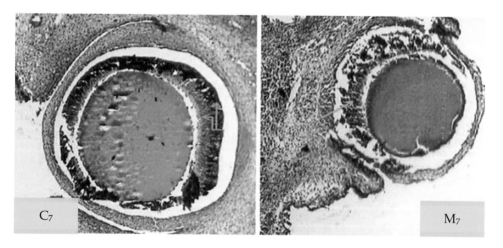

Figure 7: The retina develops as an out pocketing from the neural tube, called the optic vesicle. The inner wall of the optic cup becomes the neural retina, while the outer wall becomes the pigment epithelium (TekiehE, 2010) in pregnancy 17th day. Experimental (M7) and control (C6) groups.

2   Summary

Opioid abuse and the subsequent side effects are one of the major problems of today's world and are growing day after day. Among the most fragile drug abusers are the pregnant mothers. Based on the previous researches, the side effects of opioid drug consumption, such as morphine, will harm not only the mother but also the placenta and embryo and the abnormalities will be transmitted to the next generation. Research works conducted on rat placenta and embryo show that morphine will affect the placenta directly and also, it will cause disruption in the development of embryonic cavities, such as the amniotic cavities, by passing through the placenta barrier. Most of the embryo development disorders and abnormalities, caused by pregnant mothers' morphine consumption are related to the central nervous system. Delay in the natural development of any part of the central nervous system will lead to a disorder in the development of other parts of the nervous system. Oral morphine consumption by pregnant mothers will create several abnormalities which are dependent on the consumption period and also on the duration of development of different parts of the embryo based on the pregnancy day. Morphine will cause development disorders and natural differentiation of ectoblast cells from neural plate and neural tube, and delay in closing the front neural tube will cause anencephaly and delay in closing the back neural tube will lead to spinabifida. Besides, according to the research works, morphine will cause disorders in the formation of brain bulbs and ventricles and the choroid plexus. Disorders in the development of prosencephal bulb will lead to a delay in the natural development of the important subsequent parts, such as the embryo visual system. Since the visual system receives the external stimulations, it plays an important role in the survival of most of the beings. Visual system is a complex system with several types of tissues and cells which, is in connection with other senses.

In addition, delay in the development of rhombencephalon will cause problems in the balance center, including the cerebellum, and also visual disorders and the ability to link the sense to other senses such as olfactory and the sense of taste. Another abnormal effect of morphine on rat central nervous system is disorder in choroid plexus and neural cavities development the result of which is changes in the cerebrospinal fluid leading to disorders in nutrients supply and the natural differentiation of neuroblast cells. Natural development of different parts of the nervous system and their mutual communicative relations are of high importance. The natural functioning of the nervous system as the receiver, processor, and transmitter of the neural messages in the embryo has a major effect on the embryo's health. On the other hand, delay in the natural development of the central nervous system will lead to dysfunctions in the system and disorders in embryo's development. Since embryo's health depends on that of the mother's, the purpose of accumulating the previous research findings in this paper, is to emphasize the abnormal effects of oral morphine consumption for consumers and also to provide supplementary findings for researchers.

Review of several studies has shown that morphine consumption by pregnant mothers and its impact on the development of different parts of the fetal nervous system impairs the normal development of different parts of the fetal central nervous system. Following a delay in the normal development of central nervous system, multiple abnormalities arise in its normal function. Thus, morphine consumption with widespread effects on the opioid receptors and also modified serum corticosterone levels of the mother, placenta, and the fetus can lead to induction of widespread defection in all parts of the nervous system including the visual system, which is considered a part of the nervous system. Therefore, any failure or delay in the development of the central nervous system, especially parts of brain, in which the visual system takes the form of including prosencephalon vesicle, and diencephalon in particular, leads to impaired development and finally defective performance of the visual system.

Abbreviations

Central Nervous System= (CNS)
Blood-Brain Barrier = (BBB)
Cerebro Spinal Fluid = (CSF)
Choroid Plexus = CP

Acknowledgements

Sultan Ali Aliyary and Hamed Aliyary performed extensive literature research, prepared the manuscript and provided expertise in interpretation of data obtained from several sources. As well as numerous collaborations in cell Journal.

Authors

Masoomeh Kazemi
Neuroscience Research Center, Baqiyatallah University of Medical Sciences, Tehran, Iran

Hedayat Sahraei
Neuroscience Research Center, Baqiyatallah University of Medical Sciences, Tehran, Iran

Elaheh Tekieh
Neuroscience Research Center, Baqiyatallah University of Medical Sciences, Tehran, Iran

Hamed Aliyari
Department of Electrical, Biomedical and Mechatronics Engineering, Qazvin Branch, Islamic Azad University, Qazvin, Iran

References

Anamaria, S & Alexandra, L. J. (2007). Cerebellum morphogenesis: The foliation pattern is orchestrated by multi-cellular anchoring centers. Neural Development, 3,20-26

Andrea, M., Trescot, M.D., Sukdeb, M.D., Marion Lee, M.D. (2008). Opioid pharmacology. Pain Physician, 11, 133-153.

Anthony, B., Zhou, FC., Ogawa, T., Goodlett, CR., Ruiz, J. (2008). Alcohol exposure alters cell cycle and apoptotic events during early neurulation. Alcohol 43, 261-273.

Bachy, I., Kozyraki, R., Wassef, M. (2008). The particles of the embryonic cerebrospinal fluid: How could they influence brain development? Brain Res Bull, 75, 289–294.

Behravan,J., Piguette-Miller, M. (2007). Drug transport across the placenta, role ofthe abc drug efflux transporters. Expert Opin Drug MetabToxicol, 3,819-830.

Chahl, L.A. (1996). Opioids – mechanism of action. Aust Prescr, 19, 63-65.

Christophe,r M., Traudt,T., Kathleen, M., Ennis, L. M., Sutton, D.M., Mammel, R. R. (2012). Postnatal morphine administration alters hippocampal development in rats. J Neurosci Res, 90,307–314.

Collins, L.R., Hall, R.W., Dajani, N.K., Wendel, PJ., Lowery, CL., Kay, H.H. (2005). Prolonged morphine exposure in utero causes fetal and placental vasoconstriction: A case report. J Matern Fetal Neonatal Med, 17,417-421.

David, J.B. (2004). Delivery of therapeutic agents to the central nervous system: The problems and the possibilities. Pharmacology & Therapeutics, 29– 45.

Dehghani, L., Sahraei, H., Meamar, R., Kazemi, M. (2013). Time-dependent effect of oral morphine consumption on the development ofcytotrophoblast and -syncytotrophoblast cells of the placental layers during the three different periods of pregnancy in wistar rats. Clinical and Developmental Immunology, 974205, 6.

Doerr, J.C., Kristal, M.B. (1991). Amniotic-fluid ingestion enhances morphine analgesia during morphine tolerance and withdrawal in rat. Physiol Behav, 50,633-635.

Doverty, M., Somogyi, A.A., White, J.M., Bochner, F., Beare, C.H., Menelaou, A., Ling, W. (2001). Methadone maintenance patients are cross-tolerant to the antinociceptive effects of morphine. Pain, 93,155-163.

Dumas, O.E., Pollack, G.M (2008). Opioid tolerance development: A pharmacokinetic/pharmacodynamic perspective. The AAPS Journal, 10,537-551.

Dziegielewska, K.M., Habgood, M.D., Saunders, N.R. (2012). Barriers in the developing brain and neurotoxicology. NeuroToxicology, 33,586-604.

Edward, D.P. & Kaufman, L. M. (2003). Anatomy, development, and physiology of the visual system. Pediatr Clin North Am, 50,1-23.

Ek,CJ., Wong, A., Liddelow, SA., Johansson, P.A., Dziegielewska, K.M., Saunders, N.R. (2010). Efflux mechanisms at the developing brain barriers: Abc-transporters in the fetal and postnatal rat Toxicol Lett, 197, 51–59.

Fowden, A.L., Forhead, A.J., Coan, P.M., Burton, G.J. (2008). The placenta and intrauterine programming. J Neuroendo¬crinol, 20, 439-450.

Hao Zhang, Yu-Ning Song, Wei-Guo Liu, Xiu-Li Guo., Lu-Gang Yu. (2010). Regulation and role of organic anion-transporting polypeptides (oatps) in drug delivery at the choroid plexus. Journal of Clinical Neuroscience,23, 679–684.

Harris, M.J. & Juriloff, D.M. (2010). An update to the list of mouse mutants with neural tube closure defects and advances toward a complete genetic perspective neural tube of closure. Birth Defects Res A Clin Mol Teratol, 88, 653-669.

Hassanzadeh, K., Roshangar, L., Habibi-asl, B., Farajnia, S., Izadpanah, E., Nemati, M., Arasteh, M., Mohammadi, S. (2011). Riluzole prevents morphine-induced apoptosis in rat cerebral cortex. Pharmacol Rep, 63,697-707.

James, W., CorpeningJean, C., Doerr Mark, B. (2004). Ingested placenta blocks the effect of morphine on gut transit in long–evans rats. Brain Research, 22, 217– 221.

Joann, R. R., Yasmin, N., Gabriela, L., Vinicius, S. S., Isabel, C. M., Ana, M., Oliveira, B., Wolnei, C., Iraci, L.S. T. (2012). Morphine treatment alters nucleotidase activities in rat blood serum. Journal of Experimental Pharmacology, 202, 90050-90170.

John,M.c., Donald,B., Lambert,D.G. (2012). Opioid receptors. Continuing education in anaesthesia. Critical Care & Pain, 5,2-8

Juriloff, D.M. & Harris,M.J. (2000). Mouse models for neural tube closure defects. Hum Mol Genet, 12, 993-1000.

Kazemi,M., Sahraei, H., Azarnia, M., Bahadoran,H. (2010a). Effect of oral morphine consumption on ependym cells of choroid plexus in development of central nervous system in wistar rat embryos. J Mazandaran Univ Med Sci, 20,15-22.

Kazemi, M., Sahraei, H., Azarnia, M., Bahadoran, H. (2011a). Effect oral morphine consumption on amnioticandchronic cavities developmentin the embryo wistar rat. Journal of Shaheed Sadoughi University of Medical Sciences and Health 18,444-450.

Kazemi, M., Tekieh, E., Golabi, S., Sahraei, H. (2014). Defects in Wistar Rat's Embryo and Placenta Development: A [C]14-Morphine Study. Annual Research & Review in Biology,4,2823-2834

Kazemi, M., Sahraei, H., Azarnia, M., Bahadoran, H. (2010b). *Effect oral morphine consumption on placenta fetal and maternal portions development cells development in the wistar rat. Research & Scientific Journal ArdebilUniversity of Medical Sciences, 10,145-154*

Kazemi, M., Sahraei, H., Azarnia, M., Dehghani, L., Bahadoran, H., Tekieh, E. (2011b). *The effect of morphine consumption on plasma corticosteron concentration and placenta development in pregnant rats. Iranian Journal of Reproductive Medicine, 9, 71-76.*

Kazemi, M., Sahraei, H., Dehghani, L. (2012a). *Identification of site of action of morphine in the pregnant wistar rat's placenta: A [c]14-morphine studyCell (Yakhteh), 14,122-129.*

Kazemi,M. & Sahraei, H. (2012). *Effect oral morphine consumption onbrainvesicles prosencephslon and rhombencephal development in wistar rat embryosZanjan University of Medical Sciences & Health Service, 20,24-33.*

Kazemi,M. & Sahraei H. (2011). *The effect of oral morphine consumption on ependymal duct and spinal cord development in wistar rats embryos. Iranin Suoth Madical Journal, 14,16-19.*

Kazemi,M., Tekieh, E., Sadeghi-Gharachdaghi, S., Ghoshoni, H., Zardooz,H., Sahraei, H., Rostamkhani,F., Bahadoran, H. (2012b). *Oral morphine consumption reduces lens development in rat embryos. Basic and Clinical Neuro Sciences, 3,16-23.*

Kazemi, M., Azarnia, M., Sahraei, H., Bahadoran, H., Saeidabadi, S. (2009). *The effect oforal morphine consumption delayed lateral ventricles and chroid plexus in wistar rat embryos. Kowsar Medical Journal, 14, 11-20.*

Kazemi, M., Sahraei, H., Azarnia, M., Bahadoran, H., Salehy, M. (2010c). *The effect of oral morphine consumption delayed choroidplexus and ventricle 4thdevelopment in fourteen wistar rats embryos Goom University of Medical Sciences Journal, 89,3-9.*

Kazemi, M., Sahraei, H., Azarnia, M., Dehghani, L., Bahadoran, H. (2011c). *Effect of oral morphine consumption in female rats on development of brain cavities, central canal and choroidplexus of their embryos. Cell Journal, 12, 489-494.*

Lara-Ramírez, R., Zieger, E., Schubert M. (2013). *Retinoic acid signaling in spinal cord development. The International Journal of Biochemistry & Cell Biology, 45,1302–1313.*

Lopez-Colome, A. M. & Lopez, E. (2003). *Glutamate receptors coupled to nitric oxide synthesis in embryonic retina. Dev Neurosci, 25, 293-300.*

Maggi, R., Dondi, D., Piccolella, M., Casulari, L.A., Martini, L. (2013). *New insight on the molecular aspects of glucocorticoid effects in nervous system development. J Endocrinol Invest., 36, 775-780.*

Manchikanti, L., Fellows, B., Ailinani, H., Pampati, V. (2010). *Therapeutic use, abuse,and nonmedical use of opioids: A tenyear perspective. Pain Physician, 13,401-435.*

Mansour, A., Doyle, R., Katz, R., Valenstein, E.S. (1981). *Long-lasting changes in morphine sensitivity following amygdaloid kindling in mice. Physiology & Behavior, 27, 1117-1120.*

Mao, J., Sung, B., Ji, R.R., Lim, G. (2002). *Chronic morphine induces downregulation of spinalglutamate transporters: Implicationsinmorphine tolerance and abnormal pain sensitivity. J Neurosci, 22,8312-8323.*

Marion, L., Sanford, S., Hans, H., Vikram, P., Laxmaiah, M. (2011). *A comprehensive review of opioid-inducedhyperalgesia. Pain Physician, 14,145-161.*

Martin, C., Bueno, D., Alonso, M.I., Moro, J.A., Callejo, S. (2006). *Fgf2 plays a key role in embryonic cerebrospinal fluid trophic properties over chick embryo neuroepithelial stem cells. Parada CDev Biol, 297,402–416.*

Mashayekhi, F., Azari, M., Moghadam, L.M., Yazdankhah, M., Naji, M., Salehi, Z. (2009). *Changes in cerebrospinal fluid nerve growth factor levels during chick embryonic development. J Clin Neurosci, 16, 1334–1337.*

Mashayekhi, F., Draper, C.E., Bannister, C.M., Pourghasem, M., Owen-Lynch, P.J., Miyan, J.A. (2002). *Deficient cortical development in the hydrocephalic texas (h-tx) rat: A role for csf. Brain, 152,1859–1874.*

Mesquita, AR., Pego, J.M., Summavielle, T., Maciel, P., Almeida, O.F., Sousa, N. (2007). *Neurodevelopment milestone abnormalities in rats exposed to stress in early life. Neuroscience, 147, 1022–1033.*

Misra, A., Ganesh, S., Shahiwala, A., Shah, S.P. (2003). *Drug delivery to the central nervous system: A review. J Pharm Pharmaceut Sci, 6,252-273.*

Momb, J., Lewandowski, J.P., Bryant, J.D., Fitch, R., Surman, DR., Vokes, S.A., Applinga, D.R. (2012). *Deletion of mthfd1l causes embryonic lethality and neural tube and craniofacial defects in mice. Jessica Momb, 110 -100*

Nabiuni, M., Rasouli, J., Parivar, K., Kochesfehani, M.H., Irian, S., Miyan, J.A. (2012). *In vitro effects of fetal rat cerebrospinal fluid on viability and neuronal differentiation of pc12 cells. Fluids and Barriers of the CNS, 9, 45-52*

Nasiraei-Moghadam, S., Bahadoran, H., Saeedabady, S., Shams, J., Sahraei, H. (2009). *Oral administration of morphine delays neural plate development in rat embryos. Physiology and Pharmacology, 12,314 – 319.*

Nasiraei-Moghadam, S., Kazeminezhad,B., Dargahi, L., Ahmadiani, A. (2010). *Maternal oral consumption of morphine increases bax/bcl-2 ratio and caspase 3 activity during early neural system development in rat embryos. J Mol Neurosci 41, 156–164.*

Nasiraei-Moghadama, S., Sahraei, H., Bahadorand,H., Sadooghia, M., Salimie, S.H., Kakad, G.R., Salimie, S.H., Mahdavi-Nasabd, H., Dashtnavardd, H. (2005). *Effects of maternal oral morphine consumption on neural tube development in wistar rats. Developmental Brain Research 159,12 – 17.*

Nestler, EJ. (2001). *Molecular basis on longer plasticity underlying addiction. Nat Rev Neurosci, 2 (1), 119-128.*

Niknam, N., Azarnia, M., Bahadoran, H., Kazemi, M., Tekieh, E., Ranjbaran,M., Sahraei, H. (2013). *Evaluating the effects of oral morphine on embryonic development ofspinal cord inwistar rats. Basic and Clinical Neuroscience, 4, 24-29.*

Niu, H., Zheng, Y., Huma, T, Rizak, J.D., Li, L., Wang, G. (2013). *Lesion of olfactory epithelium attenuates expression of morphine-induced behavioral sensitization and reinstatement of drug-primed conditioned place preference in mice. Pharmacol Biochem Behav, 103, 526-534.*

Pert, C.B., Snyder,S.H. (1973). *Opiate receptor:Its demonstration in nervous tissue. Science, 179, 1011-1014.*

Puig-Domingo, M., & Vila, L. (2013). *The implications of iodine and its supplementation during pregnancy in fetal brain development. Curr Clin Pharmacol, 8,97-109.*

Qu, J., Zhou, X., Zhang, L., Ni, H., Ashwell, K., & Lu, F. (2002). *[a preliminary study on development of human visual system in fetus by dii-tracing]. Zhonghua Yan Ke Za Zhi, 38, 517-519.*

Ramazani, M., Ameli, H., Hakimi Gilani, V., Bahadoran, H., Sahraei, H. (2010a). *Reduction of cell size in amygdaloid complex of the wistar rat embryos after oral morphine consumption. Physiology and Pharmacology, 14, 181 -190.*

Ramazani, M., Hakimi, V., Ameli, H., Bahadoran, H., Sahraei, H. (2011). *Effect of oral morphine consumption during pregnancy on the tongue development in the wistar rat embryos Behbood Journal, 14, 283-289.*

Ramazani, M., Hamidi, E., Hajizadeh Moghadam, A., Bahadoran, H., Sahraei, H. (2010b). *Effect of oral morphine consumption on hippocampus developmentin wistar rats embryo. Kowsar Medical Journal., 15, 11-15.*

Ramazany, M., Tekyeh, E., Zardooz, H., Bahadoran, H., Sahraei, H. (2009). *Morphine delays fovea development in the eyes of wistar rat embryos; possible involvement of corticosterone. Physiology and Pharmacology, 13, 271-278.*

Sadraei, SH., Kaka, Gh., Dashtnavard, H., Bahadoran, H., Mofid, M.,, Sahraei, H., Mirshafiei, Gh. (2007). *Effects of maternal morphine administration on fetal cerebellum development in mice: A morphometric evaluation. Hakim Research Journal, 10, 43- 49.*

Saeedabadi, S., Sadooghi, M., Sahraei, H., Bahadoran, H., Fahanik Babaiee, J., Jalili, C. (2001). *Effects of oral morphine on the development of olfactory bulbin rat embryo. Arak University ofmedical sciences, 42, 1-8.*

Sahraei, H., Rostamkhani, F., Tekieh, E., Dehghani,L., Meamar, R., M, Kazemi. (2013). *Identification of morphine accumulation in the rat embryo central nervous system: A c14 morphine administration study. International Journal of Preventive Medicine95, 203-209.*

Sahraei, H., Rostamkhani,F., Tekieh, E., Dehghani, L., Meamar, R., M, Kazemi. (2013). *Identification of morphine accumulation in the rat embryo central nervous system: A c14 morphine administration study. International Journal of Preventive Medicine, 95, 203-209.*

Sandra, E., JuulRichard P., BeyerTheo, K., BammlerFederico,M,. Christine, A. (2011). *Effects of neonatal stress and morphine on murine hippocampal gene expression. Pediatr Res, 69, 285–292.*

Sara, E., Peng, H., Jashvant, D. (2009). *Drug interactions at the blood-brain barrier: Fact or fantasy? Pharmacol Ther, 123, 80–104.*

Sargeant, T.J., Day, D.J., Miller, J.H., Steel, R.W. (2008). *Acute in utero morphine exposure slows g2/m phase transition in radial glial and basal progenitor cells in the dorsal telencephalon of the e15.5 embryonic mouse. Eur J Neurosci, 28, 1060-1067.*

Sengpiel, F., & Kind, P.C. (2002). *The role of activity in development of the visual system. Curr Biol, 12 (23), R818-826.*

Soleimani, M., Sahraei, H., Sadooghi, M., Maleki, P. (2005). *Effects of prenatal morphine exposure on the basal ganglia development in rat embryo. J Arak University ofmedica sciences, 9, 53-61.*

Song, P., Zhao, Z.Q. (2001). *The involvement of glial cells in the development of morphine tolerance. Neurosci Res, 39, 281–286.*

Tekieh,E., Ramezani,M., Zardooz, H., Goolmanesh, L., Bahadoran, H., Sahraei, H. (2010). *Effects of oral morphine consumption during pregnancy on retina development of the wistar rat embryo. semnan University ofmedical sciences, 12, 79-85.*

Temugin B, Tong LiuYCL, Zhen-ZhongX, Ru-Rong J. (2012). *Acute morphine activates satellite glial cells and up-regulates il-1β in dorsal root ganglia in mice via matrix metalloprotease-9. Molecular Pain, 8, 18-25*

Wittwer, E., Steven,E.K. (2006). *Role of morphine's metabolites in analgesia: Concepts and controversies. AAPS Journal, 8, 39-47.*

Yuan, Feng., X. H., Yilin, Yang., D.C., Lawrence, H., Lazarus, Y.X. (2012). *Current research on opioid receptor function. Curr Drug Targets, 13, 230–246.*

Zachariou, V., Bolanos, CA., Selley, DE., Theobald, D., Cassidy, M.P., Kelz, M. (2006). *An essential role fordeltafosb in the nucleus accumbens in morphine action. DeltaFosB:Nat Neurosci, 9, 205-211.*

CPSIA information can be obtained at www.ICGtesting.com
Printed in the USA
LVIW01n1034200316
479957LV00013B/56